GYNAECOLOGY ILLUSTRATED

For Churchill Livingstone

Publisher: Timothy Horne
Indexer: Peter Butcher
Design: Design Resources Unit/Jim Farley
Production Controller: Nancy Arnott
Sales Promotion Executive: Marion Pollock

GYNAECOLOGY ILLUSTRATED

A.D.T. Govan PhD FRCP (Glas) FRCOG FRCPath
Department of Obstetrics and Gynaecology,
University of Glasgow

D. McKay Hart MD FRCS (Glas) FRCOG
Department of Obstetrics and Gynaecology,
University of Glasgow

Robin Callander FFPh FMAA AIMI
Medical Illustrator

FOURTH EDITION

CHURCHILL LIVINGSTONE
EDINBURGH LONDON MADRID MELBOURNE NEW YORK AND TOKYO 1993

CHURCHILL LIVINGSTONE
Medical Division of Longman Group UK Limited

Distributed in the United States of America by Churchill
Livingstone Inc., 650 Avenue of the Americas, New York,
N. Y. 10011, and by associated companies, branches and
representatives throughout the world.

First edition 1972
Second edition 1978
Third edition 1985
Fourth edition 1993

ISBN 0-443-04799-5

British Library Cataloguing in Publication Data
A catalogue record for this book is available from the British
Library.

Library of Congress Cataloguing in Publication Data
A catalog record for this book is available from the Library
of Congress.

The
publisher's
policy is to use
**paper manufactured
from sustainable forests**

Produced by Longman Singapore Publishers (Pte) Ltd
Printed in Singapore

PREFACE

Gynaecological practice continues to change and we have rewritten and updated this book to reflect the developments in the speciality in the seven years which have passed since the last edition. The sequence of chapters has been altered for easier reference and the contents have been changed to reflect modern practice. The importance of the menopause and hormone replacement therapy is acknowledged by the inclusion of an appropriate chapter. AIDS has replaced syphilis and tuberculosis as the most feared infectious disease and an outline of the syndrome and its management is provided. We have attempted to meet the requirements of the medical student and of the primary care doctor, stressing what is important and relevant in contemporary gynaecology.

1993

Alasdair D. T. Govan
David McK. Hart
Robin Callander

CONTENTS

CHAPTER 1

EMBRYOLOGY OF THE REPRODUCTIVE TRACT

DEVELOPMENT OF THE OVARY

The germ cells which will eventually inhabit the gonads originate from the primitive hind gut. They appear around the 25th day.

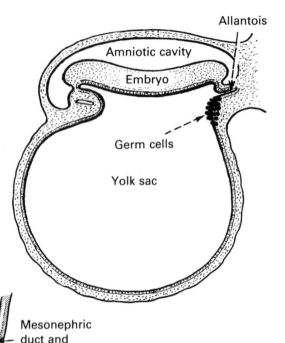

By 30 days the gut complete with mesentery is formed. The germ cells now migrate from the gut to the root of the mesentery.

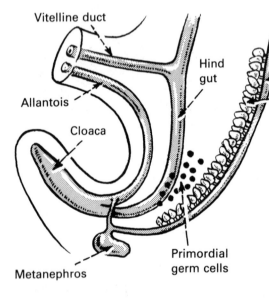

Transverse Section of Embryo

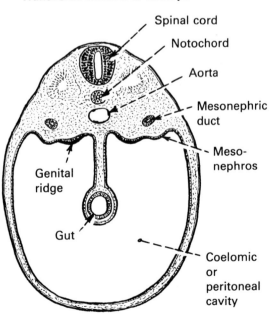

At the same time the coelomic epithelium proliferates and forms thickenings, the genital ridges, together with the underlying mesenchyme on either side of the mesenteric root near the developing kidney.

DEVELOPMENT OF THE OVARY

At this stage the primitive gonad (genital ridge) consists of mesoderm (coelomic epithelium plus mesenchyme) covered by coelomic epithelium. The germ cells now migrate from the root of the mesentery to the genital ridge.

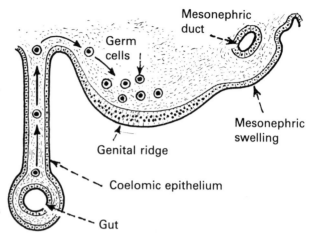

The coelomic epithelium growing into the genital ridge forms so-called sex cords which enclose each germ cell.

Up to this time, around the 7th week, the gonad is of indifferent type, male being indistinguishable from female.

The germ cells and most of the sex cord cells remain in the superficial part, the future cortex of the ovary. The cords lose contact with the surface epithelium and form small groups of cells each with its germ cell, a primitive follicle. Some of the sex cord cells grow into the medulla. These tend to regress and form rudimentary tubules, the rete.

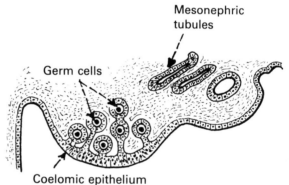

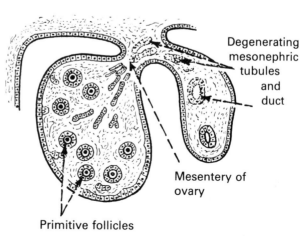

As the ovary grows it projects increasingly into the peritoneal (coelomic) cavity, thus forming a mesentery.

DEVELOPMENT OF THE OVARY

At the same time the ovary descends extraperitoneally in the abdominal cavity. Two ligaments develop and these may help to control its descent, guiding it to its final position and preventing its complete descent through the inguinal ring in contrast to the testes. The first structure is the suspensory ligament attached to the anterior (cephalic) pole of the ovary and connecting it with its site of origin, the genital ridge.

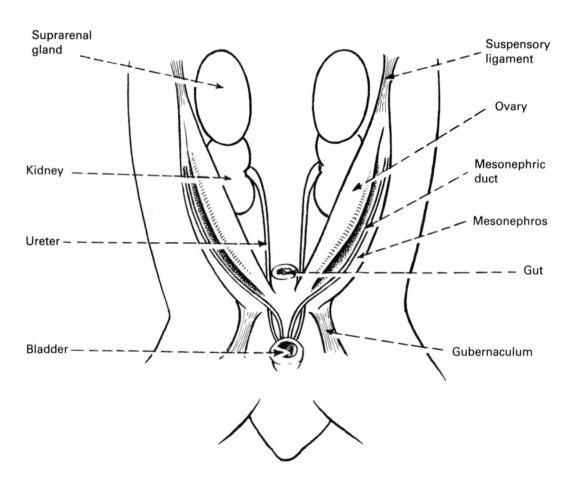

Another ligament or gubernaculum develops at the posterior or caudal end of the ovary. At first attached to the genital ridge it later becomes attached to the developing uterus and follows the latter.

DEVELOPMENT OF UTERUS AND FALLOPIAN TUBES

When the embryo reaches a size of 10mm at 35–36 days a longitudinal groove appears on the dorsal aspect of the coelomic cavity lateral to the Wolffian (mesonephric) ridge.

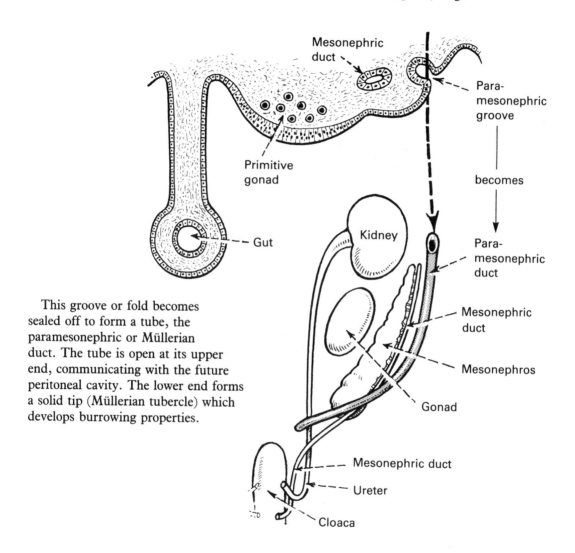

This groove or fold becomes sealed off to form a tube, the paramesonephric or Müllerian duct. The tube is open at its upper end, communicating with the future peritoneal cavity. The lower end forms a solid tip (Müllerian tubercle) which develops burrowing properties.

DEVELOPMENT OF UTERUS AND FALLOPIAN TUBES

The Müllerian ducts from either side grow in a caudal direction, extraperitoneally. They also bend medially and anteriorly and ultimately fuse in front of the hind gut. The mesonephric duct becomes involved in the walls of the paramesonephric ducts.

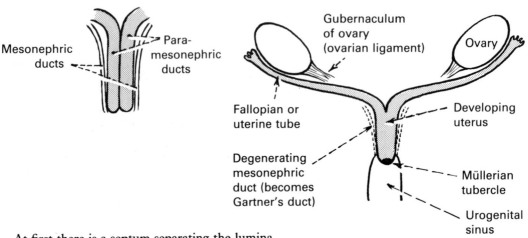

At first there is a septum separating the lumina of the two ducts. Later the septum disappears and a single cavity is formed, the uterus. The upper parts of both ducts retain their identity and form the fallopian tubes.

While this is happening the ovary is also affected. Its gubernaculum is ultimately attached to the Müllerian duct at the cornu of the developing uterus. Its effect is to pull the ovary medially so that its long axis becomes horizontal.

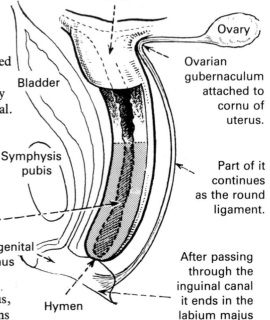

The lower end of the fused Müllerian ducts beyond the uterine lumen remains solid, proliferates and forms a solid cord. This cord will canalise to form the vagina which opens into the urogenital sinus.

At the point of entry into the urogenital sinus, part of the Müllerian tubercle persists and forms the hymen.

DEVELOPMENT OF EXTERNAL GENITALIA

At an early stage the hind gut and the various urogenital ducts open into a common cloaca.

A septum (urorectal) grows down between the allantois and the hind gut during the 5th week.

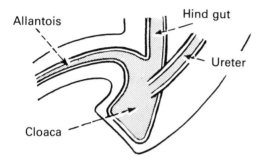 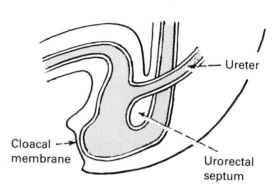

Eventually this septum fuses with the cloacal membrane dividing the cloaca into two compartments – the rectum dorsally and the urogenital sinus ventrally. At the same time the developing uterus grows down and makes contact with the urogenital sinus.

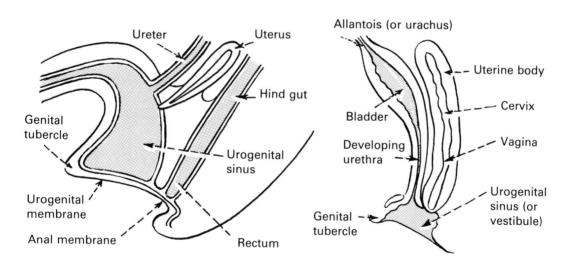

At the end of the 7th week the urogenital membrane breaks down so that the urogenital sinus opens on to the surface.

The developing uterus and vagina push downwards and cause an elongation and narrowing of the upper part of the urogenital sinus. This will form the urethra.

DEVELOPMENT OF EXTERNAL GENITALIA

Meanwhile on the surface of the embryo around the urogenital sinus five swellings appear. At the cephalic end a midline swelling grows, the genital tubercle, which will become the clitoris. Posterior to the genital tubercle and on either side of the urogenital membrane a fold is formed – urethral folds. Lateral to each of these a further swelling appears – the genital or labial swelling. These swellings approach each other at their posterior ends, fuse and form the posterior commissure. The remaining swellings become the labia minora.

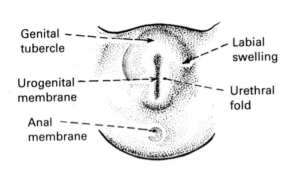

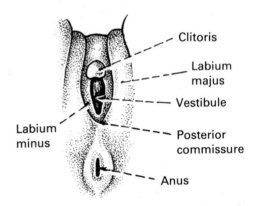

Certain small but clinically important glands are formed in and around the urogenital sinus.

In the embryo epithelial buds arise from the urethra and also from the epithelium of the urogenital sinus. In the male these two sets of buds grow together and give rise to the glands of the prostate. They remain separate in the female, the urethral buds forming the urethral glands and the urogenital buds giving rise to the para-urethral glands of Skene. The ducts of the latter open into the vestibule on either side of the urethra.

Two other small glands arise by budding from the epithelium of the posterior part of the vestibule, one on either side of the vaginal opening. These are the greater vestibular or Bartholin's glands. Similar smaller glands also arise in the anterior portion of the vestibule.

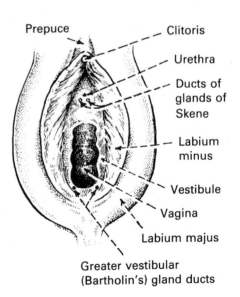

DEVELOPMENT OF TESTIS

Some consideration must be given to the development of the male genital organs in view of the anomalies which may arise either due to organisational defects, endocrine influences or genetic abnormalities.

TESTIS The early development of the organs of reproduction is the same in both male and female up to the 6th–7th week. Around this time the male gonad develops radial fibrous tissue bundles which divide the specialised tissue into cords. These cords of mesoderm enclose the germ cells, extend into the medulla and join to form the rete tubules.

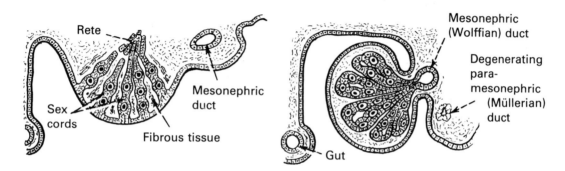

The rete tubules make contact with the mesonephric ductules and thus join with the mesonephric (Wolffian) duct which becomes the main sex duct of the male. In the meantime a paramesonephric (Müllerian) duct forms as in the female, but this subsequently degenerates and plays no functional role in the male. The mesonephric body also degenerates.

The mesonephric duct which becomes the main sex duct or ductus deferens, opens into the urogenital sinus.

The proximal part of this mesonephric duct becomes greatly elongated and convoluted to become the epididymis. At the distal end near its junction with the urogenital sinus the duct becomes dilated to form an ampulla from which the seminal vesicle arises. The ultimate portion of the duct forms the ejaculatory duct.

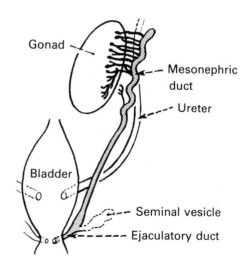

DEVELOPMENT OF TESTIS

DESCENT of TESTIS

The posterior end of the testis is continuous with a band which runs round the abdominal wall to reach the inguinal region. At this point the band becomes attached to a mass of mesenchyme which will form the inguinal canal and which is continuous with the genital swelling. This structure thus formed becomes the gubernaculum testis. Although the body elongates the gubernaculum does not and thus the testis descends in a relative sense and comes close to the inguinal region. At the sixth month a diverticulum of the coelomic lining (peritoneum) is formed – the processus vaginalis. This grows into the gubernaculum, helping to form the inguinal canal, extending downwards, distending the genital swelling to form the scrotum. The testis follows along this line pushing the processus vaginalis before it. The processus vaginalis eventually becomes the tunica vaginalis.

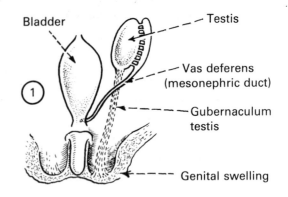

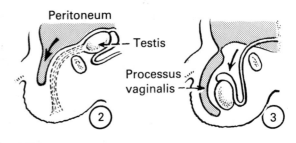

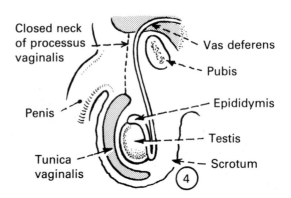

PROSTATE

The development of the prostate has already been indicated (page 8). Small epithelial buds arise from the urethra and from the urogenital sinus. Coming together they surround the urethra as it issues from the bladder. The ejaculatory ducts also pass through these buds to join the urethra. A small saccule, the prostatic utricle, develops from the region of the Müllerian tubercle which is on the dorsal wall of the urethra. This is thought by some to be the masculine equivalent of the uterus.

DEVELOPMENT OF MALE EXTERNAL GENITALIA

The earlier stages of development of the external genitalia are the same in both sexes. The same five swellings appear in the male around the cloaca (page 8).

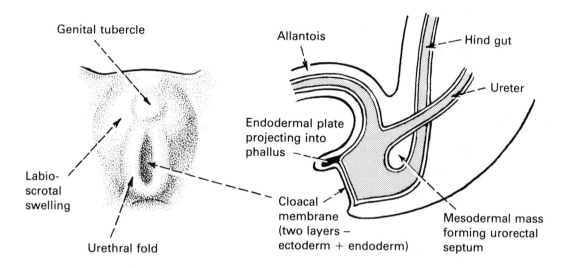

The genital tubercle elongates to form a phallus. Meanwhile a projection arises from the endoderm lining the interior of the cloaca and pushes into the mesenchyme of the phallus.

A groove appears on the under surface of the phallus – the primitive urethral groove.

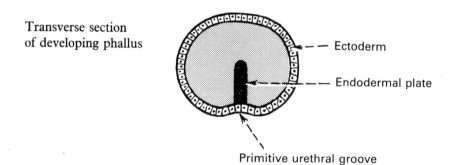

DEVELOPMENT OF MALE EXTERNAL GENITALIA

As in the female a mesodermal mass, the urorectal septum, grows downwards and separates the urogenital sinus from the rectum and anus. The urogenital portion of the cloacal membrane disintegrates so that an open gutter is formed through which the urine drains. This gutter is continuous anteriorly with the primitive urethral groove on the phallus.

The ectoderm on the under surface of the phallus disappears, exposing the underlying endodermal plate.

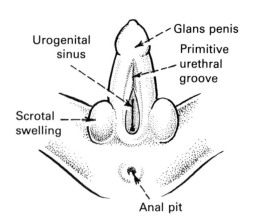

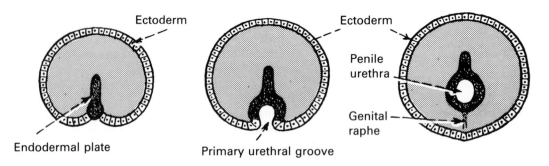

The endodermal plate becomes hollowed to form the primary urethral groove.

The hollow endodermal plate is drawn back into the body of the phallus and in the process it forms a tube. The ectodermal surface is restored.

At the same time the urethral folds are approximated and ultimately fuse.

The testes descend into the labio-scrotal swellings which become distended and move medially to form the scrotum.

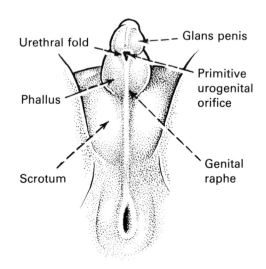

CHAPTER 2

ANATOMY OF THE REPRODUCTIVE TRACT

THE PERINEUM

The PERINEUM (Gk. 'around the natal area')

The **anatomical** or true perineum is the diamond-shaped outlet of the pelvis and the soft tissues which cover it.

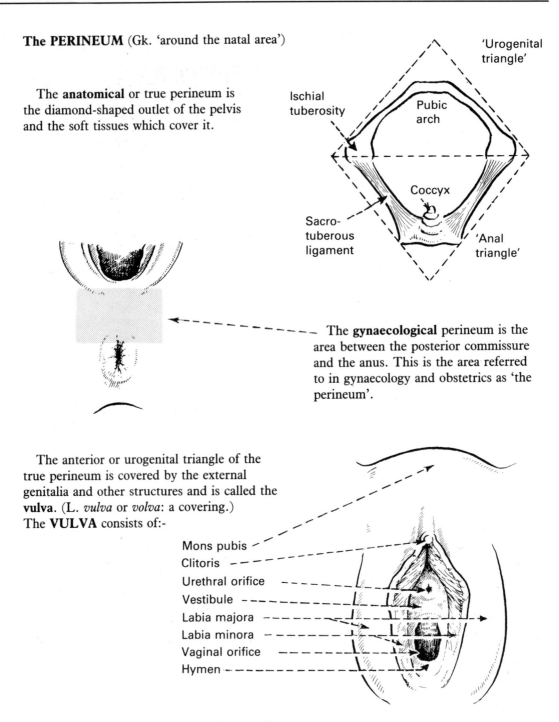

'Urogenital triangle'

Ischial tuberosity

Pubic arch

Coccyx

Sacro-tuberous ligament

'Anal triangle'

The **gynaecological** perineum is the area between the posterior commissure and the anus. This is the area referred to in gynaecology and obstetrics as 'the perineum'.

The anterior or urogenital triangle of the true perineum is covered by the external genitalia and other structures and is called the **vulva**. (L. *vulva* or *volva*: a covering.)
The **VULVA** consists of:-

Mons pubis
Clitoris
Urethral orifice
Vestibule
Labia majora
Labia minora
Vaginal orifice
Hymen

Subcutaneous: the bulb of the vestibule and the greater vestibular (Bartholin's) glands.

FiFE COLLEGE OF
HEALTH STUDIES

THE VULVA

MONS PUBIS and LABIA MAJORA

The mons pubis is a pad of fatty tissue
overlying the symphysis pubis and covered
by skin and pubic hair. The labia are
folds of skin and fat which pass from the
mons back to the perineum. The lateral
labial surfaces are pigmented and hairy,
the inner smooth and containing many
sebaceous, sweat and apocrine glands
which give off the smell peculiar to
the vulva.

The substance of the labia consists
of vascular fatty tissue with many
lymphatics, and also vestigial remnants
of the dartos muscle. (The labium is the
homologue of the scrotum.)

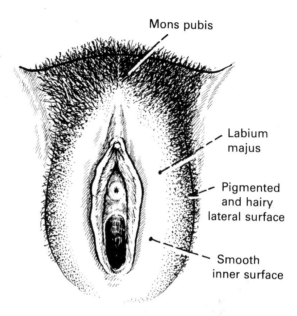

Mons pubis

Labium
majus

Pigmented
and hairy
lateral surface

Smooth
inner surface

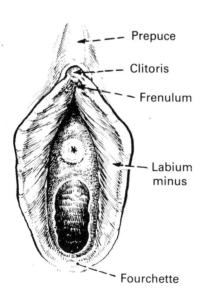

Prepuce

Clitoris

Frenulum

Labium
minus

Fourchette

CLITORIS and LABIA MINORA

The clitoris is the vestigial homologue
of the penis and is formed the same way
from two corpora cavernosa and a glans of
spongy erectile tissue which has a copious
blood supply from the clitoral artery. The
clitoris is highly innervated.

The labia minora are two cutaneous
folds enclosing the urethral and vaginal
orifices. Anteriorly each divides to form
a hood or prepuce, and a frenulum
for the clitoris. Posteriorly they unite
in a frenulum or fourchette which is
obliterated by the delivery of a baby.
The labia minora contain no fat but many
sebaceous glands.

15

THE VULVA

The **VESTIBULE** is the area between the labia minora. It is perforated by the urethral and vaginal orifices and the ducts of Bartholin's glands. The fossa navicularis between the vagina and the fourchette is, like the fourchette, obliterated by childbirth. The lesser vestibular glands are mucosal glands discharging on to the surface of the vestibule.

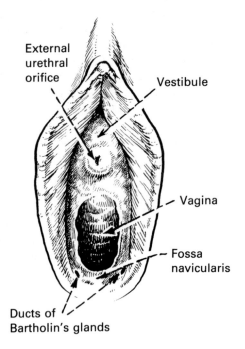

External urethral orifice

Vestibule

Vagina

Fossa navicularis

Ducts of Bartholin's glands

The **EXTERNAL URETHRAL ORIFICE** is in the healthy state a small protuberance with a vertical cleft. The tiny orifices of the paraurethral (Skene's) ducts lie just inside or outside the meatus. The paraurethral glands are homologues of the prostate and form a system of tubular glands surrounding most of the urethra.

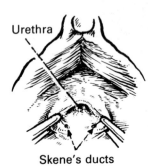

Urethra

Skene's ducts

The **VAGINAL ORIFICE** is a midline aperture incompletely closed by the **HYMEN**. The hymen is a thin fold of tissue lined by squamous epithelium with a small hole (sometimes several) for the passage of menstrual blood. It is ruptured by coitus and more or less obliterated by childbirth. A few tags of skin are left called *carunculae myrtiformes*. The appearances of the hymen are unreliable as medicolegal evidence, whether of virginity or childbirth.

Normal virgin hymen

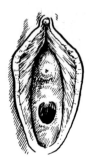

Hymen after coitus (or after using tampons)

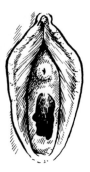

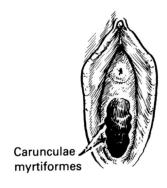

Carunculae myrtiformes

BARTHOLIN'S GLAND

The **BULB of the VESTIBULE** consists of
two masses of erectile tissue on either side
of the vagina, lying beneath the skin and
bulbospongiosus muscle but superficial to
the perineal membrane. They are connected
anteriorly by a narrow transverse strip and are
the homologue of the bulb of the penis.

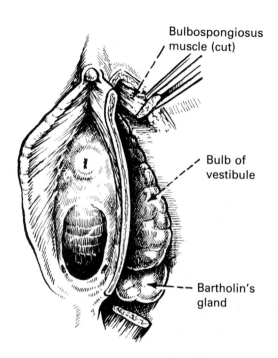

BARTHOLIN'S (Greater vestibular) glands
are the homologues of the bulbo-urethral
(Cowper's) glands in the male but lie
superficial instead of deep to the perineal
membrane. Each gland is partly covered
by the erectile tissue of the bulb and drains
by a duct about 2cm long which opens into
the vaginal orifice lateral to the hymen.
Bartholin's gland is not palpable in the
healthy state.

The erectile tissue of the bulb becomes tumescent during sexual excitement and the glands
secrete a mucoid discharge which acts as a lubricant.

Histology of Bartholin's Gland

The gland is formed of
racemose glands lined with
columnar or cuboid epithelium.
The duct demonstrates the
very intimate embryological
connection between genital and
urinary tracts by being lined
with transitional epithelium.

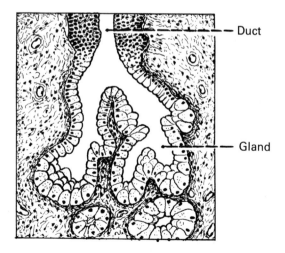

MUSCLES OF THE PERINEUM

Ischiocavernosus

This muscle compresses the root of the clitoris during sexual excitement, to produce erection by venous congestion.

Bulbospongiosus

This muscle conceals the vestibular bulb and Bartholin's glands. Its function is to diminish the vaginal orifice during coitus.

Transversus perinei superficialis

A feeble muscle which helps to fix the perineal body.

Sphincter ani externus

Normally in a state of contraction to keep the anus closed. It also helps to fix the perineal body.

The **Perineal body** is a fibromuscular node between anus and vagina with attachments to 8 muscles.

One Sphincter ani
One Bulbospongiosus
Two Transversi perinei superficiales
Two Transversi perinei profundi (deep: not shown here)
Two Levatores ani

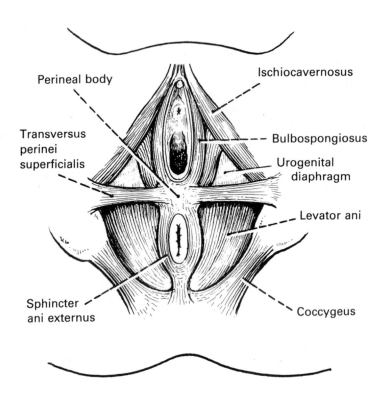

The whole mass is what gynaecologists mean when they talk about 'the perineum'. If it is damaged during parturition and not properly repaired and healed it will not function properly and the efficiency of the whole pelvic diaphragm may suffer.

THE UROGENITAL DIAPHRAGM

The UROGENITAL DIAPHRAGM (Triangular ligament)

This area of the perineum is more developed and surgically more important in the male. It consists of two sheets of fascia with a layer of muscle in between. It covers the pubic arch and is pierced by the urethra and, in the female, by the vagina.

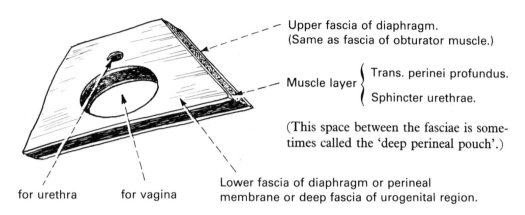

Upper fascia of diaphragm.
(Same as fascia of obturator muscle.)

Muscle layer { Trans. perinei profundus.
Sphincter urethrae.

(This space between the fasciae is sometimes called the 'deep perineal pouch'.)

Lower fascia of diaphragm or perineal membrane or deep fascia of urogenital region.

for urethra   for vagina

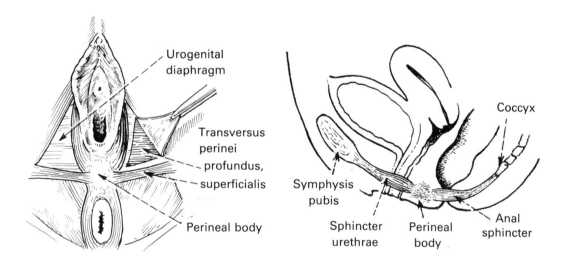

Urogenital diaphragm

Transversus perinei
profundus,
superficialis

Perineal body

Coccyx

Symphysis pubis

Sphincter urethrae

Perineal body

Anal sphincter

All the perineal muscles lie superficial to the perineal membrane except the transversus perinei profundus which helps to fix the perineal body.

(See page 353 on the function of the sphincter.)

The 'sphincter urethrae' is the system of musculature which assists the bladder muscle in closing the urethra. It is made up of the transversus perinei, the bulbospongiosus and the levator ani; the anchoring bony points are the lower border of the symphysis pubis and the coccyx.

ANATOMY OF THE PELVIS

ISCHIORECTAL FOSSA

A wedge-shaped space between the ischial tuberosity and the anus, filled with fat and crossed by vessels and nerves.

Boundaries:-

Laterally, the obturator fascia and ischial tuberosity.

Posteriorly, the sacrotuberous ligament.

Anteriorly, the urogenital diaphragm.

Medially, the sphincter ani and levator (anal) fascia.

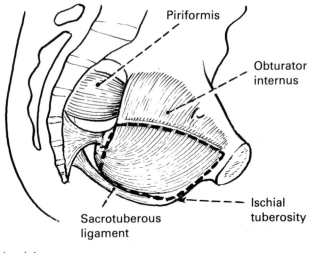

Piriformis

Obturator internus

Sacrotuberous ligament

Ischial tuberosity

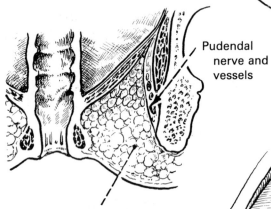

Pudendal nerve and vessels

The ischiorectal fat is traversed by the pudendal vessels and nerves and some small perineal branches of sacral nerves.

This pad of fat supports the anal canal and pelvic diaphragm.

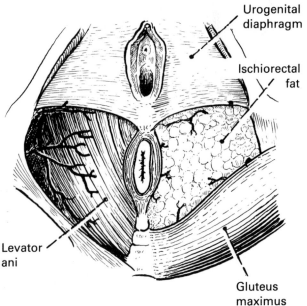

Urogenital diaphragm

Ischiorectal fat

Levator ani

Gluteus maximus

20

MUSCLES OF THE PELVIS

Levator ani ⎫
Coccygeus ⎬ Pelvic diaphragm
Obturator internus
Piriformis

The **Levator ani** arises from the back of the pubis, the obturator fascia (by a 'tendinous arch' or 'white line') and the ischial spine.

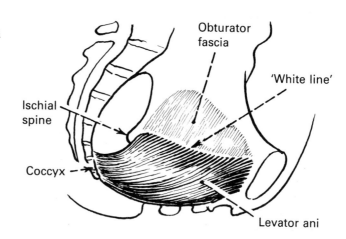

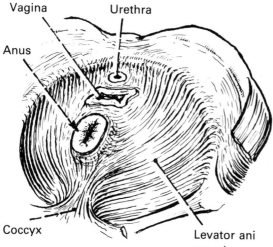

(*From below*)

The fibres pass back and medially to be inserted into the vaginal wall, the perineal body, the anal wall, the anococcygeal raphe, and the coccyx.

Nerve supply: nerve to levator ani and pudendal nerve (S4).

The **Coccygeus** is a triangular muscle, partly replaced by the sacrospinous ligament. It arises from the ischial spine and fans out to an insertion on the sides of the sacrum and coccyx.

Nerve supply: S4 and anococcygeal nerve (S5).

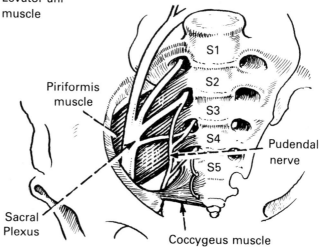

21

PELVIC DIAPHRAGM

The **Obturator internus** arises from the anterolateral wall of the pelvis (and obturator membrane) and passes backwards through the lesser sciatic foramen to be inserted into the trochanter of the femur. (L5, S1 and S2)

The **Piriformis** arises from the front of the sacrum and passes through the greater sciatic foramen to be inserted into the trochanter of the femur. (S1 and 2)

These muscles are primarily lateral rotators of the hip and postural muscles.

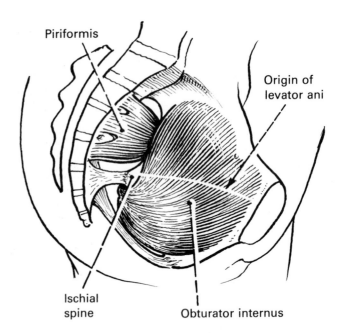

FUNCTIONS of the PELVIC DIAPHRAGM

Apart from helping to fix the perineal body and assist the vaginal and anal sphincters, the main function of the pelvic diaphragm is to support the pelvic viscera.

The muscles used to be named:

$$\left.\begin{array}{l}\text{pubococcygeus}\\\text{iliococcygeus}\end{array}\right\}=\text{levator ani}$$

$$\text{ischiococcygeus} = \text{coccygeus}$$

and in the lower animals their function is to move the tail (the coccyx). In man they have to meet the requirements of the erect position and resist the strain imposed by any increase in intra-abdominal pressure such as laughing, coughing, straining at stool etc. In addition a complete relaxation of the muscles should be possible during parturition so that the vaginal foramen may enlarge almost to the size of the bony pelvic outlet.

PELVIC FASCIA

The PELVIC FASCIA

Parietal Layer

The aponeuroses and fascial sheaths of the pelvic muscles (the 'wallpaper' of the pelvis).

Visceral Layer

The fascial sheaths of the organs and the fatty tissue filling the space between them (the 'stuffing' of the pelvis).

In certain areas this stuffing is condensed and strengthened by plain muscle fibres and elastic tissue to form the ligaments of the uterus (pages 31, 32).

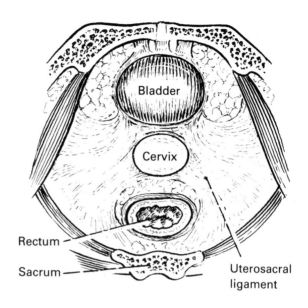

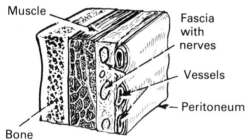

Relations of the Fascia

The nerve trunks, which leave the pelvis may be described as 'outside' the fascia which gives them fascial sheaths. The vessels are 'inside' and lie between fascia and peritoneum.

These fascial prolongations on structures leaving the pelvis form points at which pus may track from a pelvic abscess to point in the buttock or groin or above the inguinal ligament.

(The greater sciatic notch is not shown.)

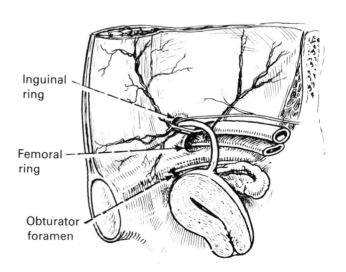

THE VAGINA

A canal of plain muscle extending from the vestibule to the uterus.

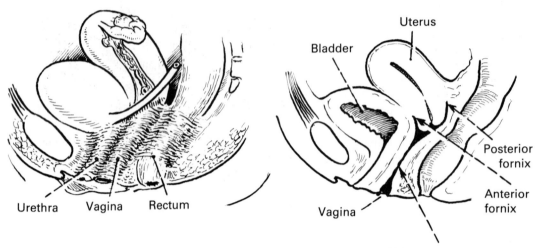

Lateral view. Note the close relationship to urethra, bladder and rectum.

Sagittal section. Note anterior and posterior walls normally in contact; also anterior and posterior fornices.

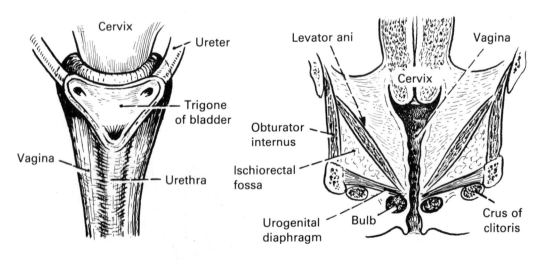

Anterior view shows the very intimate relationship with the bladder base and ureters.

Coronal section shows the relationship of vagina and pelvic floor.

THE VAGINA

In the nulliparous adult the vagina is H-shaped in section and marked by longitudinal furrows – the columns of the vagina – and numerous transverse ridges or rugae. This configuration permits great distension during parturition; and is much less marked in the parous woman.

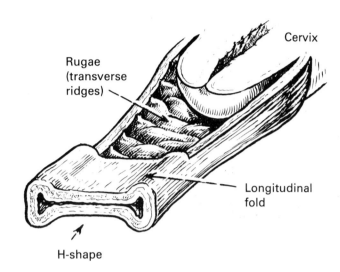

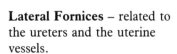

Vaginal Fornices

These are gutters at the top of the vagina, surrounding the cervix.

Anterior Fornix – related to the bladder base and the utero-vesical fossa.

Posterior Fornix – related to peritoneum of the Pouch of Douglas. This fornix is deeper than the anterior one because of the angle the cervix makes with the vagina. The male's ejaculate is deposited in the posterior fornix during coitus, where it is in close contact with the cervical os.

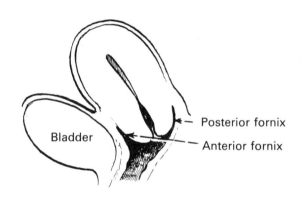

Lateral Fornices – related to the ureters and the uterine vessels.

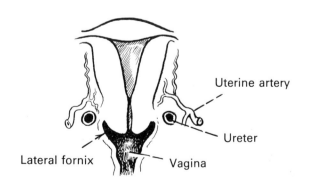

THE VAGINA

HISTOLOGY

Its length is about 9cm along the posterior wall and 7.5cm along its anterior. The width gradually increases from below upwards.

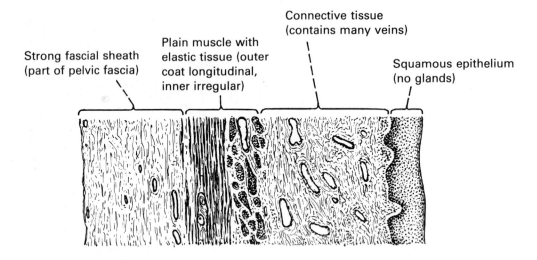

The vagina pierces the urogenital diaphragm and is encircled at its lower end by the voluntary bulbospongiosus which has some sphincteric action, although the levator ani muscle is more effective.

Vaginal secretion

This is composed of alkaline cervical secretion, desquamated epithelial cells and bacteria. The epithelium is rich in glycogen which is converted by Doderlein's bacillus into lactic acid. The vaginal pH is about 4.5 and provides a fairly effective barrier against infection.

The vaginal epithelium

This is composed of several layers of squamous cells with no keratinisation. It develops papillae which dip into the fibrous corium. It is much thinner in the child and the rugae are absent. This appearance recurs in old age. Cyclic changes are discussed on page 54.

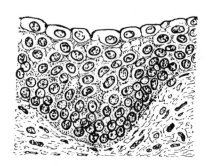

UTERUS

The uterus is a hollow viscus composed of plain muscle whose sole function is gestation.

It lies between the rectum and the bladder and is continuous with the vagina.

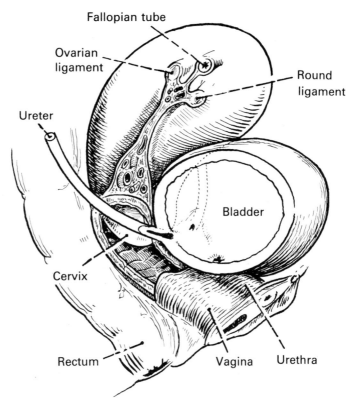

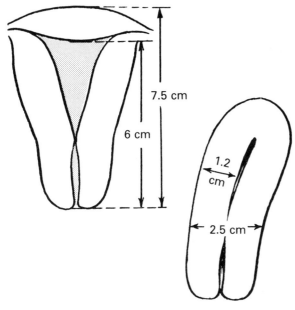

7.5 cm

6 cm

1.2 cm

2.5 cm

It is important to be familiar with the measurements of the adult nulliparous uterus because of the frequent physiological or pathological variations.

Length 7.5cm (3 in.)
Thickness 2.5cm (1 in.)
Length of cavity 6cm (2½ in.)
Thickness of muscle wall is about 1.2cm (½ in.)

27

UTERUS

CORPUS and CERVIX

The upper two-thirds of the uterus are called the corpus or body, and the lower third the cervix or neck. They are quite distinct in function and therefore in structure as well, although the transition from muscle to fibrous tissue is gradual.

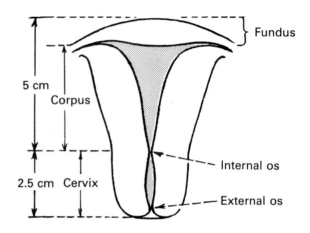

CORPUS

Its function is to provide a mucous membrane (endometrium) suitable for implantation, and thereafter to contain the growing fetus until it is mature. It is composed mainly of unstriped muscle.

CERVIX

Its function is to provide an alkaline secretion favourable to sperm penetration, and once the uterus is gravid, to act as a sphincter. It is composed mainly of fibro-elastic tissue.

ISTHMUS UTERI This name is sometimes given to the upper few millimetres of the cervical canal below the internal os, an area to which the specific function of developing into the lower segment has been ascribed. The epithelium is intermediate between corpus and cervix; but if it were not for the importance of the lower segment in the modern theory of the physiology of pregnancy, it is unlikely that anatomists would have provided either an identity or a name for the isthmus uteri.

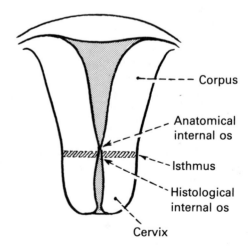

UTERUS

CAVITY of the CORPUS

The anterior and posterior walls are almost in contact but in coronal plane the cavity is triangular.

The muscle wall at each cornu is pierced by the very narrow interstitial portion of the fallopian tube.

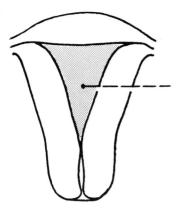

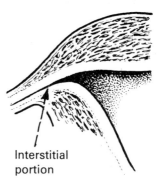

Interstitial portion

CERVIX

The external os is small before parturition and is sometimes called the os tincae (mouth of a small fish). After the birth of a child it becomes a transverse slit – 'the parous os'.

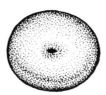

Nulliparous os

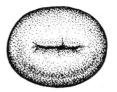

Parous os

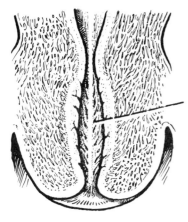

The cervical canal is fusiform and marked by curious folds called the 'arbor vitae'.

The cervix is divided into supra- and infravaginal portions by the attachments of the vagina. The infravaginal part is also called the 'portio vaginalis'.

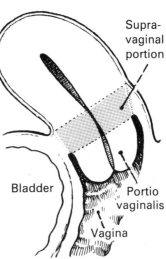

Supra-vaginal portion

Bladder

Portio vaginalis

Vagina

UTERUS

RELATIONSHIP of UTERUS and URETER

The ureter is directly related to the uterine artery and the vaginal vault but is not in direct contact with the uterus.

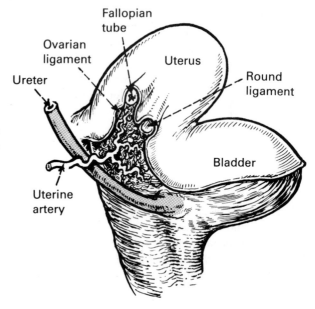

This picture shows the ureter passing under the uterine artery on its course to the bladder.

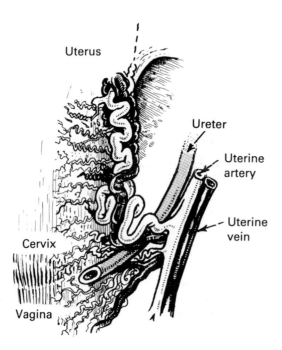

In this picture the bladder has been removed to show just how close the ureter is to the cervix. It also demonstrates the problems which are likely to be encountered in controlling haemorrhage and avoiding damage to the ureter during surgery in this area. (See pages 340–345)

UTERUS

LIGAMENTS of the UTERUS

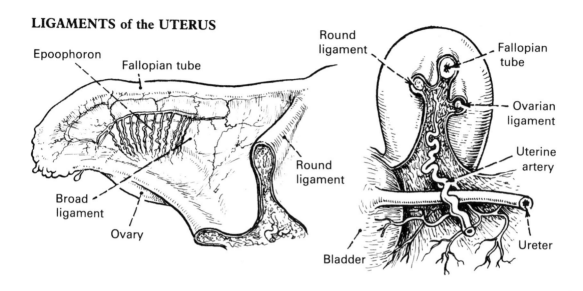

The **Broad ligament** is a fold of peritoneum passing from the uterus to the side wall of the pelvis. It contains the fallopian tube, the round and ovarian ligaments, the mesonephric remnants, the ovario-uterine anastomosis and in its base, the ureter.

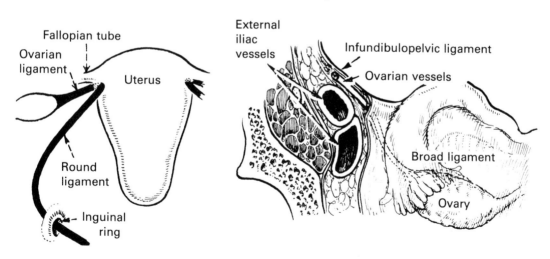

The ovarian and round ligaments are the vestigial gubernaculum. The round ligament ends in the inguinal canal and its fibres disperse in the labium majus.

The part of the broad ligament between infundibulum and pelvic wall is called the infundibulopelvic ligament and contains the ovarian vessels and nerves. Note proximity of external iliac vessels.

UTERUS

LIGAMENTS of the UTERUS – (*contd*)

The main supports of the uterus are the fibromuscular condensations of tissue in the pelvic fascia (page 23).

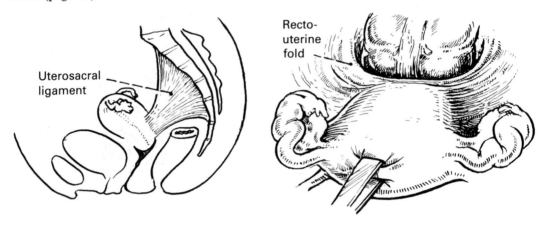

The **Uterosacral Ligaments** pass from the back of the uterus to the front of the sacrum and are easily identified by the covering recto-uterine fold of peritoneum. These ligaments maintain the anteverted position of the uterus, and they are accompanied by uterine vessels and nerves.

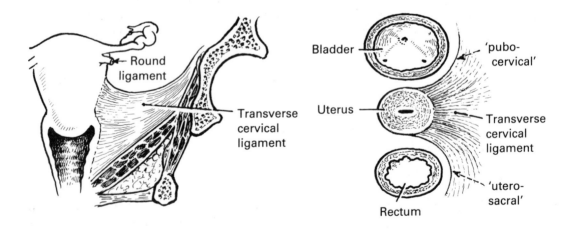

The **Transverse Cervical Ligaments** (Mackenrodt's, cardinal ligaments) pass from uterus and vagina to a wide insertion in the lateral pelvic wall. They lie below the broad ligament and contain vessels and nerves. The uterosacral ligament may be regarded as the posterior edge of the transverse cervical; its anterior edge is sometimes called the pubocervical but this is not well defined.

UTERUS

HISTOLOGY

The uterus has an incomplete peritoneal coat which is very adherent. The anterior bare area is to allow movement of the bladder. There is a complete fascial sheath continuous with the vagina and the body is made of plain muscle interspersed with fibro-elastic tissue. There is a reversion of the ratio of muscle to connective tissue as the cervix is approached; and the cervix is nearly all fibrous.

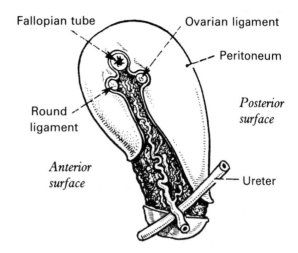

The epithelium of the cavity is called endometrium and consists of a single layer of cuboid or columnar ciliated cells on a cellular stroma. The stroma is deeply pierced by invaginations of the epithelium called uterine glands which secrete a small amount of mucus to maintain moistness.

For cyclical changes in the endometrium see page 53.

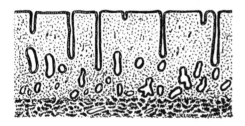

Endometrium (low power)

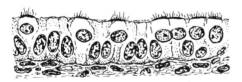

Uterine gland (high power)

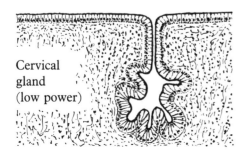

Cervical gland (low power)

The cervix is lined by a single layer of high columnar ciliated epithelium which covers the folds of the arbor vitae (page 29) and lines the cervical glands. The glands secrete an alkaline mucus which is favourable to the activity of spermatozoa.

FALLOPIAN TUBE

The tube extends from the cornu of the uterus into the peritoneal cavity and is about 10cm long. The two tubes are twice the width of the pelvis and they do more than just provide a passage for the ovum into the uterus. They must be sufficiently mobile to assist the ovum onwards by peristalsis; and sufficiently long to allow the ovum time for maturation after it has been fertilised in the ampulla and before it is ready for implantation in the uterus. The tube and ovary together are called the adnexa ('viscera adnexa' – organs next to) of the uterus.

Interstitial part	**Isthmus**	**Ampulla**	**Infundibulum**
1cm long and very narrow (less than 1mm).	2cm long, straight and cord-like. 1mm diameter.	5cm long, thin walled and convoluted.	2cm long. The terminal expansion, with fimbrial processes which help to attract the ovum.

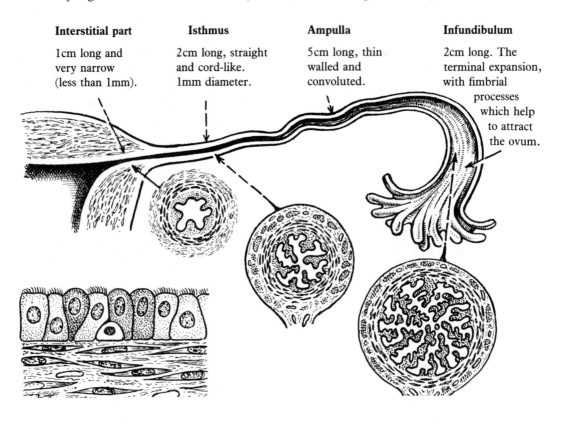

The tube has a lining of ciliated cells interspersed with non-ciliated secretory cells ('peg' cells). There is little or no submucosa. The epithelium is arranged in a complex pattern of plications which becomes more marked as the outer end is approached. (For cyclic changes see page 54.)

BROAD LIGAMENT

Blood Vessels

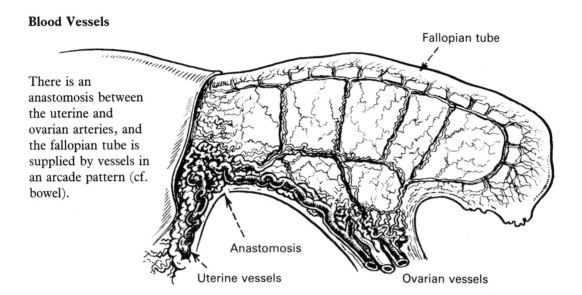

There is an anastomosis between the uterine and ovarian arteries, and the fallopian tube is supplied by vessels in an arcade pattern (cf. bowel).

Fallopian tube

Anastomosis

Uterine vessels

Ovarian vessels

Vestigial Structures

The epoophoron and the paroophoron are remnants of the mesonephros, and the duct (Gartner's duct) is the vestige of the mesonephric duct which passes into the uterine muscle about the level of the internal os and continues downwards in the vaginal wall.

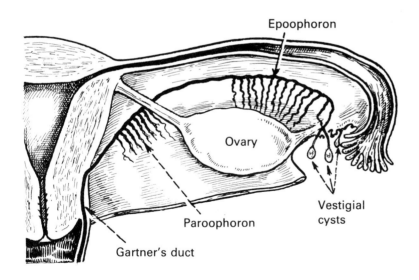

Epoophoron

Ovary

Paroophoron

Gartner's duct

Vestigial cysts

These structures may give rise to cysts (Hydatids of Morgagni, Kobelt's tubules, fimbrial cysts) whose embryonic derivation is uncertain. They are probably mesonephric and can be grouped together as 'vestigial cysts'.

OVARY

The ovary is about 3cm long and
1.5cm wide, roughly the size and shape
of a date. It has its own mesentery, the
mesovarium from the posterior leaf
of the broad ligament and is attached
to the cornu of the uterus by the
ovarian ligament which is continuous
with the round ligament, the vestigial
gubernaculum.

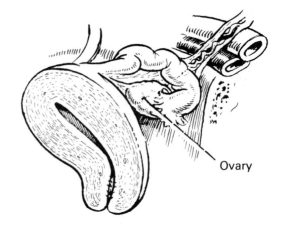

Ovary

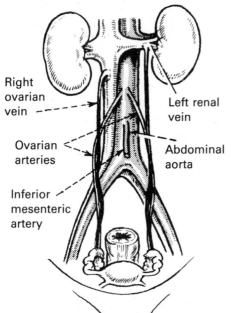

Right ovarian vein

Ovarian arteries

Inferior mesenteric artery

Left renal vein

Abdominal aorta

The ovary is developmentally an abdominal
organ and its blood supply is from the
abdominal aorta. The ovarian vessels lie in the
infundibulopelvic ligaments.
Note: The left ovarian vein empties into the left
renal vein.

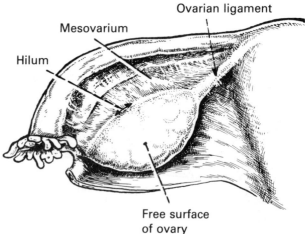

Mesovarium

Ovarian ligament

Hilum

Free surface
of ovary

The free surface of the ovary has no
peritoneal covering, only a surface epithelium.
The part attached to the mesovarium through
which all vessels and nerves pass, is called
the hilum.

OVARY

HISTOLOGY

Cross-section shows the ovary to be roughly divided into a vascular medulla and a cortex.

The cortex is composed of a specialised ovarian stroma with a cuboidal surface epithelium which, like the tubal ostium, is intraperitoneal.

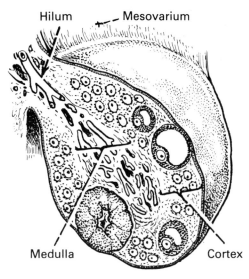

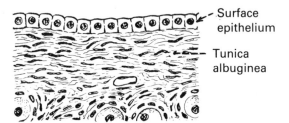

Note the condensed layer of stroma under the surface epithelium, called the tunica albuginea.

Ova are very numerous in the infant and child (at least over 100,000) but much less so in the adult.

The hilum is characterised by the presence of paroophoron tubules which are of plain muscle lined with ciliated epithelium; and by vestigial remnants of the sex cords called the rete ovarii, the analogue of the seminiferous tubules. These tissues are one reason for the extraordinary variety of ovarian tumours which can develop.

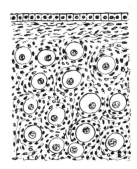

Cortex in an infant.

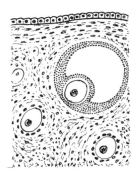

Cortex in an adult.

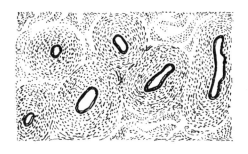

The hilum, showing cross-section of paroophoron tubules.

OVARY

The **CORPUS LUTEUM** ('Yellow body': carotene gives the mature corpus luteum a yellow colour.) During growth the Graafian follicle gradually approaches the surface of the ovary and eventually extrudes the ovum through the stigma, into the waiting fimbriae of the tube. The follicle cells then quickly become luteinised by the retention of fluid to form the corpus luteum whose function is to secrete progestins and prepare the organism for implantation of the fertilised ovum.

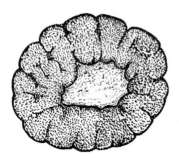

Corpus luteum (low power)

Thecal cells   Lutein cells

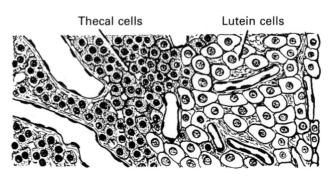

Corpus luteum (high power)

The growing corpus luteum is supplied with capillaries from the ovarian stromal vessels, and both theca and granulosa lutein cells secrete all the hormones – oestrogens, progestins (predominantly) and androgens.

Corpus albicans

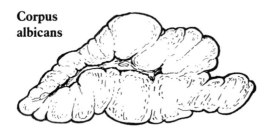

As the physiological cycle proceeds degeneration gradually occurs, and eventually the corpus luteum is hyalinised – a corpus albicans – and is absorbed in about a year. This scarring accounts for the irregular surface of the ovary in the more mature woman.

Follicular atresia

More than half the oocytes present at birth are absorbed before puberty and all are gone at the menopause. Only about 400 can ever become mature follicles, but at each cycle and probably during childhood several follicles may start to develop and for a time produce hormones. This abortive attempt ends in atresia and the atretic follicle is absorbed; but the process may account for anovular cycles and for the oestrogens produced by young pre-pubertal girls whose breasts are beginning to develop.

CHANGES IN THE GENITAL TRACT WITH AGE

Apart from normal growth the appearances of the genital tract depend entirely on the supply of oestrogens.

The Vulva

This is only a cleft in the perineum before puberty. Then the labia minora become more prominent and the fat of the mons and the labia majora is increased. Apart from the effects of coitus and parturition (page 16) the most obvious sign of ageing is the gradual increase in size of the labia minora compared with the labia majora.

The Vagina

The rugae are absent before puberty and gradually (over several years) disappear after the menopause. In old women the vagina is thin, atrophic and completely smooth.

The Ovary

This is at its largest during the reproductive stage and shrinks thereafter. All the oocytes are gone by the time of the menopause and the cortex consists of fibrous tissue.

The Uterus

Infantile: the cervix is longer than the corpus and there is no flexion.

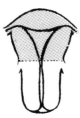

Pubertal: with the gradual increase in oestrogens the corpus grows in relation to the cervix.

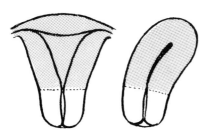

Adult: the corpus is now twice as long as the cervix and the normal degree of flexion has appeared.

After the menopause the uterus gradually atrophies and in an old woman the cavity may be less than 5cm and the cervix simply an aperture in the senile vaginal vault.

BLOOD SUPPLY OF THE PELVIS

The common iliac artery bifurcates at the level of the sacrovertebral junction into external and internal iliac arteries. The internal iliac runs for about 4cm and divides into an anterior and posterior trunk which are the main pelvic supply. The branches are subject to great variation.

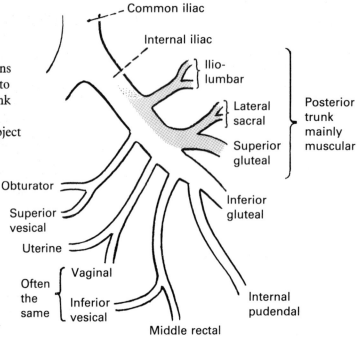

Supply to uterus, vagina and bladder.

This picture shows an arrangement often met with.

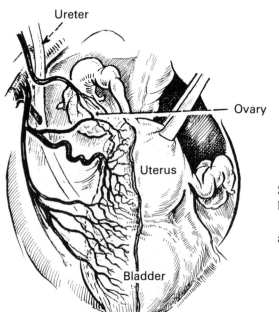

BLOOD SUPPLY OF THE PELVIS

The vessels of the uterus and vagina are much coiled to provide extra length during pregnancy. (Cf. the coiled telephone flex.) Note the nearness of the ureter.

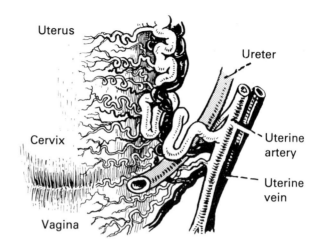

This picture shows the course of the pudendal artery passing behind the ischial spine and along the pudendal canal to the perineum.

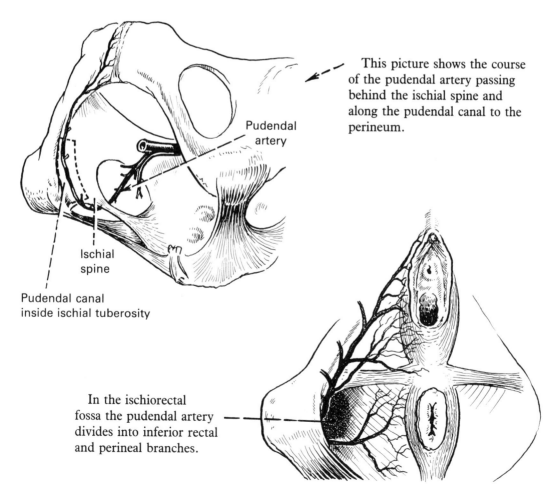

In the ischiorectal fossa the pudendal artery divides into inferior rectal and perineal branches.

BLOOD SUPPLY OF THE PELVIS

COLLATERAL BLOOD SUPPLY

If the internal iliac artery has to be ligated, the collateral circulation should be adequate. It depends on anastomoses with the abdominal aorta, external iliac and femoral arteries.

Abdominal aorta
1. Ovarian artery → uterine artery.
2. Inferior mesenteric → superior rectal → inferior rectal (pudendal).
3. Median sacral → lateral sacral.

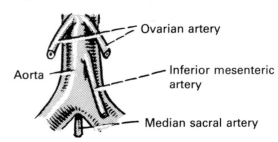

External iliac artery

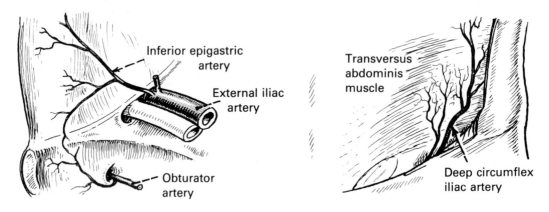

The inferior epigastric anastomoses with the obturator; the deep circumflex iliac with the iliolumbar and lumbar arteries.

The Femoral artery
The deep external pudendal anastomoses with the internal pudendal.

The superior and inferior gluteal arteries anastomose with the perforating and circumflex branches of the femoral and profunda femoris. (This is the 'cruciate' anastomosis.)

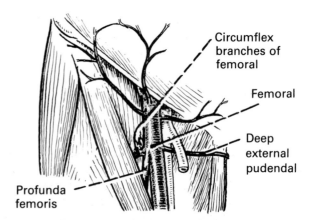

LYMPHATIC DRAINAGE OF THE GENITAL TRACT

The lymphatic plexuses accompany the blood vessels and drain into groups of glands which are constant in position and are given names.

It will be seen that while the uterus is likely to drain into the external iliac group on the lateral wall of the pelvis, the vagina drains into the internal iliac group and the ovary drains direct to the aortic glands.

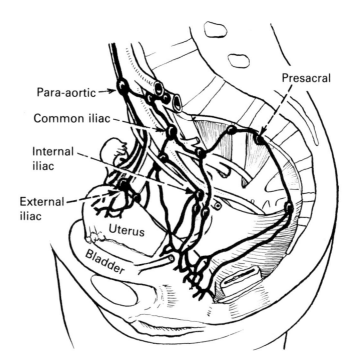

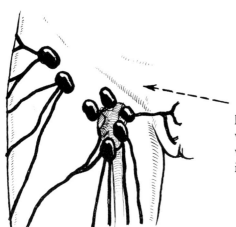

The superficial inguinal glands also receive lymph drainage from vulva and the lower vagina. (But these structures may also drain via the pudendal vessel channels into the internal iliac group.)

Because lymphatic plexuses and glands are the path of metastatic spread of cancer, treatment either by irradiation or surgery must involve an attack on the area of lymphatic drainage of the organs concerned. But the lymphatic network is so widespread and the metastatic paths are not always the same; and it is now recognised that the chance of cure is much reduced once the spread to the glands has occurred, whatever treatment is given.

NERVES OF THE PELVIS

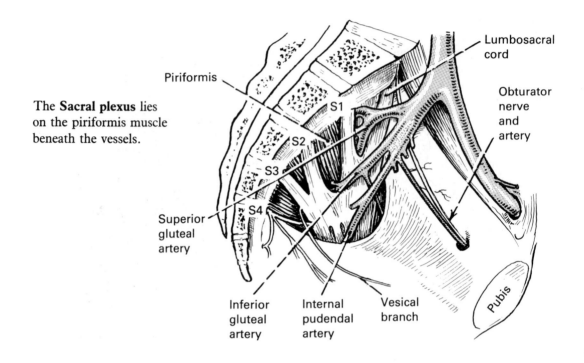

The **Sacral plexus** lies on the piriformis muscle beneath the vessels.

Piriformis

Lumbosacral cord

Obturator nerve and artery

S1

S2

S3

S4

Superior gluteal artery

Inferior gluteal artery

Internal pudendal artery

Vesical branch

Pubis

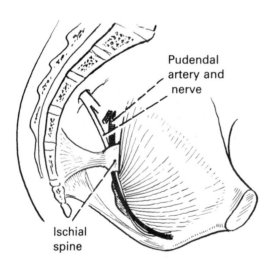

Pudendal artery and nerve

Ischial spine

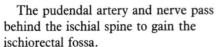

The pudendal artery and nerve pass behind the ischial spine to gain the ischiorectal fossa.

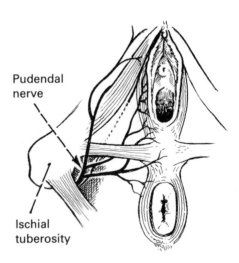

Pudendal nerve

Ischial tuberosity

The pudendal nerve crosses the ischiorectal fossa to supply the vulva and perineum.

AUTONOMIC NERVE SUPPLY OF THE PELVIS

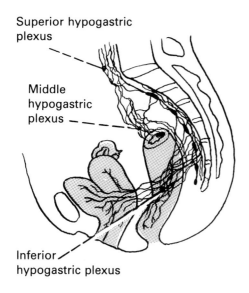

Superior hypogastric plexus

Middle hypogastric plexus

Inferior hypogastric plexus

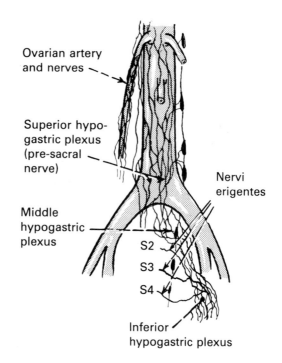

Ovarian artery and nerves

Superior hypogastric plexus (pre-sacral nerve)

Middle hypogastric plexus

Nervi erigentes

S2
S3
S4

Inferior hypogastric plexus

Sympathetic fibres enter via the lumbosacral chain and the mesenteric nerves. These are called the presacral nerve at the bifurcation of the aorta. They pass forward in the uterosacral ligaments to reach the viscera and are known there as the hypogastric plexus or plexus of Frankenhauser.

Parasympathetic nerves (nervi erigentes) join the hypogastric plexuses from sacral roots 2, 3, 4.

There is an additional sympathetic supply by the nerves accompanying the ovarian vessels.

Function of the autonomic nerves is not understood. In practice it is possible to cauterise the cervix causing only a sensation of heat. The cervix or vagina may be grasped by forceps with only a momentary pricking sensation, and a sound in the uterine cavity causes a vague 'visceral' discomfort. Yet cervical dilatation must be done under anaesthesia, and even then it has been known to cause a severe vasovagal collapse. The relief of pelvic pain by partial cordotomy has to be done well above the pelvis to be effective, and the level of choice is T.2 (see page 236).

CHAPTER 3

PHYSIOLOGY OF THE REPRODUCTIVE TRACT

OVULATION

FEMALE REPRODUCTIVE PHYSIOLOGY

The dominant process which appears to govern the physiology of the female genital organs during reproductive life is the cyclical growth and maturation of ovarian follicles.

The ovary is covered by a cuboidal "germinal" epithelium which at the hilum is continuous with that lining the peritoneal cavity. This is supported by a thin layer of fibrous tissue beneath which is the true cortex. The latter consists of a specialised stroma or parenchyma embedded in which are the primordial follicles.

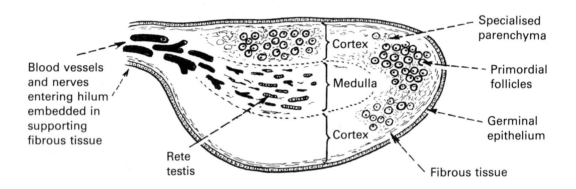

The primordial follicle consists of a primary oocyte surrounded by a single layer of flattened cells, the pre-granulosa, said to be derived from the cells of the sex cords.

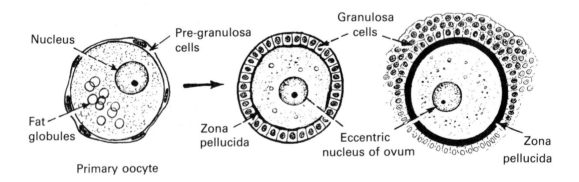

The pre-granulosa cells become cuboidal and proliferate to form a shell several layers thick. At this stage a hyaline membrane is formed immediately around the ovum – the zona pellucida.

OVULATION

The granulosa cells continue to proliferate until the follicle is approximately 200μ in diameter. Fluid spaces now appear between the granulosa cells. They coalesce to form a cavity, the antrum, pushing the ovum to one side. The granulosa cells immediately surrounding the ovum are now known as the corona radiata and the whole mass of cells in this situation is termed the cumulus.

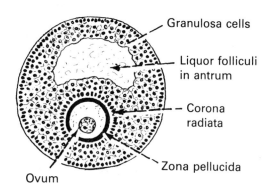

At the same time the surrounding parenchymal cells arrange themselves concentrically around the follicle and, opposite the site of the ovum, some become smaller and epithelial in appearance. As the follicle increases in size this epithelial change spreads to the parenchymal cells around the circumference of the follicle. This band of cells constitutes the theca interna. The cells are surrounded by sinusoidal capillaries thus making a structure like an endocrine gland. External to this band the parenchymal cells are also arranged concentrically but retain their fusiform shape.

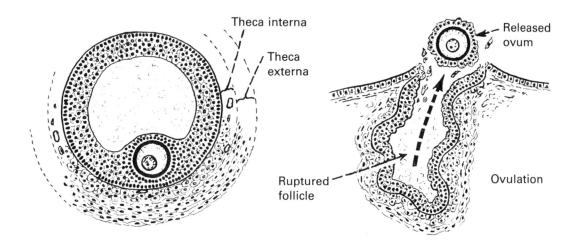

The follicle, which is called the Graafian follicle, continues to grow to a size of more than 1.0 cm. Approximately 4–5 follicles may attain this size and project on the surface of one ovary. One of these follicles ruptures on the surface, releasing the ovum surrounded by some of the granulosa cells.

49

OVULATION

From fetal life to the menopause follicular growth is continuous. Oestrogen initiates the process. Three phases can be distinguished:–

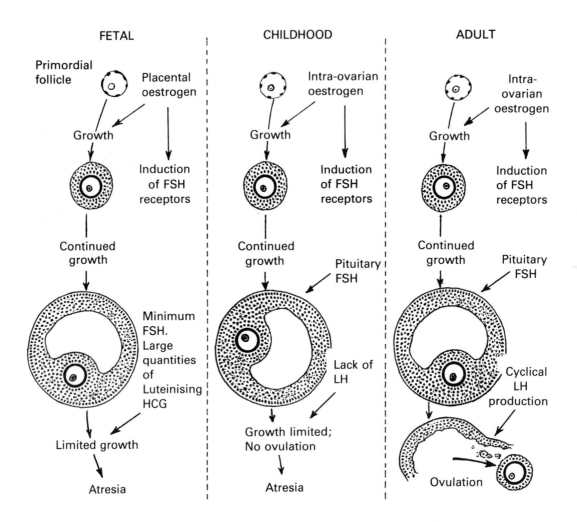

HCG = Human Chorionic Gonadotrophin.
FSH = Follicle Stimulating Hormone.
LH = Luteinising Hormone.

Normally only one follicle ovulates. Cohorts of follicles enter the growth phase in succession, thus follicles of various sizes are usually found. The follicle destined to ovulate is in a cohort stimulated to grow by FSH secreted by the pituitary during the last few days of the cycle.

OVULATION

Ovulation is the final event in a step-wise stimulatory mechanism starting in the hypothalamus which contains gonadotrophin releasing cells. These produce a gonadotrophin releasing hormone (GnRH).

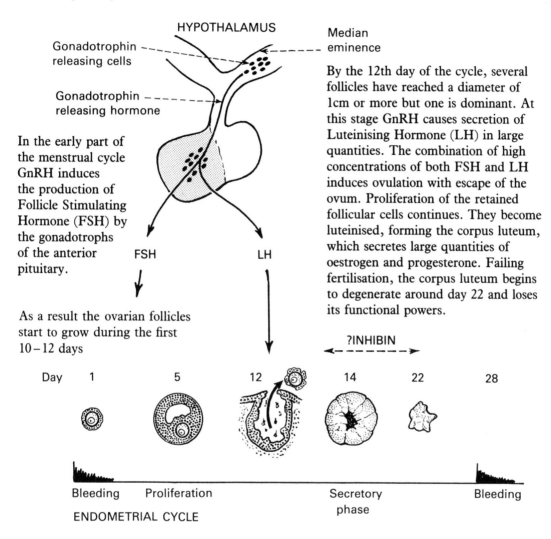

By the 12th day of the cycle, several follicles have reached a diameter of 1cm or more but one is dominant. At this stage GnRH causes secretion of Luteinising Hormone (LH) in large quantities. The combination of high concentrations of both FSH and LH induces ovulation with escape of the ovum. Proliferation of the retained follicular cells continues. They become luteinised, forming the corpus luteum, which secretes large quantities of oestrogen and progesterone. Failing fertilisation, the corpus luteum begins to degenerate around day 22 and loses its functional powers.

In the early part of the menstrual cycle GnRH induces the production of Follicle Stimulating Hormone (FSH) by the gonadotrophs of the anterior pituitary.

As a result the ovarian follicles start to grow during the first 10–12 days

RELEASING HORMONE

This substance begins to be secreted just before puberty in pulses every hour and continues in this fashion for the rest of life. There is only a single releasing hormone responsible for the production of both FSH and LH. The type of gonadotrophin secreted by the pituitary appears to be determined by other factors related to the phase of the menstrual cycle.

51

OVULATION

Inhibin

This substance, which inhibits the secretion of FSH, is produced by the corpus luteum while it is active. As a result follicular growth ceases. After the 22nd day, when the corpus luteum becomes inactive, FSH secretion and growth of follicles are resumed. Oestrogen levels begin to increase. A peak of FSH is reached by the 6th day of the succeeding menstrual cycle. At this point the rising oestrogen has a negative feedback effect and the FSH curve languishes for a day or two and then resumes its upward trend to achieve a second peak at the time of ovulation on day 12. Very low levels of LH are recorded in the early part of the cycle but a sudden surge, coinciding with the second peak of FSH induces ovulation and formation of the corpus luteum. Shortly thereafter the level of LH returns to pre-ovulatory values.

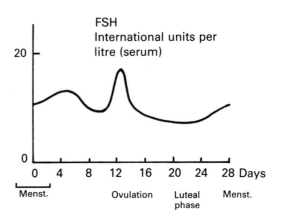

Gonadotrophin Secretion (International Units per Litre)

	Menstruation		Follicular phase		Ovulation		Luteal phase	
	Mean	Range	Mean	Range	Mean	Range	Mean	Range
FSH	10	3 – 13	8	3 – 15	20	4 – 32	5	2 – 0
LH	8	3 – 12	8	6 – 14	65	43 – 88	8	2 – 13

Control Mechanisms in Ovulation

Two forms of control operate during follicle maturation. These act in concert to produce the histological changes associated with ovulation. The first of these is indicated by a comparison of the blood concentrations of FSH and oestrogens.

These show an inverse relationship. As stated above, after the 22nd day of one cycle FSH is rising and continues to do so until the 6th day of the succeeding cycle while the curve of oestrogen only shows a significant increase a day or two before this point. FSH then declines. This is due to the negative feedback effect of rising oestrogen. The upward curve of oestrogen indicating continuing follicular growth proceeds smoothly.

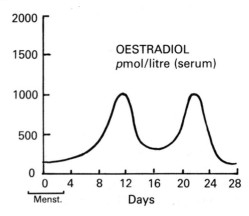

OVULATION

Control Mechanisms (*contd*)

The apparent anomaly of increasing oestrogen in the face of FSH inhibition is related to the second system of control, which involves the dominant follicle about to ovulate. At each stage of gonadotrophin production and follicular growth specific proteins are formed which are involved in the transport and reception of the various hormones from the releasing hormone onward e.g.:

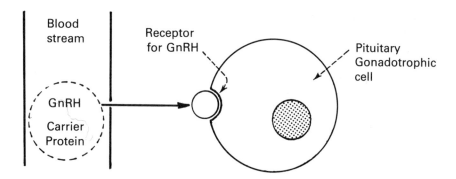

Having accepted GnRH the pituitary cell will then secrete the appropriate hormone. The same mechanism will then operate in regard to the carriage of the pituitary hormone and the reception by the ovarian follicle. The key to the continuing growth of the follicle and production of oestrogen is the amount of receptor protein in the follicular cell. The larger the follicle the greater the concentration of receptor protein and therefore the greater the amount of pituitary hormone the ovarian cell is able to accept and store. Thus although the blood FSH is temporarily reduced after the 6th day the larger follicles have accumulated sufficient FSH to maintain growth and oestrogen production.

As the blood concentration of oestrogen continues to increase it appears to reach a critical level at the 12th day, and in place of its usual negative feedback effect on the pituitary it suddenly exerts a positive feedback effect with consequent rise in FSH (the second peak) and secretion of LH.

Luteinising Hormone

LH is present throughout the menstrual cycle but, apart from a short period at ovulation, it remains at a low level. The rapid increase at ovulation coincides with the second peak of FSH secretion.

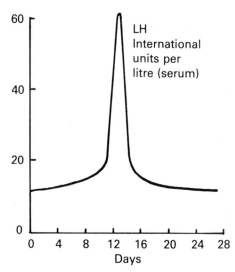

ENDOMETRIAL CYCLE

By the 5th day of the menstrual cycle the endometrium shows proliferation of its stroma and glands, the latter elongating. The cells lining the glands are cuboidal with definite limiting membranes and the stromal cells are thin and spindly – early proliferative phase.

In a week's time (12th day) the glands are very large and are now dilated – late proliferative phase. The blood vessels are also more prominent and capillaries are dilated.

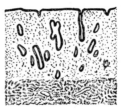

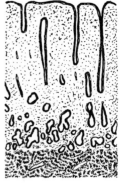

Early
proliferative
phase

Late
proliferative
phase

These proliferative changes are due to the influence of oestrogen secreted by the ovary at this time.

Following ovulation the corpus luteum produces large quantities of progesterone which induce secretory changes in the glands and swelling of the stromal cells. There is a rich blood supply and the capillaries become sinusoidal.

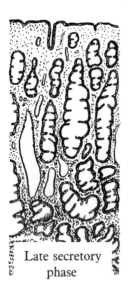

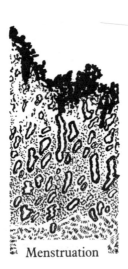

Late secretory
phase

Menstruation

Towards the end of the 28-day cycle the stroma becomes even more vascular and oedematous, small haemorrhages and thrombi appear and the endometrium ultimately breaks down due to withdrawal of the hormonal support.

The superficial layers of endometrium together with blood and leucocytes are shed and discharged – menstruation. Within a day or two the raw surface is healed over by epithelium proliferating from the basal portions of glands.

CYCLIC CHANGES IN VAGINA AND TUBE

Changes also occur in other parts of the genital tract.

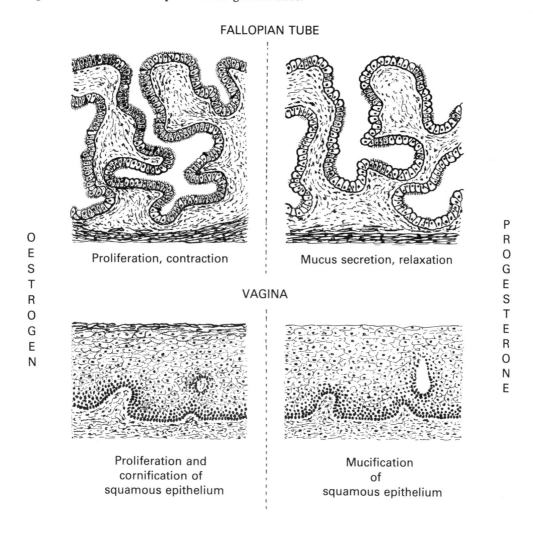

FALLOPIAN TUBE

O E S T R O G E N

Proliferation, contraction

Mucus secretion, relaxation

P R O G E S T E R O N E

VAGINA

Proliferation and
cornification of
squamous epithelium

Mucification
of
squamous epithelium

It is generally considered that a primordial follicle reaches the stage of ovulation in the first 12 days of a menstrual cycle but we have no accurate knowledge of the time-scale involved in the earliest changes in the follicle such as halving the number of chromosomes etc. It is therefore possible that it requires more than one cycle for the dominant follicle to reach maturity. The important factor however is the increase in hormonal production during the cycle.

CYCLIC OVARIAN HORMONAL CHANGES

OESTROGENS

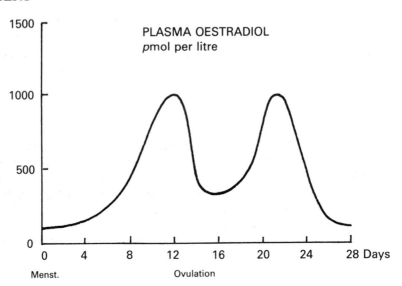

The plasma values of the three main oestrogens, oestradiol, oestrone and oestriol, are almost parallel throughout the cycle. Oestrone and oestradiol show a ratio of 2:1 but oestriol output has no strict mathematical relationship to the others. The levels are low during menstruation and very gradually increase. Significant changes are noted around the 7th–8th day of the cycle, rising to a maximum around the 12th day – ovulation peak. A fall occurs 24 hours later followed by a further increase a week later – the maximum phase of corpus luteum activity.

PROGESTERONE

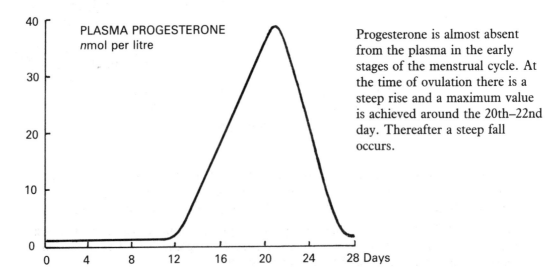

Progesterone is almost absent from the plasma in the early stages of the menstrual cycle. At the time of ovulation there is a steep rise and a maximum value is achieved around the 20th–22nd day. Thereafter a steep fall occurs.

ACTION OF OVARIAN HORMONES

OESTROGEN

Its biological purpose is to develop the child into the adult female and prepare her for the function of mating.

PROGESTERONE

This hormone prepares the fertilised female for the long ordeal of gestation and has no homologue in the male. In a clinical sense, it has an anti-oestrogen action.

TARGET TISSUES

HYPOTHALAMUS
BREASTS
GENITAL TRACT

Tissues of these structures are particularly sensitive to oestrogen stimulation. The cytoplasm of their cells contains a specific oestrogen receptor molecule which has an affinity for oestrogen 100,000 times greater than the carrier protein which retains the hormone in the bloodstream.

Progesterone receptors appear in the cytoplasm only after the cell has been primed by oestrogen.

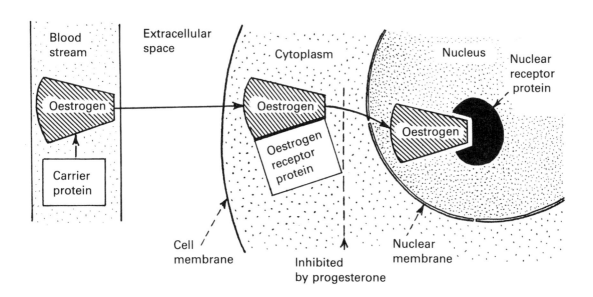

Transfer of the oestrogen molecule to the cell nucleus occurs more readily during the FSH phase of the cycle than during the LH phase, when progesterone levels are highest. The number of oestrogen receptors is reduced after the menopause, but they never disappear.

The steroids being lipids are transported by quite separate lipophilic proteins and the tissues stimulated by the steroids have their receptors in the cell cytoplasm instead of on the cell surface as in the preceding steps of the ovulatory process.

EFFECTS OF OVARIAN HORMONES

GENITAL TRACT

Oestrogen stimulates growth and vascularisation, while progesterone increases endometrial gland secretion. In the cervix, secretion is considerably increased by oestrogen (to produce a favourable medium for spermatozoa) while progesterone dries it up. In the vagina, oestrogen causes cornification of cells and enlargement of nuclei with increased deposits of glycogen.

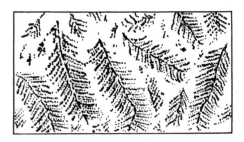

'Ferning' pattern in vaginal smear due to oestrogen stimulation.

BREAST

Oestrogen stimulates growth of the stroma, duct system and pigmentation, while progesterone stimulates growth of gland alveoli. Secondary sex characteristics are controlled by oestrogen.

HYPOTHALAMUS

The hypothalamic-pituitary axis mediates the effects of ovarian hormones and through FSH and LH controls the menstrual cycle.

CARDIOVASCULAR SYSTEM

Oestrogen relaxes smooth muscle of the vascular tree and causes vasodilatation, tending to improve circulation and prevent hypertension. Oestrogen and to a lesser extent progesterone cause water and salt retention.

SKELETON

Oestrogen helps to retain calcium in the bones and at puberty produces the growth spurt and then closure of long bone epiphyses.

PSYCHOLOGICAL CHARACTERISTICS

Femininity is a great deal more than a mere manifestation of circulating hormone levels, but the fluctuations of the menstrual cycle do to some extent affect the individual's attitude and mood. During the oestrogen phase, the woman is on the whole more confident and active, more cheerful, outward looking and energetic. Progesterone brings about a reduction in physical activity, a quietening of mood, even some depression.

PUBERTY

Puberty is the period of rapid growth when the child develops the physical characteristics of the adult. In addition to growth in stature, enlargement and changes in function of internal organs occur. Sexual changes are the most obvious. The mechanisms are poorly understood but the main feature is an awakening of centres in the hypothalamus.

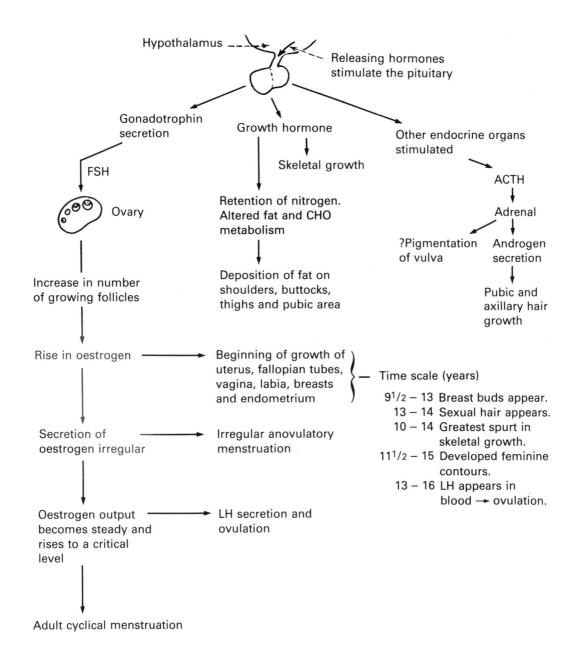

THE MENOPAUSE

Menopause is the name given to the stage in life when the woman gradually loses her cyclical ovarian activity. In many ways it is a reversal of the changes occurring at puberty. It usually takes place between the ages of 47 and 52.

Menstruation rarely ceases abruptly but tends to become somewhat irregular and less frequent over a year or a little longer. The cessation does not appear to be due to a complete disappearance of ovarian follicles. Primordial follicles have been found in the ovaries of old women. It would appear that there has to be a critical number of actively growing follicles before the menstrual cycle can operate.

For details of the patho-physiology and clinical features etc. of the menopause, see pages 472 et seq.

CHAPTER 4

GENETIC and CONGENITAL ABNORMALITIES

MATURATION OF GERM CELLS AND GENETIC ABNORMALITIES

Before fertilisation of the ovum can occur there has to be a rearrangement of the genetic material within the nuclei of the germ cells of both male and female. In the female this occurs during fetal life but in the male it is delayed until puberty.

Every cell in the adult contains 46 chromosomes, two of which are of sex type, XX in the female, XY in the male.

Prior to fertilisation the chromosomes must be reduced from 46 to 23 in both ovum and sperm, and each will possess one sex chromosome. This reduction division process is termed MEIOSIS.

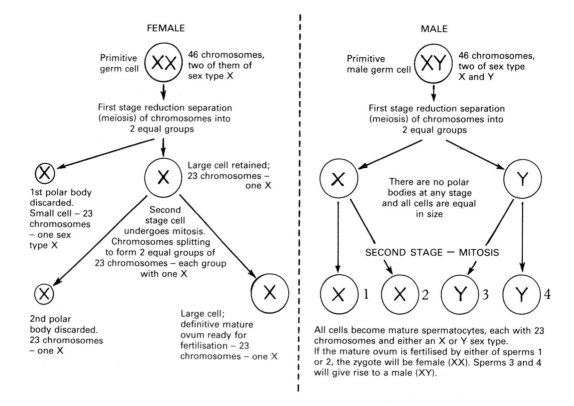

FEMALE

Primitive germ cell — XX — 46 chromosomes, two of them of sex type X

First stage reduction separation (meiosis) of chromosomes into 2 equal groups

X — Large cell retained; 23 chromosomes – one X

1st polar body discarded. Small cell – 23 chromosomes – one sex type X

Second stage cell undergoes mitosis. Chromosomes splitting to form 2 equal groups of 23 chromosomes – each group with one X

2nd polar body discarded. 23 chromosomes – one X

Large cell; definitive mature ovum ready for fertilisation – 23 chromosomes – one X

MALE

Primitive male germ cell — XY — 46 chromosomes, two of sex type X and Y

First stage reduction separation (meiosis) of chromosomes into 2 equal groups

X   Y

There are no polar bodies at any stage and all cells are equal in size

SECOND STAGE — MITOSIS

X 1   X 2   Y 3   Y 4

All cells become mature spermatocytes, each with 23 chromosomes and either an X or Y sex type. If the mature ovum is fertilised by either of sperms 1 or 2, the zygote will be female (XX). Sperms 3 and 4 will give rise to a male (XY).

MATURATION OF GERM CELLS AND GENETIC ABNORMALITIES

Genetic abnormalities in relation to sex and gender are the result of a defect in meiosis in which there is failure in the separation of the two sex chromosomes commencing in stage 1 and continued in stage 2. In the FEMALE, the result depends on whether both sex chromosomes are transferred to the polar bodies or to the definitive maturing ovum:

A. Deletion of sex chromosomes

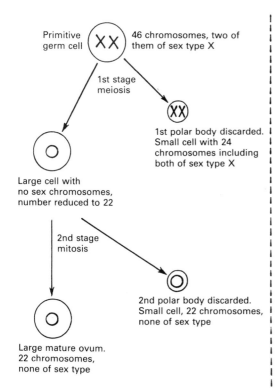

Primitive germ cell — XX — 46 chromosomes, two of them of sex type X

1st stage meiosis

XX — 1st polar body discarded. Small cell with 24 chromosomes including both of sex type X

Large cell with no sex chromosomes, number reduced to 22

2nd stage mitosis

2nd polar body discarded. Small cell, 22 chromosomes, none of sex type

Large mature ovum. 22 chromosomes, none of sex type

If the mature ovum is fertilised it will result in a zygote with 45 chromosomes and a sex chromosome make-up of XO. Sperm with Y chromosomes either do not fertilise this type of ovum or, if they do, the resulting combination YO is lethal.

B. Acquisition of a sex chromosome

In this case both X chromosomes are transferred to the cell which will become the definitive mature ovum.

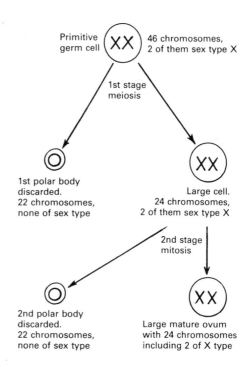

Primitive germ cell — XX — 46 chromosomes, 2 of them sex type X

1st stage meiosis

1st polar body discarded. 22 chromosomes, none of sex type

Large cell. 24 chromosomes, 2 of them sex type X

2nd stage mitosis

2nd polar body discarded. 22 chromosomes, none of sex type

XX — Large mature ovum with 24 chromosomes including 2 of X type

Fertilisation of this ovum will result in a zygote with 47 chromosomes and a sex chromosome make-up of XXY.

MATURATION OF GERM CELLS AND GENETIC ABNORMALITIES

In the MALE there is a slightly more complex situation due to the absence of polar bodies.

A. **Deletion of sex chromosomes**

B. **Acquisition of sex chromosomes**

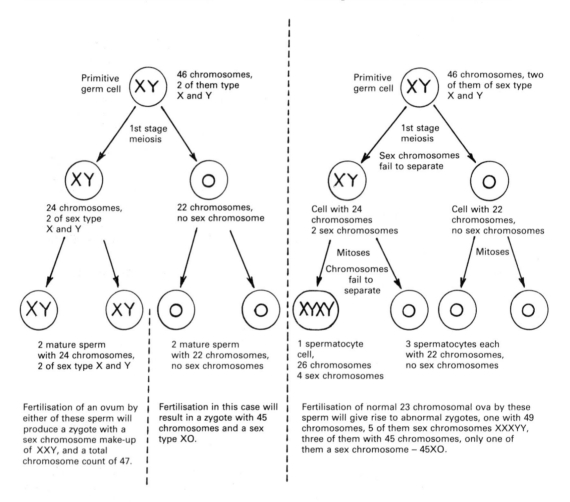

A. Deletion of sex chromosomes

Primitive germ cell (XY) — 46 chromosomes, 2 of them type X and Y

1st stage meiosis

(XY) 24 chromosomes, 2 of sex type X and Y

(O) 22 chromosomes, no sex chromosome

(XY) (XY) 2 mature sperm with 24 chromosomes, 2 of sex type X and Y

(O) (O) 2 mature sperm with 22 chromosomes, no sex chromosomes

Fertilisation of an ovum by either of these sperm will produce a zygote with a sex chromosome make-up of XXY, and a total chromosome count of 47.

Fertilisation in this case will result in a zygote with 45 chromosomes and a sex type XO.

B. Acquisition of sex chromosomes

Primitive germ cell (XY) — 46 chromosomes, two of them of sex type X and Y

1st stage meiosis

Sex chromosomes fail to separate

(XY) Cell with 24 chromosomes 2 sex chromosomes

(O) Cell with 22 chromosomes, no sex chromosomes

Mitoses — Chromosomes fail to separate

Mitoses

(XXXY) 1 spermatocyte cell, 26 chromosomes 4 sex chromosomes

(O) (O) (O) 3 spermatocytes each with 22 chromosomes, no sex chromosomes

Fertilisation of normal 23 chromosomal ova by these sperm will give rise to abnormal zygotes, one with 49 chromosomes, 5 of them sex chromosomes XXXYY, three of them with 45 chromosomes, only one of them a sex chromosome – 45XO.

MATURATION OF GERM CELLS AND GENETIC ABNORMALITIES

Partial deletion

In this situation only part of a sex chromosome is passed on during meiosis.

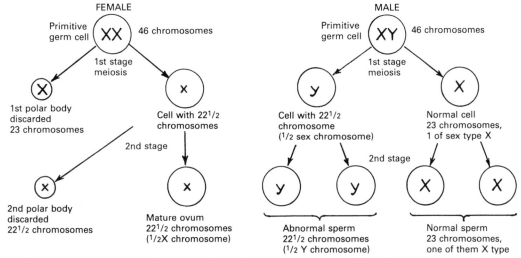

Fertilisation of the abnormal ovum will produce a zygote with $45\frac{1}{2}$ chromosomes and a sex chromosome pattern of either Xx or Yx.

Fertilisation of a normal ovum by the abnormal sperm produced by partial deletion will result in a zygote with $45\frac{1}{2}$ chromosomes, sex pattern Xy.

Mosaics

During early development of the zygote there may be failure to pass on a normal complement of chromosomes to all cells and separate clones of cells may appear in the fully developed embryo. These defects may affect the sex chromosomes.

Possible variations

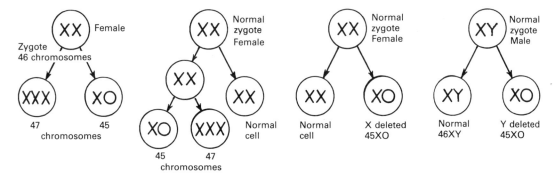

Study of these charts shows that, in the main, faults in the meiotic mechanism, no matter whether they are due to deletion or acquisition of chromosomes in either male or female, result in zygotes in one of three abnormal sex chromosome patterns – 45XO, 47XXY, 49XXXYY.

GENETIC ABNORMALITIES

Clinical syndromes

The clinical results of these chromosomal abnormalities are not quite as straightforward as one might expect. The X chromosome favours development of female characteristics but full development is only possible if there are two such chromosomes. Any alteration in this number leads to abnormalities. Development of the testis is entirely dependent on the presence of a Y chromosome. The testis, in addition to forming testosterone which aids the development of male characteristics, also produces a Müllerian inhibitory factor. In the absence of a testis the whole Müllerian tract will develop but curiously this does not depend on the presence of ovaries. These inter-relationships result in syndromes with variations in individual cases.

Investigations of genetic defects

In all cases it is important to obtain a family history as complete as possible. Siblings and relatives of patients frequently give a history of amenorrhoea and infertility.

Laboratory studies

Examination of cells, e.g. a buccal smear, from a normal female, stained suitably will show a small pyramidal mass of chromatin at the edge of the nuclear membrane. The cells are stated to be 'chromatin positive' and the mass of chromatin is called a 'Barr body'.

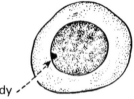
Barr body

The presence of such a chromatin mass indicates that the individual possesses two X chromosomes, but this is no guarantee that the patient is genetically normal. The sex chromosome pattern could well be XXY or some other variant. It merely indicates the presence of two X chromosomes. If the individual possesses more than two X chromosomes, e.g. XXX, there will be two Barr bodies, i.e. there is always one Barr body less than the number of X chromosomes.

Absence of the Barr body indicates that the patient has only one X chromosome. This is the situation in the normal male (XY) but if it is associated with some malformation of the genitalia the individual may be an incomplete female (XO).

Another cellular feature of females is to be found in polymorphonuclear leucocytes. These cells commonly have a small mass of chromatin projecting from the nucleus in the form of a drumstick.

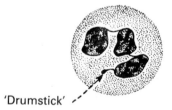
'Drumstick'

Chromosome analysis

While tests for Barr bodies can be useful, in many instances it may be necessary to establish the complete chromosome pattern. This is done by culturing cells from the patient, either lymphocytes separated from a blood sample or fibrocytes from a biopsy of fibrous tissue. The cells are grown in the presence of colchicine which terminates the mitotic process at the metaphase. The resulting chromosomes are separated, counted, arranged in their groups and studied.

GENETIC ABNORMALITIES

TURNER'S SYNDROME – Sex chromosome deletion (X)

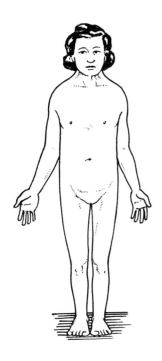

Amenorrhoea

Normal intelligence

Webbing of neck

Coarctation of aorta

Secondary sex characteristics absent

Infantile figure of female phenotype

Small stature, poor hip development

Streak gonad, failure of ovarian development

Uterus and fallopian tubes, infantile

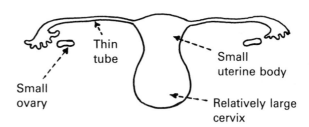

Thin tube

Small ovary

Small uterine body

Relatively large cervix

In 'typical' Turner's syndrome the chromosomal pattern is 45XO. Some patients may exhibit a few of the stigmata – so-called atypical cases, and in these subjects there is usually partial deletion of an X chromosome giving an Xx pattern. Mosaicism, e.g. XO/XX, may result in the appearance of some of the features of Turner's syndrome but the presence of cells with an XX configuration can be associated with perfectly formed ovaries and menstruation may occur.

In males some of the somatic stigmata of Turner's may appear. This may be due to partial deletion of the Y chromosome – Xy, or to mosaicism – XO/XY.

Treatment

It is essential that diagnosis should be established as early as possible. Blood should be sent for chromosome analysis in any female child of exceptionally small stature. At the age of 11 or 12 years, ethinyl oestradiol 0.025 to 0.05mg should be given daily for 3 to 6 months to stimulate growth of uterus and breasts. Following this, oestrogen may be given daily with cyclical progestogen in the form of a standard sequential HRT preparation. This results in a 'menstrual' cycle. Occasionally it may be necessary to give anabolic steroids to help breast development.

GENETIC ABNORMALITIES

KLINEFELTER'S SYNDROME (Sex chromosome acquisition – X)

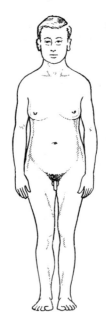

This clinical condition is associated with an increase in the number of X chromosomes. The pattern may be XXY, XXXY, XXXYY or XXXXXY. Despite the X chromosomes which cause the cells of the individual to be chromatin positive usually associated with female sex, the influence of the X chromosomes is nullified by the Y chromosome. Physically, the appearance is that of a male. At puberty, however, the testes fail to enlarge. Facial hair is scanty and pubic hair has a female distribution and there may be some breast development. There is infertility. Increase in the number of X chromosomes is associated with increasing mental retardation.

SUPER-FEMALE (Sex chromosome acquisition – X, sometimes at both stages of meiosis)

This is a term sometimes used when the subject possesses extra X chromosomes but no Y chromosome. The pattern may be XXX, XXXX or even XXXXX. Physically these individuals are normal females, but the important point is that there is usually some mental retardation and the degree of this increases with each extra X chromosome. Diagnosis is made by examination of a buccal smear, which will reveal multiple Barr bodies, the number being equal to the number of X chromosomes -1.

CONGENITAL ABNORMALITIES

TESTICULAR FEMINISATION (Total androgen insensitivity)

This is a condition which may be mistaken for a sex chromosome abnormality. It is due to the insensitivity of the fetal tissues to hormones. The chromosomal pattern is 46XY but although the individual possesses testes he is an apparent female. Androgens are secreted but tissues appear to be insensitive and develop along female lines. Usually the diagnosis is made in early adult life when the patient complains of amenorrhoea.

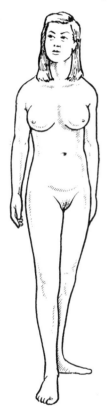

Female phenotype with tendency to eunuchoid proportions.

Normal or large breasts with small nipples.

Absent or scanty (sometimes normal) pubic hair.

Absent or scanty axillary hair.

Female external genitalia with blind vagina.

Absent or rudimentary internal genitalia.

Undescended testes anywhere along course of normal descent (20% become malignant in 4th decade).

Testes secrete oestrogens and androgens. Probably Leydig cells produce feminising hormones.

Hereditary from mother:
  One quarter of female offspring are carriers.
  One quarter of male offspring are feminised.
  The remainder are normal.
  Carriers may show scanty pubic and axillary hair and may have delayed menarche.

The almost complete absence of Müllerian structures would suggest that the testes are still producing the Müllerian inhibitory factor.

Until full growth is achieved no therapy should be attempted. When the epiphyses have fused the gonads should be excised. This is a precautionary measure in view of the increased incidence of tumours in such gonads. Following this treatment the patient is liable to have menopausal symptoms and should be given hormone replacement therapy, continuously in the beginning until the vaginal smear is fully oestrogenised, and then cyclically.

All of these foregoing syndromes, whether genetic or not, can pose social, psychological and sexual problems. The patient may have to make a great deal of mental adjustment and in such cases sensitive counselling will be required.

CONGENITAL ABNORMALITIES

A number of other developmental abnormalities of the female sex organs occasionally arise, some of which may suggest sex chromosome abnormalities. It is essential to diagnose these conditions as early as possible since treatment can often allow the infant to develop normally.

ADRENOGENITAL SYNDROME

Adrenal dysfunction due to congenital deficiency of the enzyme 21-hydroxylase. It should be detected and treated at birth.

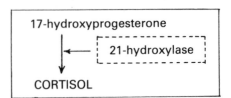

1. Deficiency of 21-hydroxylase leads to low cortisol secretion.
2. Low cortisol leads to unopposed high ACTH secretion.
3. High ACTH secretion leads to adrenal hypertrophy.
4. Adrenal hypertrophy leads to high 17-hydroxyprogesterone secretion.
5. Since the pathway to cortisol is blocked the alternative pathway to androgen formation is taken.
6. The fetus and neonate show signs of virilism, and if the baby survives she will suffer from primary amenorrhoea.

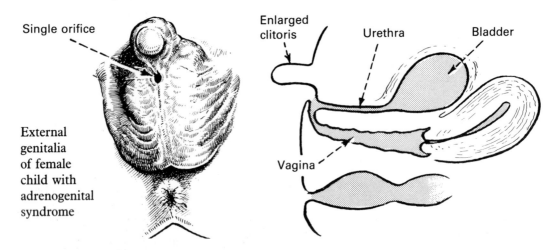

External genitalia of female child with adrenogenital syndrome

Treatment

Chromosome analysis will reveal XX karyotype. Addisonian crisis may develop at any time and may be fatal. The diagnosis must be recognised as soon as possible and treatment given immediately with corticosteroids which will reverse the changes in the endocrine organs, reducing the ACTH level and ultimately the adrenal hypertrophy. Virilisation will regress. Prompt recognition and treatment will allow the infant to grow into a normal female. The abnormal genitalia should alert the attendant at the birth and help should be sought from a paediatrician.

ABNORMALITIES OF OVARY AND TUBE

Congenital abnormalities arise from:-

1. Incomplete development of the Müllerian ducts.
2. Imperfect development of the gonad.
3. Imperfect development of the cloacal region.
4. Sex chromosome abnormalities.

Many abnormalities in many combinations may be met with, but only those compatible with life and growth are of interest to the gynaecologist. Because of the close relationship between the genital and urinary tracts, intravenous pyelography should always be carried out when a genital abnormality is found.

ABNORMALITIES of the OVARY

1. Absence of one ovary may occur in an otherwise normal woman. Before operating on one ovary, always look at the other.

2. This is seen in cases of ovarian dysgenesis. In place of the ovary there is a strip of whitish connective tissue continuous with the ovarian ligament. It may contain vestiges of a rete, and occasional cells which may be of germ cell type, but no follicles. These 'streak' ovaries are sometimes the seat of tumour growth such as gonadoblastoma and dysgerminoma and should always be removed.

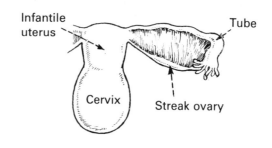

ABNORMALITIES of the FALLOPIAN TUBE

Absence is rare. The tube may be imperfectly developed.

This illustration shows a condition in which the proximal half of the left tube has failed to develop. The right adnexa are normal. All of these conditions are rare but their importance lies in their association with infertility.

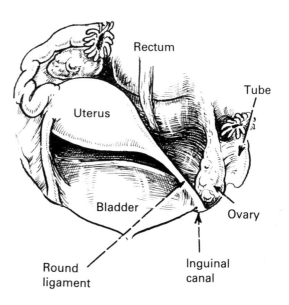

71

ABNORMALITIES OF THE UTERUS

1. Absent or rudimentary uterus
The uterus consists of two nodules connected by a membrane ('ribbon' uterus). The other structures are normal. The patient may be asymptomatic apart from infertility. If a cavity exists in a nodule, cryptomenorrhoea and dysmenorrhoea may arise and retrograde flow lead to pelvic endometriosis.

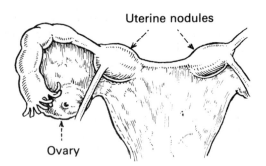

Uterine nodules

Ovary

2. Double uterus (Bicornuate uterus)
One or other variant of this condition is the commonest abnormality. It is due to failure of fusion of the Müllerian ducts, or failure of one to develop. Examples:

(a) Uterus Didelphys
Double uterus and cervix, usually with double vagina. Some writers call this 'pseudo-didelphys' unless there is also a double vulva.

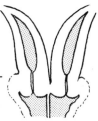

(b) Uterus Bicornis
Note the ligament which usually passes from rectum to bladder.

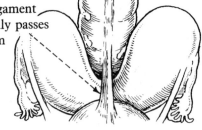

(c) Uterus Bicornis Bicollis
Two corpora with fused cervices.

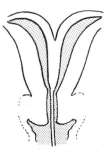

(d) Uterus with accessory horn
The accessory horn has no cervix. If it menstruates, cryptomenorrhoea will follow. Spermatozoa can reach the horn by crossing the peritoneal cavity.

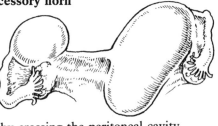

3. Uterus Unicornis
One duct has failed to develop.

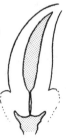

These abnormalities may be associated with infertility. If pregnancy occurs in 2(a), (b) and (c), the non-pregnant horn may continue to menstruate, simulating abortion. More frequently abortion does occur. In 2(d) cryptomenorrhoea may arise in the accessory horn. Endometriosis and dysmenorrhoea may follow due to retrograde flow.

ABNORMALITIES OF THE VAGINA

Gynatresia (Occlusion of the genital canal) may be due to complete absence of the vagina, or incomplete development, or the presence of a transverse septum producing the same effect as an imperforate hymen. There may also be a longitudinal septum producing a double vagina, usually in association with a double uterus. A few examples are shown.

a. Absence of the whole genital tract except for the lower one third of the vagina. Coitus is possible but there is no possibility of pregnancy.

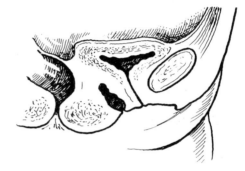

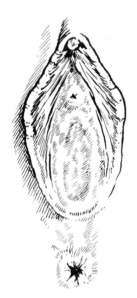

b. Complete absence of vagina. There is a slight depression over the hymen. Normal coitus is not possible.

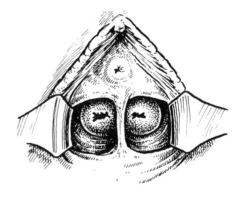

c. Septate (double) vagina showing also two cervices.
Normal pregnancy and delivery are possible.

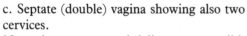

Vaginal abnormalities can occur alone, but are usually associated with abnormal internal genitalia, and inspection by laparoscopy or laparotomy with gonadal biopsy is called for. If the internal genitalia are relatively normal cryptomenorrhoea with dysmenorrhoea and possibly endometriosis will occur in (a) and (b).

ABNORMALITIES OF THE VULVA

1. Complete absence of the vulva has never been found in a liveborn child. Double vulva is excessively rare, but cases have been reported of complete duplication of the whole genital tract and bladder with normal function.

2. Ectopia Vesicae

This is an extreme defect seen in the newborn, but one which is susceptible to surgical treatment. There is failure of development of the symphysis pubis, mons, lower abdominal wall and anterior wall of bladder. The tissues exposed are the posterior wall of the bladder, the ureteric orifices and the floor of the urethra.

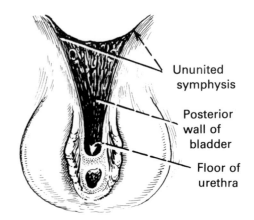

Ununited symphysis

Posterior wall of bladder

Floor of urethra

CONGENITAL ABNORMALITIES of CLOACAL ORIGIN

These are due to failure of the cloacal septum to divide the cloaca perfectly into hindgut and urogenital sinus. The less serious degrees may persist unnoticed in adults as some form of ectopic anus.

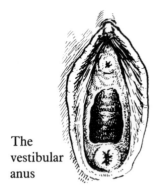

Patients with these abnormalities can defaecate through vestibule or vagina apparently without suffering from incontinence.

The vestibular anus

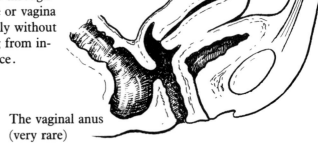

The vaginal anus (very rare)

In all of these vulval abnormalities infection is a problem – of the urinary tract in ectopia vesicae and of the genital tract in the other two.

GENITAL ABNORMALITIES

The results of these conditions as they relate to gynaecological practice have already been mentioned in the section dealing with amenorrhoea.

CHAPTER 5

EXAMINATION OF THE PATIENT

TAKING THE HISTORY

The ancient Greeks believed that hysteria was related to diseases of the womb (Gk: hystera, a womb). A woman discussing gynaecological problems will often show signs of distress – embarrassment, fear, shame. The gynaecological patient must have . . .

. . . Privacy

The consultation should be held in a closed room. Permission should be sought for the presence of a nurse or student.

. . . Time

She should be allowed to tell her own story before any attempt is made to elicit specific symptoms.

. . . Sympathy

The doctor's manner must be one of interest and understanding.

Once a rapport is established, enquire about age, parity, menstrual history and past history with special reference to previous gynaecological treatment.

OBSTETRIC HISTORY

Record the number of pregnancies followed by the number of abortions e.g. 5^{+2}.

Note the year of each pregnancy, the type of delivery, any history of trauma, excessively long labour or any other complication.

Puerperal infection? This may be the origin of a chronic pelvic inflammation.

Infertility? If so, is it voluntary or involuntary? Methods of contraception should be asked about.

Abortions? The degree of haemorrhage should be established, and whether curettage was done. There is a tendency to attribute any irregular and unexpected bleeding to a 'very early miscarriage'. Distinguish between spontaneous and therapeutic abortion.

GENERAL HISTORY

The gynaecologist should know if his patient has ever suffered from tuberculosis, cardiac or endocrine disease or psychiatric illness. Previous surgical procedures should be noted.

GYNAECOLOGICAL HISTORY

Previous gynaecological treatment is best learnt about from clinical records if obtainable. Patients' recollections may be incorrect or misleading.

Enquire about vaginal discharge (see page 146 et seq.).

MENSTRUAL HISTORY

This can vary very much from patient to patient and still be within normal limits. Vague complaints are unlikely to be due to gynaecological disease.

Menarche

This is the age of onset of menstruation and varies between 10 and 16 years.

Rhythm of cycle and duration of flow

These are conveniently expressed together as a numerical fraction. Thus 5/28 means that the patient menstruates for 5 days every 28 days. The normal cycle lasts between 21 and 30 days and the bleeding lasts for between 3 and 9 days. Make sure that you are told the number of days of bleeding and the number of days from day one of a period to day one of the next. Ask if a menstrual diary is kept. Poor memory or irregular cycles may produce fractions such as 5–10/21–35.

Irregular bleeding

This can be caused by ovulation, hormonal fluctuation or organic disease, and the history is in fact often misleading.

Bleeding after intercourse (post-coital bleeding) and post-menopausal bleeding are always taken to suggest the possibility of malignant disease: yet the cause is more often benign.

Volume of blood loss

This can vary between 30 and 200ml. Blood should be liquid, but parous women may pass small clots. Large clots mean that the loss is abnormal and the fibrinolytic system cannot break down all the blood that is shed.

15g haemoglobin represents 50mg elemental iron, so a menstrual loss of 80ml would mean a loss of about 40mg iron. About a dozen internal tampons might be used for one menstruation. The patient's estimate of loss may be unreliable, especially if she uses phrases like 'torrential' or 'welling up'.

Menstrual molimina

(Lat: *molimen*, great exertion)
These are the secondary effects of the menstrual cycle. Some discomfort is normal, and there may be irritability, depression, breast discomfort, backache, pelvic pain. These symptoms should stop short of pre-menstrual tension and the pain should not be so severe as to keep the patient off her work.

Menopause

The cessation of menstruation.

It usually occurs between 48 and 53 years. Menorrhagia at this time is not normal. The patient should be asked about the extent of vasomotor disturbance ('hot flushes') and other symptoms.

COMPLAINTS OF PAIN

PAIN

The patient is asked where pain is felt, and whether it is intermittent, related to the period or continuous. The 'ordinary' period pain is felt in the back, lower abdomen and down the thighs. It must be distinguished from other abdominal causes of pain such as appendicitis.

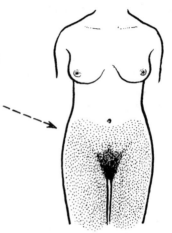

Areas of referred pain during menstruation

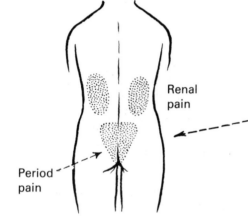

Renal pain

Period pain

The backache of period pain ('like a steel plate pressing inwards') is referred to the sacral area and should be distinguished from the loin pain of renal disease which can be exacerbated by the congestion of menstruation.

Pain associated with intercourse (dyspareunia) may not be mentioned spontaneously, and the doctor should ask if pain is caused or worsened by intercourse.

The severity of pain can be judged to some extent by its effect on the patient's behaviour. She should not have to go off her work for 'normal' dysmenorrhoea: if it is so severe as to cause fainting or nausea, tubal pregnancy must be considered. Torsion of an ovarian cyst produces intense, continuous pain.

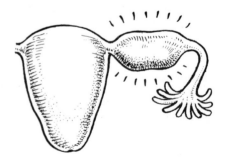

Tubal pregnancy

EXAMINATION OF THE BREASTS

A gynaecological examination provides
a suitable opportunity for examining the
breasts. Signs of pregnancy or lactation may
be observed or a lump may be palpated. The
breast is a much commoner site of cancer
than the genital tract.

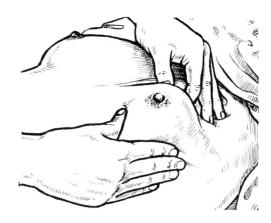

The examination can be made with the
patient lying on her back. The breast is gently
but thoroughly palpated with the fingers, and
the axilla is also palpated.

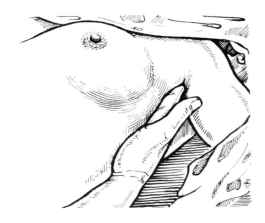

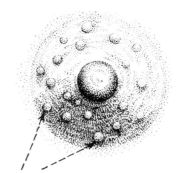

Montgomery's Tubercles, a reliable
sign of early pregnancy.

Method of testing for colostrum or
milk. The hands gently squeeze
the whole breast.

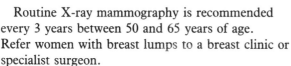

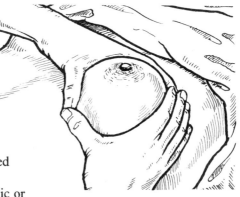

Routine X-ray mammography is recommended
every 3 years between 50 and 65 years of age.
Refer women with breast lumps to a breast clinic or
specialist surgeon.

ABDOMINAL EXAMINATION

This must never be omitted, whatever the patient's complaint. Many gynaecological tumours form large swellings which leave the pelvis altogether; and an undisclosed pregnancy may be present. Always examine the upper abdomen. Be certain that the bladder is empty. Instruct the patient to tell you if you are hurting her.

Ovarian cysts often have long pedicles. This ovarian cyst is completely abdominal, and would not be palpable on bimanual pelvic examination.

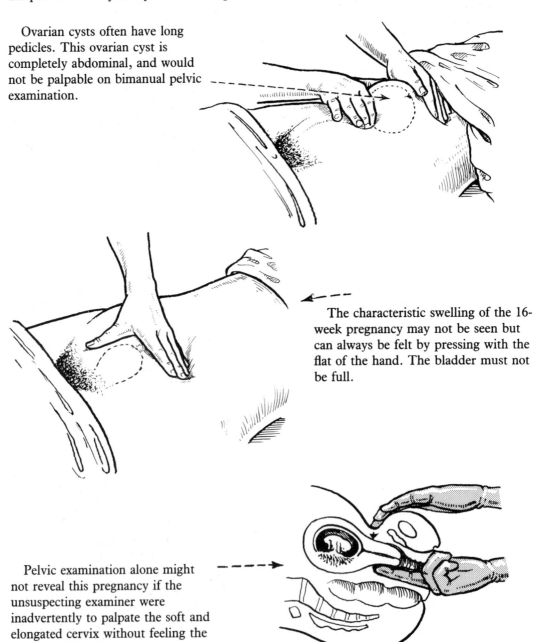

The characteristic swelling of the 16-week pregnancy may not be seen but can always be felt by pressing with the flat of the hand. The bladder must not be full.

Pelvic examination alone might not reveal this pregnancy if the unsuspecting examiner were inadvertently to palpate the soft and elongated cervix without feeling the enlarged corpus (cf. Hegar's sign).

ABDOMINAL EXAMINATION

All the classical techniques of inspection, palpation, and auscultation (for a fetal heart) are advised, but the most important is gentle palpation with the flat of the hand to detect solid or semi-solid tumours.

The examiner must bear in mind the various intra-abdominal structures which may give rise to swellings.

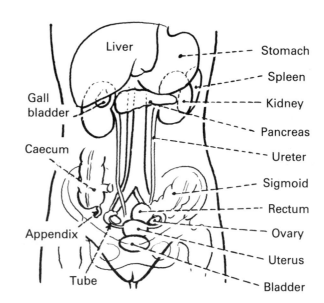

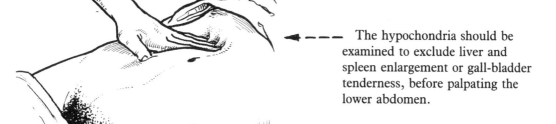

The hypochondria should be examined to exclude liver and spleen enlargement or gall-bladder tenderness, before palpating the lower abdomen.

An attempt to palpate the kidneys should be made. Tenderness may be elicited in the loin, suggesting urinary tract infection.

ABDOMINAL EXAMINATION

Inspection may show the characteristic shape of a large ovarian cyst. The outline is rounded and uniform, the skin is stretched and a fluid thrill may be elicited.

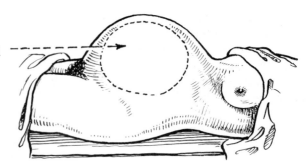

Tympanitic (due to bowel gas)

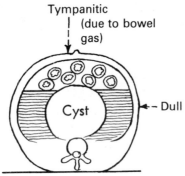

Cyst

– Dull

If ascites is present (and this means that the cyst is probably malignant) the outline tends to be cylindrical, with some flattening at the top. The umbilicus is everted and the percussion note is dull in the flanks but tympanitic above because of the upward floating of the intestines.

Tympanitic

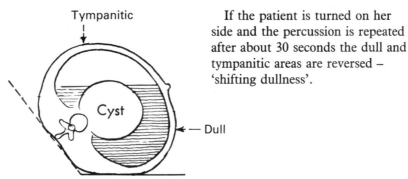

Cyst

— Dull

If the patient is turned on her side and the percussion is repeated after about 30 seconds the dull and tympanitic areas are reversed – 'shifting dullness'.

The very fat abdomen is not uncommon in gynaecology. Palpation is extremely difficult and examination under anaesthesia and more elaborate investigations will be necessary (ultrasonography, X-rays, laparoscopy if feasible).

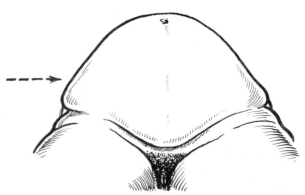

EXAMINATION OF THE VULVA

The dorsal position is most convenient for patient and doctor although some prefer the patient to be in the lateral position. During palpation, the condition of the labia, clitoris, anus and surrounding skin should be noted. Thus excoriation suggests irritating discharge and pruritus, purplish discoloration might be a sign of diabetes.

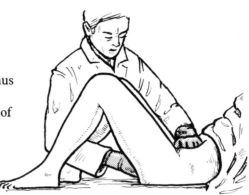

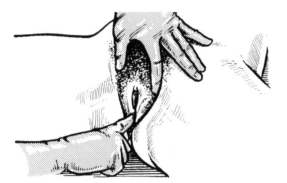

1. A single finger presses on the perineum, avoiding the sensitive vestibule, and accustoming the patient to the examiner's touch.

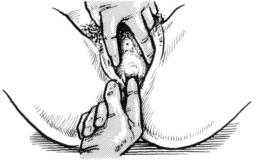

2. Urethral meatus and vestibule are exposed. Pressure from the finger will squeeze any pus from the peri-urethral glands.

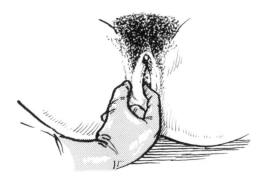

3. Bartholin's gland is palpated (on both sides). It is difficult to feel the normal gland.

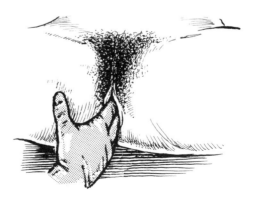

4. If there is room, a second finger is inserted and the perineal floor is palpated by stretching.

83

BIMANUAL PELVIC EXAMINATION

This technique needs practice. The external hand is the more important and supplies more information. It is customary to use two fingers in the vagina, but an adequate outpatient examination may be made with only one finger. Very little information is gained if the patient finds the examination painful. In a virgin or a child only rectal examination should be carried out.

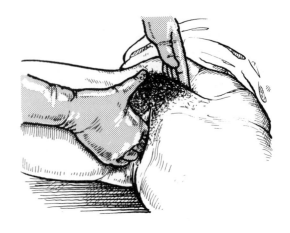

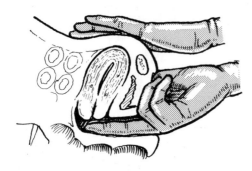

1. The cervix is palpated and any hardness or irregularity noted.

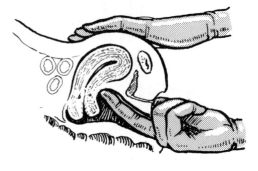

2. The whole uterus is identified, and size, shape, position, mobility and tenderness are noted.

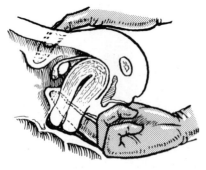

3. The lateral pelvis is palpated and any swelling noted. Normal adnexa are difficult to feel unless the ovary contains a corpus luteum.

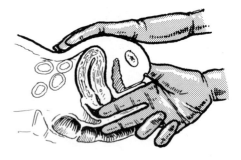

4. Sometimes rectovaginal examination is helpful, if the vagina admits only one finger or if the rectovaginal septum is to be examined.

SPECULUM EXAMINATION

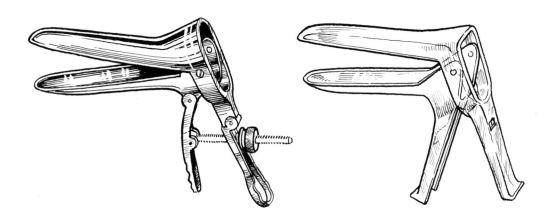

The bi-valve speculum is the most useful (Cusco's pattern is shown here). It is made either of steel or perspex (disposable) and is designed to open after insertion so that the cervix can be seen and a cytological smear or bacteriological swab taken as required. The steel speculum has a screw for retaining it in the open position.

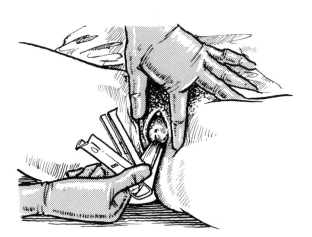

1. The speculum is applied to the vulva at an angle of 45 degrees from the vertical. This allows the easiest insertion.

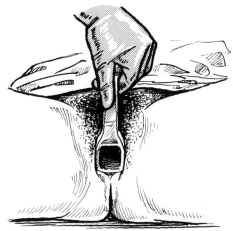

2. When fully inserted it is gently opened out and held in position with the cervix between the blades. A good light is needed for inspection.

SPECULUM EXAMINATION

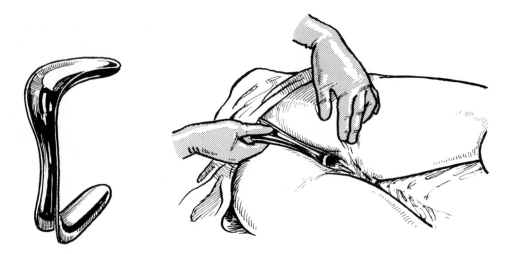

SIMS' SPECULUM (the duckbill speculum) is designed to hold back the posterior vaginal wall so that air enters and the anterior wall and cervix are exposed.

In this picture the patient is in Sims' position (semi-prone) which is useful if the anterior wall is to be studied (e.g. if fistula is suspected).

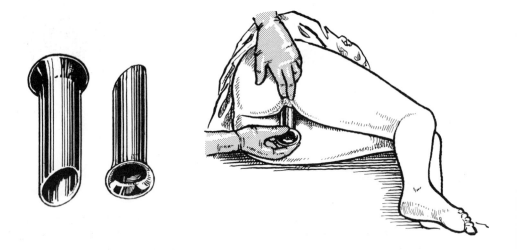

FERGUSON'S SPECULUM is essentially a metal tube and, although obsolescent, can prove useful in cases of marked vaginal prolapse when the bi-valve speculum cannot contain the vaginal wall sufficiently to allow a view of the cervix. In this picture the patient is in the lateral position, which is sometimes used if the cervix cannot be seen in the dorsal position.

LAPAROSCOPY

Inspection of the pelvic cavity through an endoscope passed through the abdominal wall. This investigation is now very frequently performed, but it does carry risks which must be taken into account.

Technique

The patient is anaesthetised, the bladder emptied, the uterus curetted and a cannula and forceps fixed to the cervix. This allows the uterus to be moved about once the endoscope is passed, and dye can be injected through the cannula to test the patency of the tubes.

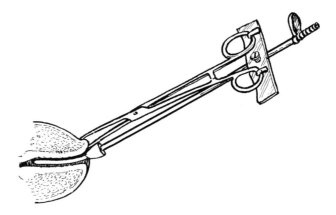

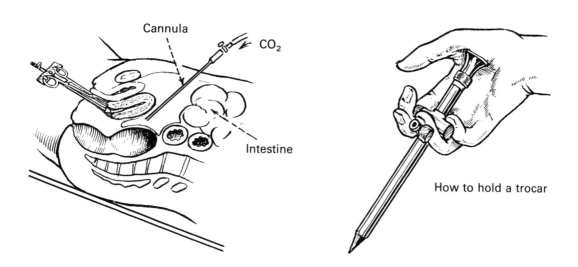

How to hold a trocar

The table is tilted to encourage the intestines to fall away from the pelvis and about 2 litres of CO_2 injected through a thin cannula. A small incision is made through skin, fat and rectus sheath just below the umbilicus and a trocar and cannula large enough to accommodate the endoscope is forced through the abdominal wall which should by now be elevated away from the viscera.

LAPAROSCOPY

The coldlight endoscope is passed through the cannula and the inspection made. An assistant or the operator himself can move the uterus about by means of the forceps on the cervix and a dilator or Spackman's cannula in the uterus.

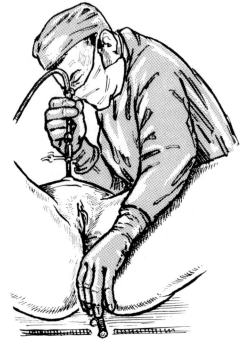

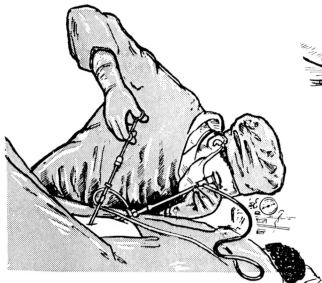

A special biopsy forceps can be passed through another cannula and used to lift up any tissue that may be obstructing the view or to take ovarian biopsies. Some adhesions may be divided using laparoscopy scissors.

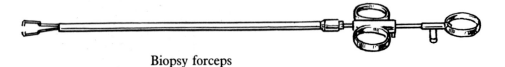

Biopsy forceps

LAPAROSCOPY

Complications

1. Perforation of a viscus especially bowel. An adequate amount of CO_2 must be instilled to raise the abdominal wall, and the table must be acutely tilted so that the bowel falls back from the pelvis.
2. Haemorrhage from damage to vessels, or from a trochar puncture.

Infection is very rare and nearly always the result of unnoticed bowel damage.

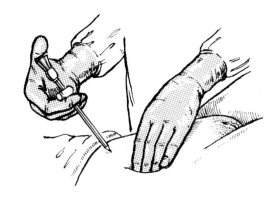

Indications

1. Diagnostic. Such conditions as salpingitis, endometriosis, early tubal pregnancy, can be identified or excluded.
Laparoscopy is particularly important in investigating complaints of vague pain.
2. Infertility Investigation. Besides inspection, the patency of fallopian tubes can be demonstrated by observing the passage of dye injected through the cervix (hydrotubation).
3. Sterilisation. See page 328.

Special care required

1. Previous abdominal operation. Bowel or omentum may be adherent to the scar or to pelvic structures.
2. Very fat women.

CULDOSCOPY

In culdoscopy the endosope was passed through the posterior fornix. This technique has been superseded by laparoscopy.

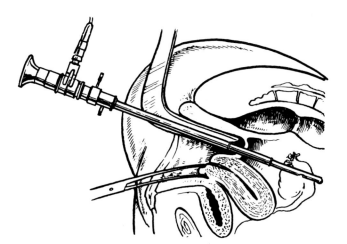

CHAPTER 6

ABNORMALITIES OF MENSTRUATION

AMENORRHOEA

The absence of menstruation occurs under very varying circumstances. What may be termed 'physiological amenorrhoea' is normal at four distinct phases of life – the early stage of the menarche, during pregnancy, lactation and following the menopause.

Menarche

The menarche may appear superficially to be an abrupt process but in reality the changes occur quite gradually. They involve an 'awakening' of the hypothalamic releasing centre, the pituitary secretion of gonadotrophins, growth hormones, and the development of Graafian follicles in the ovary. The number of follicles entering the growth phase and the degree of growth achieved is limited. Oestrogen secretion is low and progesterone is absent. Endometrial growth is very limited. Ultimately the growth of follicles is increased and becomes cyclical and menstruation occurs although ovulation is not achieved during the early cycles. There is therefore a phase when the system is beginning to function but there is amenorrhoea.

Pregnancy

Amenorrhoea is the natural result of fertilisation of an ovum. The secretion of chorionic gonadotrophin maintains the activity of the corpus luteum in the early part of pregnancy. The levels of oestrogen and progesterone remain high, thus ensuring the integrity of the endometrium. Later in pregnancy the production of oestrogen and progesterone is taken over by the placenta. Another factor about which we know little but which may play a part is the secretion of inhibin during pregnancy. This may stop FSH production.

Lactation

Soon after delivery prolactin is secreted in large quantities by the anterior pituitary. There is partial suppression of LH production so that ovarian follicles may grow, but ovulation does not occur and amenorrhoea is the result. If the mother does not breast feed, menstruation will return in 2 to 3 months, but if she does breast feed the period of amenorrhoea will be prolonged. This prolongation of amenorrhoea however is limited, and despite continued breast feeding menstruation will resume.

Menopause

The changes at this period of life are very similar to those occurring at the menarche but in the reverse order. In a proportion of women menstruation ceases abruptly, but in many the menstrual cycles alter. Frequently they become shorter initially but later they lengthen and tend to be irregular before ceasing entirely. The basic mechanism is the progressive reduction in the number of active Graafian follicles and thus a fall in oestrogen levels. This fall in oestrogen production is accompanied by a progressive rise in FSH levels which continues for a considerable time.

PATHOLOGICAL AMENORRHOEA

Pathological amenorrhoea means an absence of menstruation due to a recognisable abnormality. Amenorrhoea is a symptom and not a disease, but it is an indication of abnormal circumstances. A division has been made between adult patients who have never menstruated – Primary amenorrhoea (a rare condition) – and patients who have ceased to menstruate after periods have been established – Secondary amenorrhoea (a not uncommon circumstance, with many causes).

PRIMARY AMENORRHOEA

In gynaecological practice the criteria used in investigating the possibility of this diagnosis are:

1. No period by the age of 14 years with absence of secondary sexual characteristics.
2. No period by the age of 16 years regardless of normal growth and development and secondary sexual characteristics.

Other diagnoses should be considered and as far as possible excluded.

Examination

1. After confirming the absence of signs of puberty –
2. The possibility of a genetic defect should be considered:
    (a) Look for the stigmata of Turner's syndrome.
    (b) Take blood to determine the genetic sex.
3. Test for the presence of an endocrine condition.
    Request assays of LH, FSH, TSH, GH, cortisol (as a measure of ACTH).
    Growth hormone assays are an infrequent request but should be kept in mind especially if the patient is smallish.
4. Coned X-ray Tomography (or CAT SCAN) of pituitary fossa to exclude tumour.
5. Examination under anaesthesia to exclude genital abnormality. In some cases a laparoscopy and gonadal biopsy may be required.

Treatment

This is best left to the endocrinologist. Especial care must be taken to eliminate the possibility of growth hormone deficiency since such children are extremely sensitive to steroid therapy. Inexpert treatment can destroy any chance of achieving adequate growth. If menstruation is the main concern, cyclical replacement therapy with oestrogen and progestogen or cyclical oral contraception may be employed.

PRIMARY AMENORRHOEA

CRYPTOMENORRHOEA

This is another example of apparent primary amenorrhoea. There is no visible bleeding although the usual cyclical molimina are present. In that there is no flow of blood the term amenorrhoea can be used, but the cause is an obstruction by a vaginal septum or an imperforate hymen rather than a functional abnormality.

Three degrees are recognised.

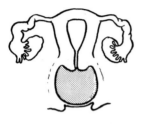 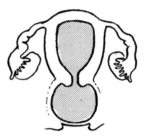 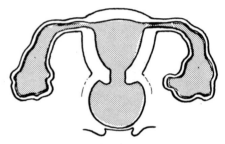

Haematocolpos. Only the vagina is distended by altered blood.

Haematometra. The uterus is also distended.

Haematosalpinx. In longstanding cases the tubes are also involved.

Clinical Features

The patient is usually a girl of 17 or so, complaining of primary amenorrhoea and pelvic pain of increasing severity. In longstanding cases the pressure of the distended vagina may cause urinary retention. Pregnancy must be excluded.

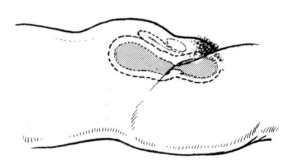

Examination

A pelvic mass is palpated and may even be visible. The vaginal membrane or hymen is bulging.

Treatment

Incision and drainage. Very large amounts of inspissated blood may be released, and if the septum is particularly thick, some form of plastic operation may subsequently be required.

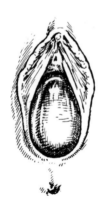 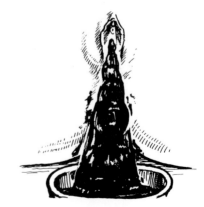

PRIMARY AMENORRHOEA

GENETIC AMENORRHOEA

For full development and function of the female reproductive organs two X chromosomes are required. Any reduction in that number results in Turner's syndrome, of which there are several variants.

Turner's syndrome (see page 67).

CONGENITAL ABNORMALITIES and AMENORRHOEA

There are two important conditions which are associated with amenorrhoea and which may be mistaken for genetic abnormalities.

1. **Testicular Feminisation** (Total androgen insensitivity).

This is a dysgenetic condition of the testes which results in an individual whose genetic sex is male (XY) but whose appearance is phenotypically female. The uterus is absent. (See page 69.)

2. **Adrenogenital syndrome.**

This syndrome, another congenital condition, is important to the gynaecologist not only as a cause of amenorrhoea but because it may be present at birth.

There are several forms, but the important one for present purposes is that which gives rise to masculinisation of the female infant. Increased pigmentation of the skin, particularly in the genital region, is usually present. The labia are fused and resemble a scrotum and at the anterior end of the raphé there is an orifice. This together with an apparent but small penis suggests hypospadias. Testes cannot be palpated in the scrotum. (See page 70.)

PRIMARY OVARIAN FAILURE

This is a rare condition which may occur in early childhood causing primary amenorrhoea or be delayed till after puberty resulting in secondary amenorrhoea. The cause appears to be a reduction in the number of germ cells migrating to the ovary. These undergo a progressive atresia during childhood until either all have been destroyed or the number remaining is insufficient to initiate the normal functional cycle.

Another and more severe form of the same failure of germ cell migration is sometimes seen. In this case no germ cells reach the ovary and 'streak' ovaries are the result. The mesenchyme of the ovary develops in the usual site complete with suspensory ligament but no germ cells are present.

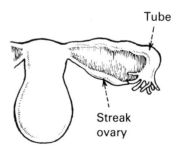

Tube

Streak
ovary

PRIMARY AMENORRHOEA

PRIMARY PITUITARY FAILURE

There are two distinct syndromes of pituitary dwarfism with amenorrhoea.

1. **Fröhlich's Dwarfism** (Dystrophia Adiposo-Genitalis).

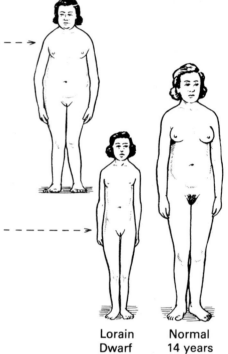

In this condition the features are:
Stunting of growth.
Feminine distribution of body fat.
Genital hypoplasia.
Diminished intelligence.
Decreased production of pituitary hormones.
Amenorrhoea.

The cause is usually tumour growth in the region of the hypothalamus or pituitary, or both e.g. chromophobe adenoma, glioma, meningioma or craniopharyngioma.

2. **Lorain-Levi Syndrome**

There is a deficiency of growth and gonadotrophic hormones in this case, resulting in dwarfism and amenorrhoea. The child is slender with 'boyish' contours. Pubertal changes do not occur; there is lack of genital hair. Intelligence is normal. Bones are slender and fragile. Attacks of hypoglycaemia are common. No causal lesion can be found in the region of the pituitary.

Lorain
Dwarf

Normal
14 years

FAILURE OF UTERINE DEVELOPMENT

There are varying degrees of this condition resulting in double uterus or uterus unicornis (page 72). Provided there is a cavity lined by endometrium, function can be normal. Amenorrhoea occurs when the developmental abnormality results in a uterus consisting of a mass of muscle without a cavity and therefore no endometrium and no menstruation.

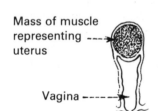

Mass of muscle representing uterus

Vagina

Sometimes there are two masses representing a bicornuate uterus but without a uterine cavity in either.

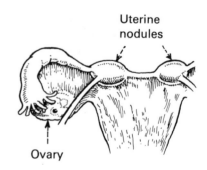

Uterine nodules

Ovary

SECONDARY AMENORRHOEA

There are multiple causes of secondary amenorrhoea, the commonest being pregnancy and missed abortion. These must always be considered no matter what the patient may say about the possibility of pregnancy.

Other causes of secondary amenorrhoea:

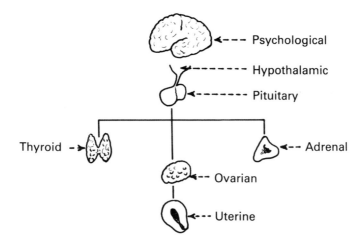

PSYCHOLOGICAL STATES

It is claimed that approximately 60% of cases of secondary amenorrhoea are the result of mental stress due to various causes e.g. marital or family discord, illness, depression, pseudopregnancy. In the last case the patient has the signs and symptoms of early pregnancy and develops an hysterical state due to a desire for or fear of pregnancy. The treatment of these conditions does not come within the ambit of the gynaecologist. Psychological help is necessary. The gynaecologist's role is, however, important i.e. to make sure that the amenorrhoea is not due to a physical lesion. The cause of the amenorrhoea in psychological states is thought to be an inhibition of hypothalamic releasing hormone production leading to absence of FSH and LH.

Dietary or Metabolic Amenorrhoea

This is a condition which may be considered psychological. It occurs in women in whom the desire to slim becomes obsessional. Fasting affects hypothalamic function in some way not understood and amenorrhoea results. It is sometimes seen in ballet dancers. Another instance is the young adult who tries to reject the physiological changes of adult sexuality and starves herself – a condition called ANOREXIA NERVOSA. This rejection displays itself as a fear of normal body weight, and probably of the sexual implications of menstruation.

SECONDARY AMENORRHOEA

ANOREXIA NERVOSA (*contd*)

Weight loss is first achieved by abstinence from recognised 'fattening' foods, and gradually all food is refused except fruit, peanut butter, etc. The girl will occasionally indulge in eating binges (bulimia) but afterwards, or if forced to eat, she will induce vomiting, thrusting her fingers down her throat if necessary. Weight fluctuates but a stage of emaciation is eventually reached which is in contrast to the patient's mental alertness.

Amenorrhoea. Pituitary sensitivity to LH/FSH releasing factor seems particularly dependent on body weight. In anorexia nervosa, when the weight falls below 45 kg, the LH/FSH output is diminished and the LH/FSH ratio reversed, which is the pre-pubertal pattern. Clomiphene is ineffective and cyclic bleeding will not resume until normal weight is regained.

Aetiology is unknown, but two-thirds of the patients are from social classes I and II, and there is very often a disturbed family relationship especially with the parents, who are unable to help the patient to resolve her adolescent conflicts.

Treatment is almost entirely in the hands of the psychiatrist except when starvation and weight loss are so severe as to require treatment in an acute medical ward.

Gynaecological Aspects

Many girls develop a transient mild degree of anorexia which may be represented by the parents as a desire to 'slim' and avoid 'puppy fat'. Amenorrhoea will be the presenting symptom and, if anorexia is suspected, no investigation is immediately required. Instead there should be reassurance and explanation, and continued observation until weight gain is satisfactory and menstruation has returned.

Anorexia nervosa must be regarded as a serious condition requiring prolonged observation. In one well-known study* of the progress of 100 patients followed for 4–8 years, only 48 were considered to have had a good outcome, and there were two deaths from inanition.

Other types of Metabolic Amenorrhoea

Any condition which alters metabolism profoundly will tend to cause amenorrhoea. In hypo- and hyperthyroidism and severe diabetes amenorrhoea is a common complication.

The same may be said of general illness, acute or chronic.

* Hsu L, Crisp A., Harding B., Lancet (1979) 1, 61.

PREMATURE MENOPAUSE

In this condition (about 10% of cases of amenorrhoea) the patient who is usually under 35 complains of the absence of periods and of oestrogen deprivation symptoms such as hot flushes, mood instability, loss of libido.

INVESTIGATION

A full investigation for other causes of amenorrhoea must be carried out, but the only abnormal finding is a raised serum FSH level. An ovarian biopsy should be taken as well, and if there are no primordial follicles a diagnosis of premature menopause may be made. An FSH level over 20U/l is strongly suggestive.

FSH in the Normal Cycle

During the follicular phase FSH is not raised above 13U/l, and the mid-cycle peak does not exceed 32U/l. For several years, as the natural menopause approaches, FSH/LH levels tend to rise and remain high after the periods have stopped. In the peri-menopausal years there may be episodes of raised FSH secretion causing transient amenorrhoea which is followed by ovulation and normal cyclic bleeding.

Ovarian biopsy

This is essential if an accurate prognosis for future ovulation and conception is asked for, and if any follicles are present the patient is quite likely to resume normal menstrual function. Where follicles are present the condition is considered to be one of ovarian resistance to gonadotrophins for reasons unknown. It may be that in some women the total number of germ cells is reduced and 'used up' at an early age.

Treatment

There is no treatment which will overcome the ovarian resistance or the raised FSH, but symptoms of oestrogen withdrawal must be treated with oestrogens.

Donated ovum IVF is now a possibility in premature menopause subjects.

PSEUDOPREGNANCY

This is a curious hysterical condition in which the patient either yearns for or fears a pregnancy. Besides missing periods, she develops symptoms such as nausea and vomiting, breast discomfort and tightness of her clothes due to abdominal swelling. Apprehensive patients may require the reassurance of repeated negative urine pregnancy tests, but the unfortunate woman who yearns for motherhood is more difficult to convince, and treatment may involve a suggestion of 'missed abortion' followed by curettage.

SECONDARY AMENORRHOEA

ENDOCRINE CAUSES

HYPERPROLACTINAEMIA

Prolactin occurs as an episodic secretion from the anterior pituitary, and the normal blood level is between 150 and 400mU/l depending on the laboratory. During pregnancy there is a tenfold increase.

It has long been known that persisting or 'inappropriate' hyperprolactinaemia, occurring when the woman is non-pregnant, can cause amenorrhoea or galactorrhoea (inappropriate lactation) or both.

The principal causes are:

1. **Pituitary tumour**, usually a micro-adenoma (<10mm diameter).

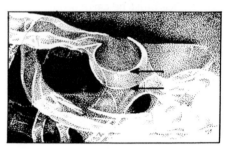

'Double floor' appearance of the pituitary fossa due to tumour

2. **Primary hypothyroidism**, due to the increase in thyroid releasing hormone.
   The increased thyroid releasing hormone acts on the galactophore cells of the pituitary. This results in:

Raised prolactin
↓
Suppression of oestrogen production
↓
Failure of secretion of gonadotrophin
releasing hormone by hypothalamus
↓
Absence of LH surge necessary for
ovulation
↓
Amenorrhoea

3. **Drugs**. Normally, increase in prolactin is prevented by an inhibitory factor which resembles dopamine. Certain drugs interfere with this action e.g. phenothiazines can block receptors for dopamine. Other drugs such as reserpine and methyldopa deplete the amount of dopamine.
   Contraceptive pills may cause amenorrhoea. Possibly the progestogen creates a pregnancy-like condition.

4. Cases of functional hyperprolactinaemia occur where no causal mechanism can be discovered.

Hyperprolactinaemia is said to be responsible for 20% of all cases of secondary amenorrhoea. In an increasing number of amenorrhoeic patients hyperprolactinaemia is being detected.

SECONDARY AMENORRHOEA

HYPERPROLACTINAEMIA (*contd*)

Treatment

Bromocriptine

This is a semi-synthetic ergot alkaloid which directly opposes prolactin secretion probably by acting in the same manner as dopamine which is believed to be the hypothalamic prolactin-release-inhibiting factor (PRIF). [The serotonin antagonist, metergoline, has the same effect.] When the amenorrhoea is due to hypogonadism induced by hyperprolactinaemia (with or without galactorrhoea – formerly called the lactation-amenorrhoea syndrome), bromocriptine will reduce the prolactin level to normal and conception may follow unless some method of contraception is used. The dose is of the order of 2.5mg thrice daily, reached gradually, and side-effects include nausea and giddiness with fainting (syncope).

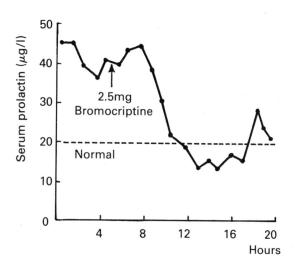

Effect of bromocriptine on serum prolactin. Duration 12–16 hours.

If the hyperprolactinaemia results from a microadenoma of pituitary there is a risk of pituitary expansion during pregnancy and preliminary irradiation of the gland or even surgery have been advised to limit cell growth, before pregnancy is contemplated.

SECONDARY AMENORRHOEA

PITUITARY DISORDERS

SIMMOND's DISEASE (Sheehan's syndrome) occurs in women and is due to ischaemic necrosis of the pituitary following post-partum haemorrhage. The normally low pressure in the pituitary portal vascular supply increases the susceptibility of the gland. The results vary with the extent of necrosis and may include the following:

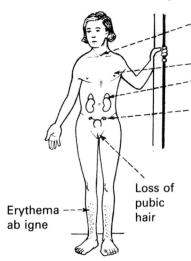

Lack of TSH – low BMR, features of hypothyroidism, sensitivity to cold, coarsening and loss of hair.

Lack of prolactin – failure of lactation, and later breast atrophy.

Lack of ACTH – deficiency of glucocorticoids – weakness, low BP, hypoglycaemia, coma may occur.

Lack of gonadotrophins – amenorrhoea, sterility, loss of libido.

Erythema ab igne

Loss of pubic hair

Treatment consists of hormone replacement therapy – hydrocortisone, thyroxine and oestrogen/progestogen.

Where the necrosis is extensive, death may occur due to the complete loss of control of metabolism. With lesser degrees, lack of one or other of the pituitary hormones may be the dominating feature. In time, the peripheral endocrine organs – thyroid, adrenals, ovaries – show atrophy.

CUSHING's SYNDROME

This is an excess production of cortisol and other steroids by:
(a) An adenoma or carcinoma of the adrenal cortex
or (b) Excess production of ACTH by a pituitary tumour
or (c) Ectopic production of these substances by tumours of other organs such as bronchial carcinoma or carcinoid tumours.

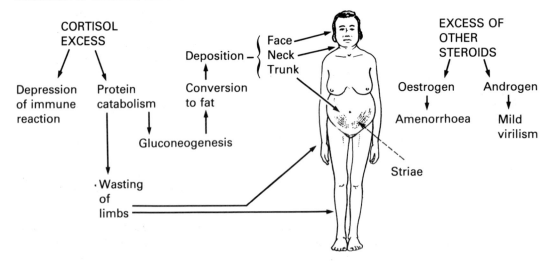

SECONDARY AMENORRHOEA

ADRENAL HYPOFUNCTION (ADDISON's DISEASE)

Previously mainly due to destruction of the adrenals by tuberculosis this disease in industrialised countries is almost entirely caused by auto-immune reactions.

The effects are due to loss of secretion of cortisol and aldosterone, but there is also loss of other steroid substances.

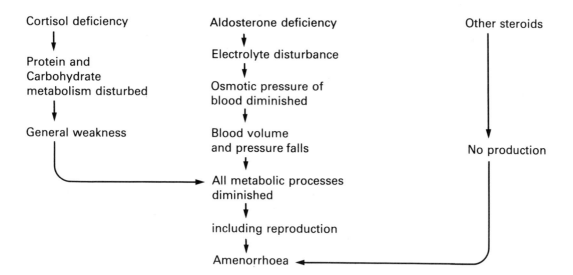

OVARIAN CAUSES OF SECONDARY AMENORRHOEA

There are several conditions in adult life in which ovarian follicular growth is defective.

1. Mention has already been made of the disappearance of primordial follicles during childhood resulting in failure of pubertal development, causing (a) one form of primary amenorrhoea. This is thought to be due to diminution in the total number of germ cells migrating to the ovary and atresia of those which have migrated. The same set of circumstances may operate later in life either in the teenage years causing (b) secondary amenorrhoea or even later when it is termed (c) premature menopause. Gonadotrophin levels (FSH) are raised as in the normal menopause.

2. **Resistant ovarian syndrome**.

   This condition is characterised histologically by the presence of numerous primordial follicles but no follicular development.

   The cause of the condition is unknown. There may be some defect in the transport or receptor mechanisms of gonadotrophins.

3. **Autoimmune oophoritis**.

   This is a rare condition involving a peri-follicular lymphoplasmacytic inflammatory reaction.

Because of the rarity of all these conditions and the difficulty in diagnosis, specific treatment is non-existent. Treatment for the secondary results such as osteoporosis may be necessary.

SECONDARY AMENORRHOEA

FOLLICULAR CYSTIC DISEASE and AMENORRHOEA

There are at least three syndromes associated with the presence of cystic follicles in the ovary. The clinical effects vary.

1. **Persistent cystic follicle**

   This may be associated with a high blood oestrogen level which does not fluctuate. The endometrium remains intact and there is no menstruation. Histological examination shows the cyst to be lined by granulosa cells, thecal cells being inconspicuous. Eventually the cystic follicles may undergo atresia, oestrogen falls and bleeding occurs.

2. **Stein Leventhal Syndrome**

   The original description of this condition was that of a clearly defined syndrome of a degree of virilism in the form of male type hirsutism, obesity, infertility and amenorrhoea associated with multiple small follicular cysts around 0.3cm in diameter. Histologically the cysts showed a normal or thin layer of granulosa cells but an excessively thick layer of luteinised thecal cells.

   Changes in the ovary

   The ovary is enlarged ('oyster' or 'potato' ovary) due to the cortical hyperplasia which is characteristic of the disease. Under the microscope the cortex shows thecal hyperplasia with large numbers of follicles. There are no corpora lutea.

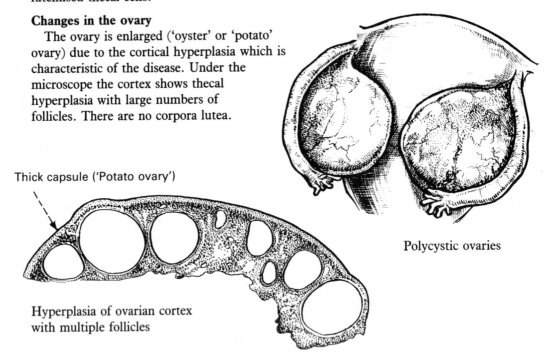

Thick capsule ('Potato ovary')

Hyperplasia of ovarian cortex
with multiple follicles

Polycystic ovaries

Biochemically there is an increased blood LH and low FSH in some cases. Oestrogen levels may be normal but androstenedione and testosterone are increased.

SECONDARY AMENORRHOEA

FOLLICULAR DISEASE of the OVARIES (*contd*)

3. Persistent cystic follicle with high blood LH and low FSH

This is a variant of the Stein Leventhal syndrome. Androstenedione and testosterone levels are raised. The patient has the same clinical features but is not obese.

There appear to be several clinical conditions associated with cystic follicles which may be due to variations in the relative populations of granulosal and thecal cells.

Treatment

There are four problems to be tackled:
1. The endocrine disturbance involving the pituitary hormones.
2. Obesity.
3. Hirsutes.
4. Infertility.

1. To suppress the hypothalamic releasing hormone an oral contraceptive containing oestrogen may be tried. This can be followed by clomiphene which may induce ovulation and restore the menstrual cycle to normality. If there is no sign of an LH surge chorionic gonadotrophin, 5000 units, should be given a week later.
   Pituitary gonadotrophins must not be used to treat the amenorrhoea. Patients with polycystic ovaries are extremely sensitive to pituitary gonadotrophins. They can be used to treat infertility but with the greatest of care.

2. A regime of diet and exercise is the safest treatment for the obesity. Proprietary slimming preparations are to be avoided.

3. There are various methods of treating hirsutes. If it is not gross, shaving, depilatory creams or electrolysis may be used.
   When the menstrual cycle is under control cyproterone acetate 160mg can be given daily from day 5 to day 14 plus ethinyl oestradiol 30μg from day 5 to day 25 to maintain control of the cycle and prevent conception. This should be maintained for 9 months when the cyproterone can be stopped. The result is reasonably effective but there is a 20% failure rate. An alternative treatment is spironolactone which blocks the binding sites of testosterone.

4. While the above treatment with clomiphene can restore fertility sometimes additional factors must be looked at such as prolactinaemia.
   Bromocriptine. The prolactin level is raised in about 13% of patients and, if no abnormality of the pituitary gland is detected, bromocriptine should be given (about 2.5mg twice daily).
   Dexamethasone. This is given to suppress adrenocortical activity, but should not be used unless there is evidence of hyperfunction of the gland.

SECONDARY AMENORRHOEA

AMENORRHOEA and OVARIAN TUMOURS

Disturbance of menstruation is unusual with the commoner forms of ovarian tumour such as cystadenomas. Amenorrhoea is much more likely to occur in cases of functioning tumours producing steroids.

HORMONE-PRODUCING TUMOURS

The commonest tumours of this kind are steroid-producing, particularly sex steroids. Both androgenic and oestrogenic effects have been described with every histological variety but certain tumours of well defined histological structures are commonly associated with the production of one type of steroid.

OESTROGEN-PRODUCING TUMOURS

These belong to the granulosa-theca cell group and are found at all ages. They account for 3% of all solid tumours of the ovary.
Oestrogen excess causes:
1. Hyperplasia of myometrium ⟶ enlarged uterus.
2. Hyperplasia of endometrium ⟶ irregular bleeding. Occasionally amenorrhoea occurs if the production of oestrogen does not fluctuate.
3. Hyperplasia of mammary gland tissue ⟶ enlargement, tenderness of breasts.
4. Oestrogenic vaginal smear.

In childhood there is accelerated skeletal growth and appearance of sex hair.
5% occur in children ⟶ precocious puberty.
60% occur in childbearing years ⟶ irregular menstruation.
30% occur in post-menopausal women ⟶ post-menopausal bleeding.

Diagnosis
Granulosa cell tumour in childhood is the usual cause of female precocity and diagnosis is obvious. In childbearing and post-menopausal years diagnosis is difficult owing to multiplicity of causes of irregular vaginal bleeding. Laparoscopy and ovarian biopsy may be useful.

Pathology
These tumours vary very much in function. Large tumours may be virtually functionless. In childhood and early adult life the tumours are composed mainly of granulosa cells. In later life they are usually thecomata. The granulosa cell type of growth should be considered as carcinoma. Recurrence may occur many years after removal of the primary growth. It is not possible to correlate accurately malignancy with histological appearances. In 14% of cases endometrial hyperplasia becomes atypical and carcinoma develops.

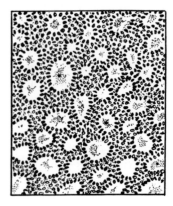

ANDROGEN-PRODUCING TUMOURS

Three distinct types of masculinising ovarian tumour are recognised: (a) Sertoli-Leydig cell tumour (Arrhenoblastoma), (b) Hilar cell tumour, (c) Lipoid cell tumour. All three cause amenorrhoea.

SERTOLI-LEYDIG CELL TUMOUR (Arrhenoblastoma)

This is a rare tumour and forms less than 1% of all ovarian tumours. It occurs in young adult females. Clinically two stages are recognised:

1. Period of defeminisation   **2. Period of masculinisation**

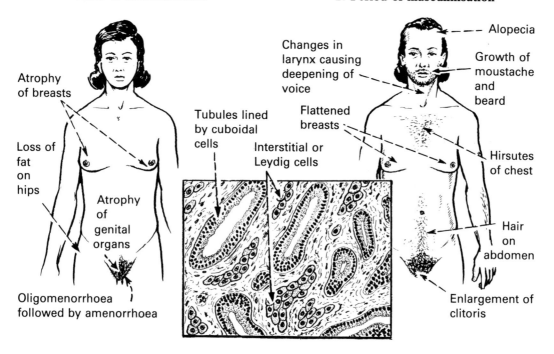

Atrophy of breasts

Loss of fat on hips

Atrophy of genital organs

Oligomenorrhoea followed by amenorrhoea

Tubules lined by cuboidal cells

Interstitial or Leydig cells

Changes in larynx causing deepening of voice

Flattened breasts

Alopecia

Growth of moustache and beard

Hirsutes of chest

Hair on abdomen

Enlargement of clitoris

Pathology

Usually appears as a small white or yellowish tumour within the ovarian substance. Cystic degeneration may occur. In 20% the tumour is malignant and behaves like a carcinoma producing widespread metastases.

Histologically it consists of primitive tubules surrounded by Leydig cells which contain crystalloids of Reinke. These are rod-shaped structures in the cytoplasm of Leydig cells and said to be diagnostic of these cells.

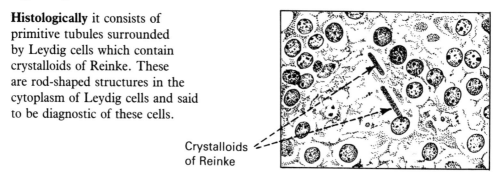

Crystalloids of Reinke

ANDROGEN-PRODUCING TUMOURS

SERTOLI-LEYDIG CELL TUMOUR (*contd*)

Biochemistry

The symptoms are due to the secretion of testosterone. The quantities are small and therefore the output of metabolites such as 17-ketosteroids is within the normal range. Direct estimations of blood testosterone can be made but this requires very sophisticated laboratory procedures.

Removal of the tumour results in regression of symptoms in the same order as their appearance. Menstruation returns within a month or two. Voice changes tend to be permanent.

HILAR CELL TUMOUR

This is a very rare tumour found in post-menopausal women. Defeminisation occurs but signs of virilism are usually mild, consisting of hirsutes, alopecia and enlargement of the clitoris.

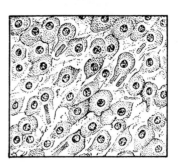

Pathology

Hilar cell tumours are small, brown, simple tumours in the ovarian hilum consisting of polyhedral Leydig cells. Crystalloids of Reinke are occasionally present. 17-ketosteroids are usually within the normal post-menopausal range. Small quantities of androgen are produced.

LIPOID CELL TUMOUR (ovoblastoma, masculinovoblastoma, adrenal-like tumour)

This is also a rare tumour causing masculinisation and producing symptoms and signs of hyper-corticoidism such as skin striae, obesity, polycythaemia, a diabetic glucose tolerance curve and hypertension.

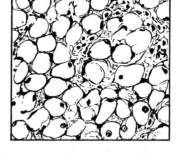

Pathology

The tumour consists of cells with a high content of lipoid and is commonly large and yellowish.

Unlike other virilising tumours the 17-ketosteroid output is greatly increased and the excretion of 17-hydroxycorticosteroids is also raised. ACTH or chorionic gonadotrophin will cause a further increase, but dexamethasone does not diminish the output, thus helping to differentiate the condition from virilism of adrenal origin.

INVESTIGATION OF AMENORRHOEA

In most instances the failure to menstruate is due to some abnormality in the control mechanism involving the hypothalamic-pituitary pathway.

A careful history and physical examination will provide pointers to likely defects in the majority of cases. Weight loss, diet and possible psychological factors should be probed. Equally questions should be posed regarding recent changes in the breasts and the presence of slight galactorrhoea. The possibility of hirsutes which the patient may be treating should be raised. All of these are conditions which the patient is apt to find embarrassing.

The physical examination will reveal congenital anomalies and ambiguous genitalia. In the case of the latter a blood sample should be examined to establish the genetic sex of the individual.

Further investigation will involve laboratory tests and the extent of these will depend on whether the patient desires to become pregnant or merely wishes the return of menstruation.

Menstruation

Since some 60% of cases of amenorrhoea are associated with increased blood prolactin this must be the first line of enquiry.

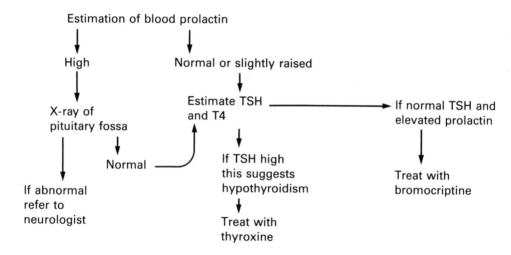

If the results of these tests are inconclusive it suggests that the cause lies between the pituitary and ovaries and further laboratory exploration must be undertaken e.g.

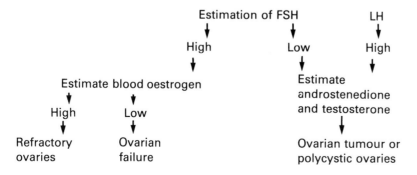

INVESTIGATION OF AMENORRHOEA

Menstruation (*contd*)

If pregnancy is desired, the menstrual cycle must first of all be normalised so far as possible. This does not guarantee that the endometrium is in a satisfactory state or will react to the sex steroids in the normal fashion. It is customary to carry out a progestogen stimulation test. This is a test of the adequacy of endogenous oestrogen production. A progestogen – say 5mg norethisterone – is given daily for a week and then stopped. If withdrawal bleeding occurs it is evidence of adequate oestrogen priming of the endometrium. Failure to bleed would indicate the need for a search for a cause of oestrogen failure or excessive androgen production.

VIRILISM

VIRILISM means signs of excessive androgen stimulation in the muscles, larynx, genitalia and hair. It is always a pathological condition.

Causes
1. Ovarian tumour.
2. Delayed onset of adrenal hyperplasia.
3. Adrenal tumour.
4. Hypothalamic or pituitary disease.
5. Chromosomal abnormality (Mosaicism or some cases of testicular feminisation.

Clinical features

The affected end-organs vary with the individual, and there is no regular pattern for the appearance of signs. The patient may first notice an increase in hair, or a reduction or cessation of menstruation. The breasts atrophy or fail to develop, the clitoris is enlarged and the voice deepens. In extreme cases a definite male muscular development is apparent and there is marked enlargement of the thyroid cartilage.

Investigations
1. Examination under anaesthesia to allow a full inspection of the genitalia. If a uterus is present an endometrial biopsy is taken. A vaginal smear will give some idea of oestrogenic secretion.
2. Laparoscopic inspection and ovarian biopsy are indicated if no mass is palpated.
3. Blood is sent for chromosomal analysis.
4. X-ray investigation may detect a cerebral tumour or adrenal enlargement.
5. Hormone investigations: There may be only a slight rise in plasma testosterone since very little excess is required to produce clinical signs of virilism, and the 17-ketosteroid level is usually normal. If it is raised, adrenal function tests must be carried out since the adrenal is virtually the only source of 17-ketosteroids in the female. Stimulation of cortisol secretion by metyrapone and inhibition by dexamethasone are effective tests in adrenal hyperplasia but not in cases of pituitary tumour.

Most patients suffering from virilism are likely to be seen for the first time at a gynaecological clinic. Because of the association of virilism with tumours, and the irreversibility of voice changes once they have occurred, the gynaecologist must always keep in mind the possibility of encountering a patient with this rare condition.

HIRSUTISM

HIRSUTISM in the female means an excessive production of hair with a tendency to male distribution. 'Excessive' is defined as beyond social acceptability or causing embarrassment to the patient.

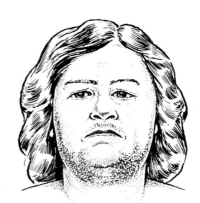

Normal pattern Hair is of two types –
(i) fine downy, vellus hair which is non-pigmented.
(ii) coarser pigmented terminal hair as in the axilla and pubis.

About one-third of women have some visible pigmented hair on the upper lip, and 5% have it on the chin and sides of the face.

Aetiology 1. Rise in secretion of free androgens.
2. Reduction in sex hormone binding globulin (SHBG).
SHBG level falls when testosterone production increases, and probably also in the case of drug- induced hirsutism.

Physiology of Testosterone
The three principal androgens are dihydrotestosterone, testosterone, and androstenedione which is the least potent but is converted to dihydrotestosterone in the follicle cells.

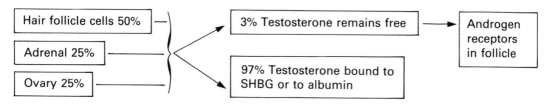

Causes:

1. Idiopathic Hirsutism
By far the commonest, it has no apparent androgen increase, and is probably due to increased local testosterone production at the target organ.

2. Polycystic Ovary Disease
There is usually slight testosterone increase.

3. Ovarian or Adrenal Disease
This includes rare conditions such as androgen-producing tumours and Cushing's disease, and must be excluded.

4. Drugs such as:-
phenytoin (Epanutin) ⎫ epilepsy
diazoxide (Eudemine) ⎬ hypertension
minoxidil (Loniten) ⎭

androgen-containing compounds

HIRSUTISM

INVESTIGATION

Most of the information necessary for deciding on treatment will be obtained from the history, but some biochemical assays are required to exclude serious disease. The testosterone secretion level is nearly always normal or at most slightly raised, and a marked increase suggests ovarian or adrenal tumour. Adrenal function can be simply assessed by estimation of the urinary excretion of 17-ketosteroids. A raised LH/FSH ratio suggests polycystic ovarian disease, and if ovarian function is in question, laparoscopy and biopsy and even laparotomy may be necessary.

LOCAL TREATMENT

Shaving
This is the best method but has ineradicable associations with virility.

Abrasives
Pads or gloves of fine sandpaper have the same effect as shaving but are as hard on the skin and have no advantage.

Electrolysis
Decomposition of the hair follicle by the passage of an electric current. Low galvanic current is used through a fine electrode. The hair is electrolysed after about 10 seconds and plucked out painlessly.

Diathermy
The follicle is coagulated instantly and the hair pulled out.

Electrical destruction of individual hairs is permanent but prolonged treatment is tedious and expensive.

Depilatory Creams
These are alkaline solutions which dissolve the hairs and allow them to be wiped away. They will injure the skin if left on too long.

Depilatory Waxes
The wax is melted and spread on to the skin. When it sets it is pulled off, plucking the hairs with it. This is painful and leaves the skin tender and reddened.

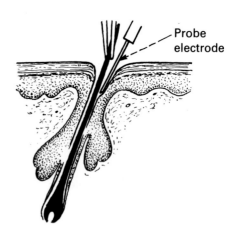

Probe electrode

HIRSUTISM

DRUG TREATMENT

Three groups are used alone or in combination:-
1. Adrenal steroid drugs such as prednisolone or dexamethasone.
2. Oestrogen/progestogen combinations.
3. Anti-androgens such as cyproterone acetate.

Adrenal Suppression

Dexamethasone 0.5mg daily has a suppressive effect on adrenal and ovarian androgen secretion but should not affect function. It must be continued for about a year, and about 1 in 5 patients respond.

Oestrogen Treatment

Oral contraceptives have been found successful in some patients. The oestrogen increases SHBG synthesis in the liver, and the progestogen inhibits LH and therefore androgen secretion.

Combined prednisolone/oestrogen/progestogen treatment

Prednisolone 2.5mg twice daily is taken along with one of the contraceptive pill compounds. This treatment is continued for up to a year and is claimed to be much more beneficial than either drug used alone.

Cyproterone acetate (Androcur)

This is an anti-androgen which acts peripherally, competing with testosterone at the androgen receptors of the follicle cells, and repeated trials have shown it to be effective. It is usually combined with an oestrogen which regulates the cycle and increases the effect:

100mg cyproterone is given from day 5 to day 14;
0.05mg ethinyl oestradiol is given from day 5 also but is continued until day 25.

There is no significant fall in circulating androgens, but side-effects include weight gain and lassitude (hypothalamic activity is reduced), and as the drug crosses the placenta and feminises the male fetus, the patient must not conceive during treatment.

Most patients are improved by cyproterone and severe acne also responds, but unfortunately relapse is very likely after treatment is stopped.

ABNORMAL MENSTRUAL BLEEDING

This is a common complaint. In most cases it is due to a local gynaecological lesion. During the reproductive phase of life three forms of bleeding have been recognised:

1. **Menorrhagia.** Regular 28 day cycles with excessive loss of blood.
2. **Polymenorrhoea.** Regular cycles of short duration and therefore more frequent, resulting in excessive loss of blood over a period of time.
3. **Metrorrhagia.** Irregular, non-cyclical, bleeding usually excessive.

Causes

These are numerous. Attempts have been made to classify the lesions according to the three patterns of bleeding. This is unsatisfactory since the same lesion can be associated with any one of the three patterns.

Causes of abnormal bleeding patterns

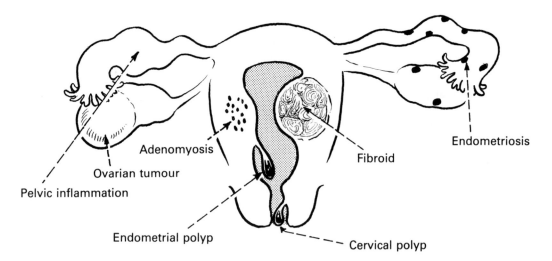

Other causes of abnormal bleeding include vaginitis, prolapse, cervicitis and cervical ectopy, urethral caruncle and cancer of the cervix or uterine body. In many cases of abnormal uterine bleeding no satisfactory etiology will be found, and the condition is then classed as 'dysfunctional uterine bleeding'.

ABNORMAL MENSTRUAL BLEEDING

GENERAL DISEASE and MENORRHAGIA

This is an uncommon association. More frequently menstrual disturbance takes the form of amenorrhoea or oligomenorrhoea in general disease.

Occasionally it may be associated with leukaemia or rare congenital bleeding conditions such as purpura. Endocrine abnormalities other than those of the pituitary-ovarian axis rarely affect the menstrual cycle. Early thyroid deficiency can result in menorrhagia but when myxoedema is established amenorrhoea is more usual. It is thought that the depression of metabolic activity influences pituitary function.

While not regarded as a disease in the ordinary sense, mental stress may upset menstruation. The result can be amenorrhoea or menorrhagia. A suggested mechanism is as follows:

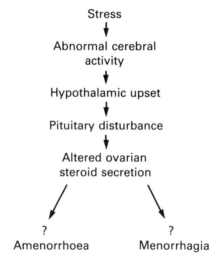

DYSFUNCTIONAL UTERINE BLEEDING

Dysfunctional uterine bleeding is the term applied to cases of excessive bleeding where no organic lesion such as those already mentioned can be found and it is concluded that the cause lies in an abnormal function of the control mechanisms associated with the menstrual cycle. It is a diagnosis very frequently made, too frequent in the opinion of many observers. Although there may be no abnormal physical signs on ordinary gynaecological examination every effort must be made by all means available – curettage, hysteroscopy, ultrasound scan, tests for chorionic gonadotrophin – to confirm that there is indeed no local lesion.

DYSFUNCTIONAL UTERINE BLEEDING

Clinical features

The patient will complain of irregular and/or heavy bleeding, often using emotive descriptions like 'flooding' or 'coming up like a well'. Any departure from a normal menstrual pattern is liable to cause anxiety and allowance must be made for this.

The patient should be asked about the number of pads or tampons used, but such evidence is not very reliable. What is normal to one woman may be regarded as abnormal by another. The important feature is the complaint of change in the pattern of bleeding rather than the absolute quantity.

Estimation of blood loss

The passage of large clots is a sign of excessive loss, but the venous blood does not often show features of anaemia. An estimation of serum ferritin may show a depletion in iron stores.

Endometrial Biopsy This is necessary to exclude malignant disease.

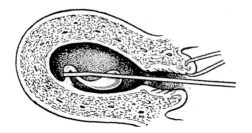 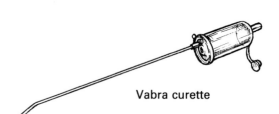

Vabra curette

Conventional Curettage

Curettage under anaesthesia will allow thorough examination and will usually reveal pathology such as polyps. It means admission at least as a day patient.

Suction Curettage

This method of obtaining material for histological examination can be done in the out-patient clinic. Adequate specimens can be obtained, but the procedure is painful.

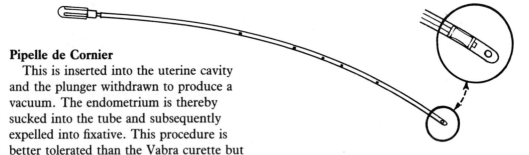

Pipelle de Cornier

This is inserted into the uterine cavity and the plunger withdrawn to produce a vacuum. The endometrium is thereby sucked into the tube and subsequently expelled into fixative. This procedure is better tolerated than the Vabra curette but does not always produce sufficient tissue to evaluate histologically.

If out-patient methods of examining endometrium do not provide reliable information, conventional curettage must be carried out.

CERVICAL DILATATION

This is the commonest method of obtaining endometrial tissue for examination and of excluding intra-uterine pathology. It is often necessary to dilate the cervical canal in order to pass the curette.

DILATATION is achieved by the application of the mechanical principle of the wedge. Each dilator is a steel tube with a conical tip which is 3mm diameter less than the shaft. Dilators are graduated in size going from 3/6mm up to at least 14/17mm.

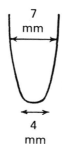

7 mm

4 mm

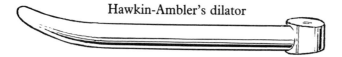

Hawkin-Ambler's dilator

Sims Uterine Curette

Galabin's uterine sound

This sound is simply a measuring rod, used to gauge the length of the uterine cavity.

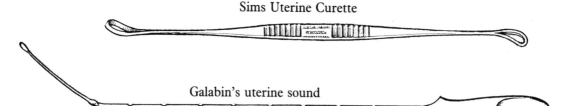

Technique

The dilator must be held firmly in one hand and pressed into the canal against traction in the opposite direction exerted by the other hand. Resistance must be overcome slowly, and the dilator must not be passed farther than the length of the uterine cavity measured by the sound.

CURETTAGE is commonly associated with dilatation of the cervix. See the preceding page.

COMPLICATIONS OF DILATATION

1. **Tight Cervix**

   Resistance can be reduced by lubricating the dilators.

   Dilators increasing by half-millimetre graduations are also available.

2. **Splitting the cervix**

   This may occur without warning even at the hands of an experienced operator. The injury may not be perceived until the curette passes through the tear and injures vessels or bowel. If the operator realises what has happened and there is no bleeding, the patient should be given antibiotic cover and observed for 24 hours. If there are then symptoms of internal or external bleeding, laparotomy must be carried out and the tear sutured.

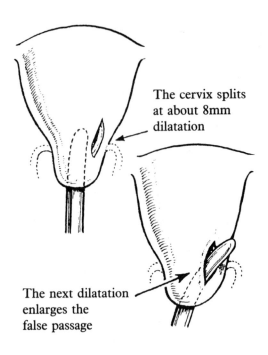

The cervix splits at about 8mm dilatation

The next dilatation enlarges the false passage

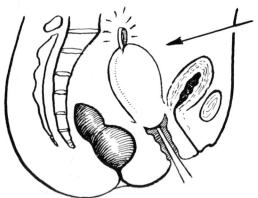

3. **Perforation of the uterus**

   This is not an uncommon occurrence and usually no ill-effects result. The usual site is the mid-line of the fundus and it becomes evident when the curette passes in further than the length of the cavity as shown by the uterine sound. Immediate laparotomy is required if there is any suspicion of damage to extra-uterine viscera, or if the curettage has been carried out to complete an abortion, when bleeding is likely to be too heavy to ignore.

4. **Trauma to cervix**

   The volsellum forceps may tear the anterior lip of cervix if pulled on too forcibly.

5. **Uterine synechiae**

   Over-vigorous curettage may remove all the endometrium from areas of anterior and posterior walls, permitting the myometrium to heal together forming adhesions – Asherman's syndrome.

DYSFUNCTIONAL UTERINE BLEEDING

TOTAL HYSTERECTOMY

This is the best treatment for the woman over 40 who has not been cured by medical treatment. She is freed from the constant loss of blood and also from the risk of uterine or cervical cancer. In general there is an improvement in the mood and activity after hysterectomy for dysfunctional bleeding, ovarian function is unimpaired and there is no reduction in the frequency of intercourse or the frequency of orgasm.

The disadvantages are:-

1. The immediate risks of any operation – sepsis and thromboembolism.
2. The risk of ureter damage. Total hysterectomy can present technical difficulties, especially in obese women.
3. The ovaries may cease to function despite being conserved.

Total Hysterectomy (Removal of uterus and cervix)

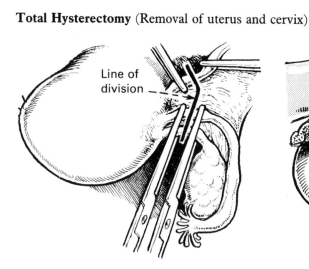

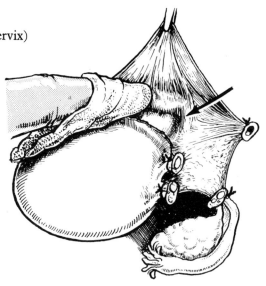

1. Division of adnexa. The ovarian ligament, fallopian tube and round ligament are clamped and divided.

2. Vesico-uterine peritoneum is opened up and bladder is being dissected off cervix. (The 'lateral vesico-uterine ligament' – marked by the arrow – conceals the ureter.)

119

TOTAL HYSTERECTOMY

Total Hysterectomy (*contd*)

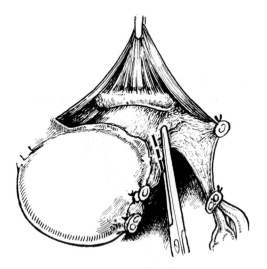

3. Parametrium containing the uterine arteries is clamped and divided.

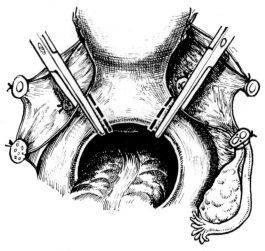

4. The uterosacral ligaments are clamped and divided.

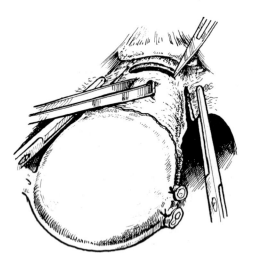

5. The top of the vagina is now clear of bladder and ureters and can be opened to allow excision of uterus and cervix.

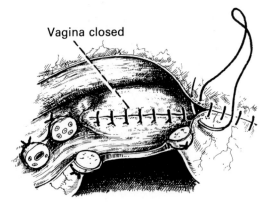

Vagina closed

6. After closing the vagina the raw area is reperitonised.

SUBTOTAL HYSTERECTOMY

Subtotal Hysterectomy – Removal of the body of the uterus only, leaving the cervix.

This operation is easier and safer than total hysterectomy but is little practised today because it does not give protection from the risk of cervical cancer. It would be indicated for technical reasons (pelvic infection, obesity) or if the patient wished to retain her cervix.

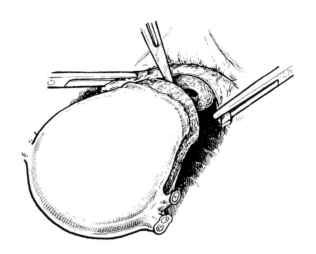

Excision of the Ovaries

This is an even simpler operation which would cure dysfunctional bleeding quite as well as total hysterectomy but it would cause severe withdrawal symptoms and does not have the same prophylactic value as removal of the entire uterus. It would only be indicated in a patient unfit for anything else.

RADIATION MENOPAUSE

A small amount of external radiation, say 500r in divided doses will, in most women, put an end to ovarian function. This is rarely employed nowadays.

Advantage

It avoids the risks and discomforts of surgery except for the curettage which must first be done to exclude organic disease of the uterus.

Disadvantages

1. Except in a woman near a natural menopause, the oestrogen withdrawal symptoms are likely to be distressing.
2. It is impossible by this method to exclude an ovarian cause for the bleeding such as a granulosa cell tumour.
3. There is no prophylaxis against uterine cancer.

MINIMALLY INVASIVE SURGERY

It has been claimed that progestogen-releasing intra-uterine contraceptive devices may give equally good control of abnormal uterine bleeding. Long-term evaluation of endometrial ablation techniques is required.

In laparoscopically assisted hysterectomy the broad ligaments, including the ovarian vessels, the round ligaments and the uterine arteries may be 'clamped and cut' by an endoscopic device which inserts multiple rows of stainless steel staples and divides the tissues. The uterus is then removed vaginally and the vaginal vault closed per vaginam.

The cost of treatment can be reduced by decreasing the number of days as an in-patient, with consequent reduction in costly nursing and ancillary care. Inconvenience to patients and relatives is also reduced by 'minimally invasive surgery' and there is increasing pressure from administrators and patients to make modern alternatives to orthodox abdominal and vaginal hysterectomy more widely available.

TRANS-CERVICAL RESECTION of ENDOMETRIUM (TCRE) is the most widely available.

Using an operating hysteroscope, the uterine cavity is distended with a glycine solution and either a wire loop diathermy instrument is used to cut strips of endometrium and underlying myometrium or a 'roller ball' electrode is used to coagulate the endometrium.

Fluid can be perfused into uterine veins during the procedure while the uterine cavity is being flushed out with the glycine solution, and an extremely careful watch must be kept on fluid balance. Care must be taken not to perforate the uterus. Only a few days of in-patient care are usually required.

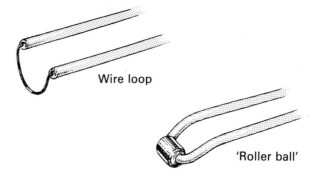

Wire loop

'Roller ball'

HYSTEROSCOPIC ENDOMETRIAL ABLATION by LASER (HEAL) involves destruction of the endometrium using a fibre-optic transmitted YAG-Neodynium laser. This apparatus is more expensive, but is less likely to perforate the uterus.

RADIO FREQUENCY ENDOMETRIAL ABLATION (RaFEA) involves destruction of the endometrium by radio waves.

None of the above techniques is guaranteed to destroy all of the endometrium and some menstrual loss may persist. They do not abolish period pain. Usually the endometrium is made atrophic with Danazol or LHRH analogue prior to the procedure.

DYSFUNCTIONAL UTERINE BLEEDING

Pathology

In the majority of cases of dysfunctional uterine bleeding the cause appears to lie in defects of ovarian steroid production. Some are associated with evidence of ovulation, others with anovulation, but in many there is no definite guide to what is happening. In a considerable number function returns to normal without treatment and provided the patient's general health is not suffering it is worth postponing treatment for 3 months or so.

ENDOMETRIAL PATTERNS and STEROID VALUES

Anovulatory with low oestrogen values

There is irregular bleeding. Sometimes the name 'threshold bleeding' is used to describe the condition. The endometrium shows an atrophic pattern. The glands are small, infrequent and show little activity. Oestrogen values in general are low but fluctuate. Progesterone values are also low. It is suggested that the fluctuation of oestrogen levels is the cause of the bleeding. When they fall they are unable to maintain the endometrium, which crumbles, causing haemorrhage.

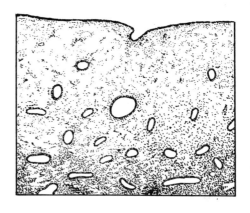

Anovulatory with high oestrogen values

This is a variation of the same process. FSH is secreted as in the normal cycle. Oestrogen increases, causing endometrial hyperplasia. Ultimately the oestrogen increase inhibits FSH production. Oestrogen then falls and bleeding, usually excessive, occurs from the bulky endometrium. The glands tend to be cystic and show mitotic activity.

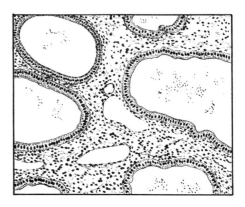

DYSFUNCTIONAL UTERINE BLEEDING

Endometrial patterns and steroid values (*contd*)

Anovulatory with high oestrogen and high FSH

This produces a histological picture known as cystic glandular hyperplasia. The glandular epithelium shows mitotic activity. There is no inhibitory feedback to the pituitary and the anomalous position of high oestrogen, high FSH continues for 2 or more months during which there is no amenorrhoea. Ultimately the oestrogen level fluctuates and the fall produces excessive, prolonged bleeding. The defect may lie in the inhibitory mechanism of the pituitary. More important than the bleeding is the fact that a considerable number of cases end in carcinoma of the endometrium.

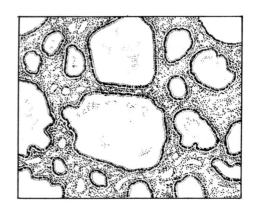

OVULATORY PATTERNS

Prolonged proliferative phase, short luteal phase

The illustration shows an endometrium in the early secretory phase although the specimen was taken on the 27th day. The prolonged oestrogenic phase has built up a thick endometrium. Progesterone is low. The cause is unknown. It may be an ovarian defect – poor reaction to pituitary LH, or a pituitary dysfunction, or insensitivity of endometrium. The mixed endocrine situation results in excessive bleeding when the oestrogen values decline and the endometrium is shed.

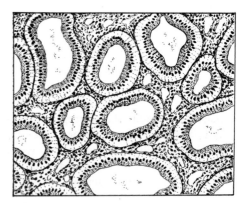

DYSFUNCTIONAL UTERINE BLEEDING

Ovulatory patterns (*contd*)

Prolonged luteal phase

In this case the corpus luteum persists beyond the usual span and menstruation is delayed. Sometimes there is irregular shedding of the endometrium resulting in short repeated periods of bleeding. The patient may describe this as 'stopping and starting'.

Specimens of endometrium show a general secretory pattern interspersed with small areas of oedema, necrosis and bleeding. In some cases it is associated with a cystic corpus luteum.

Areas of proliferative activity often exist side by side with late secretory glands.

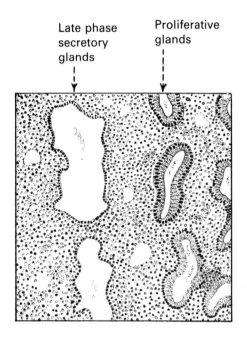

Late phase secretory glands

Proliferative glands

It is claimed that no apparent cause for bleeding can be found in 50% of cases diagnosed as dysfunctional bleeding. This may not be entirely correct. Much will depend on the timing of the curettage and steroid estimations. Many cases of dysfunctional bleeding are diagnosed in the age group 45 to 50, i.e. the climacteric. Variations in menstrual and endometrial patterns are often found at this time. Amenorrhoea may alternate with menstruation in which a normal secretory endometrium is found. Indeed, unexpected pregnancy may occur. The onset of puberty is often accompanied by menstrual disturbances with menorrhagia of anovulatory type which could be considered as a form of dysfunctional bleeding.

Treatment

A spontaneous remission in symptoms can be expected in perhaps a half of the patients investigated, so it is usual to advise conservative treatment in the first place, especially in patients nearing the menopause. Drug treatment cannot be maintained indefinitely however and for the patient over 40 whose family is complete, hysterectomy is usually required.

Trans-cervical resection of endometrium or laser ablation of endometrium are less radical alternatives which are being evaluated at present.

DYSFUNCTIONAL UTERINE BLEEDING

Treatment (*contd*)

Antifibrinolytic Agents

Tranexamic acid is a drug which is given orally during menstruation on the assumption that an overactive fibrinolytic system is preventing closure of the basal endometrial arteries by thrombosis.

Ethamsylate which reduces capillary fragility is prescribed on empirical grounds, but its effectiveness is still questioned.

Oestrogen/Progestogen

The combined oestrogen/progestogen oral contraceptive preparations are now the most effective treatment for dysfunctional bleeding, but their side effects (weight gain, depression, an increased liability to thrombosis) reduce their advantage, especially in women over 35 in whom dysfunctional bleeding is found. Progestogens alone (such as norethisterone) are also used but they are now suspected of increasing the risk of coronary infarction and stroke. Most gynaecologists have reservations about prolonged steroid hormone therapy.

Prostaglandin Synthetase Inhibitors

> Mefenamic acid.
> Flurbiprofen.
> Indomethacin.

These drugs inhibit the vasodilator effect of prostaglandin E2 and also have a useful analgesic effect.

Ovulation Stimulators

Clomiphene will restore a normal ovulatory pattern, but it increases the possibility of pregnancy which may not be wanted.

Danazol

This drug is a derivative of 17-alpha-ethinyl testosterone and is used principally in the treatment of endometriosis (q.v.). In a dose of 400mg daily it will achieve a marked reduction in blood loss and in some cases amenorrhoea. Danazol has no effect on coagulation and is safe in that respect, but when stopped the dysfunctional bleeding soon returns.

In some cases of dysfunctional uterine bleeding the bleeding is so persistent that hysterectomy is advised, especially if pregnancy is not desired. An alternative is vaporisation of the endometrium by a laser. This can be adjusted very accurately so that only the endometrial layer is destroyed. Trans-cervical resection of endometrium using diathermy loop or roller-ball is another alternative to hysterectomy.

Progestogen-bearing intrauterine contraceptive devices, not at present available in the UK, are a promising and less invasive treatment for dysfunctional bleeding.

ADENOMYOSIS

This is an infiltration of the myometrium by ectopic deposits of endometrium. It is frequently referred to as endometriosis interna to distinguish it from ectopic deposits of endometrium on the peritoneum and pelvic organs – endometriosis externa.

Pathology

The gross appearances are quite striking.

The uterus is usually enlarged and this may be quite marked.

Commonly the enlargement is most marked on one aspect of the uterus – usually the posterior. It gives rise to a tumour-like mass but there is no capsule. Often a myoma is present which confuses the situation.

The cut surface shows the typical small blood spots due to bleeding from the endometrial deposits.

In many cases the uterus is adherent to the rectum or adnexa.

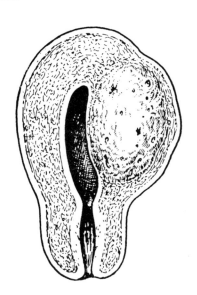

Microscopic appearances

The appearance of these endometrial deposits varies. In many cases they consist of typical glands and stroma although the stroma may be more prominent than the glands. Cyclical changes may be observed but this is not common. More often the endometrium is of immature type and if it does react it usually shows only proliferative changes suggesting oestrogen stimulation. Progestogen secretory appearances are rarely seen. Despite this, if the patient becomes pregnant, the deposits may show decidual transformation.

Examination of the adhesions between the uterus and the other pelvic structures shows that they are the result of endometriosis externa.

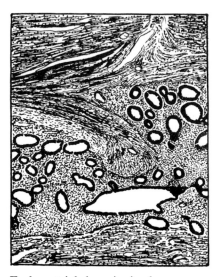

Endometrial deposits in the myometrium. Note the non-secretory gland epithelium. The surrounding myometrium undergoes moderate hyperplasia.

127

ADENOMYOSIS

Clinical Features

It is said that adenomyosis is a disease of parous women but pregnancy tends to occur after a long period of infertility. In 30% of patients the condition is only discovered accidentally during examination or treatment for some other complaint. These patients have no symptoms referable to the adenomyosis.

Pain and menstrual upset are the usual symptoms. The pain is related to menstruation and increases in severity with successive periods. Curiously the severity is not related to the extent of the adenomyosis. The same is true of the menstrual upset which usually consists of menorrhagia or polymenorrhoea. Since peritoneal endometriosis is also present in 15% of cases it is often difficult to assign the cause of the pain to adenomyosis. In other words, both conditions can be symptomless and both can be painful making diagnosis difficult. The same is true of upset menstruation, which usually takes the same form of increased blood loss.

Diagnosis

This is difficult for the reasons given above. Laparoscopy can be helpful in eliminating peritoneal endometriosis but in most cases of adenomyosis the diagnosis of adenomyosis is a matter of probability, confirmed by histology after hysterectomy.

Histogenesis

There have been several theories regarding the origin of the endometrial deposits which permeate the myometrium in adenomyosis, but the question has been resolved by careful serial sectioning of the uterine tissue. It is clear that the deposits originate from a down growth of the basal layer of the endometrium. What initiates this growth is not clear but, once started, the distribution of the deposits suggests a spread via lymphatics or capillaries. Due to haemorrhage and subsequent healing many of the deposits are 'nipped' and lose contact with the original infiltrating column of endometrial tissue.

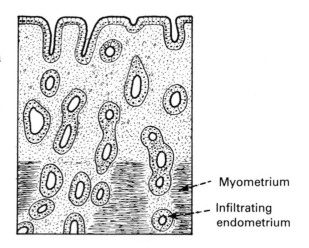

Myometrium

Infiltrating endometrium

Treatment

If symptoms are mild or absent no treatment is necessary. Severe symptoms obviously demand treatment, and hysterectomy is advised. The endometrial deposits are not responsive to hormones, but since they seem to react occasionally during the proliferative oestrogenic phase hormones may be tried, the object being to induce ovarian inactivity.

ENDOMETRIOSIS

This is a very common gynaecological lesion, consisting of ectopic deposits of endometrium in the lower part of the peritoneal cavity. It is sometimes referred to as 'external endometriosis' to distinguish it from adenomyosis. Its manifestations are very variable and can be a diagnostic difficulty.

Pathology

The gross appearance shows ectopic deposits which can vary in number from a few in one locality to large numbers distributed over the pelvic organs and peritoneum.

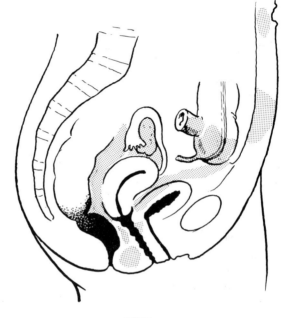

The commonest sites of these deposits are:
1. Ovary.
2. Peritoneum of the recto-vaginal cul-de-sac of the Pouch of Douglas.
3. Sigmoid colon.
4. Broad ligament.
5. Utero-sacral ligaments.

Less common are:
1. Cervix.
2. Round ligament.
3. Bladder.
4. Umbilicus.
5. Appendix.
6. Laparotomy scars.

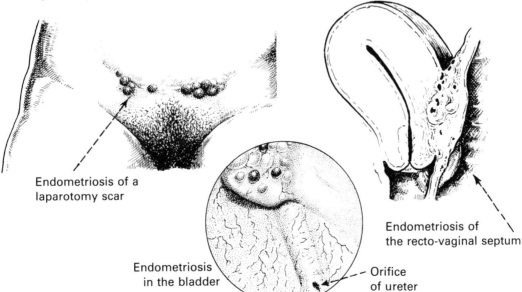

Endometriosis of a laparotomy scar

Endometriosis in the bladder

Endometriosis of the recto-vaginal septum

Orifice of ureter

129

ENDOMETRIOSIS

The commonest appearance of a typical lesion is that of a round protruding vesicle which shows a succession of colours from blue to black to brown. The variation in colour is due to haemorrhage with subsequent breakdown of the haemoglobin. Ultimately the area of haemorrhage heals by the formation of scar tissue. The result is a puckered area on the peritoneum. Commonly however the haemorrhage results in adhesion to surrounding structures. These adhesions are more apt to form between fixed structures such as the broad ligament, ovary, sigmoid colon or the posterior surfaces of the vagina and cervix.

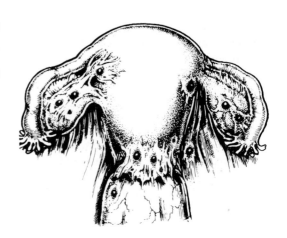

The ectopic deposits of endometrial tissue vary in size from pin-point to 5mm or more. It is these larger deposits which tend to rupture leading to adhesions. These adhesions over the ovary can lead to the formation of quite large haemorrhagic cysts due to continued bleeding from deposits, the blood being unable to escape.

Investigation has shown that many lesions do not have a 'typical' appearance. The following is a list of other appearances which have been described.
1. White, slightly raised opacities due to retro-peritoneal deposits.
2. Red flame-like or vascular swellings, more common in the broad ligament or utero-sacral ligament.
3. Small excrescences like the surface of normal endometrium.
4. Adhesions under the ovary or between the ovary and the ovarian fossa peritoneum.
5. Cafe-au-lait patches often in the Pouch of Douglas, broad ligament or peritoneal surface of the bladder.
6. Peritoneal defects on utero-sacral ligament or broad ligament.
7. Areas of petechiae or hypervascularisation usually on the bladder and the broad ligament.

Secondary Pathology

This is due to the adhesions between the endometriotic deposits and adjacent organs. In long-standing cases the pelvic cavity is obliterated by these adhesions. Retroversion of the uterus can be produced.

Histology

While the deposits consist of endometrial elements rarely do they mirror the appearance of normal endometrium especially in their architecture. In place of the compact orderly arrangement of glands and stroma there are scattered patches of gland formations with some surrounding stroma. Sometimes gland formations predominate, occasionally only stromal cells can be seen.

Sometimes the deposits show evidence of cyclical activity but the activity does not always coincide with what is happening in the uterine endometrium.

ENDOMETRIOSIS

Clinical Findings

Patients with symptomatic endometriosis seem to form a group with certain characteristics in common.

1. They are commonly in the higher socio-economic group.
2. Usually the patient is single and in her thirties.
3. If married, this status has often been acquired late in reproductive years.
4. They have few or no children.

Study of these characteristics suggests that oestrogen is likely to be the main hormonal influence in these patients or that the parous women gain protection from the establishment of endometriotic deposits by the high continuous level of progesterone during their pregnancies.

It has been estimated that endometriosis occurs in 3 to 7% of women but the true incidence is unknown. Quite often deposits are found incidentally in women who have no symptoms of endometriosis and are undergoing laparoscopy or laparotomy for some other condition. In addition, as indicated in the section on pathology, many peritoneal changes now known to be due to endometriosis were undiagnosed in the past.

Symptomatology

A. The chief symptom is PAIN and it affects more than 80% of women with endometriotic deposits. The pain tends to begin pre-menstrually reaching a peak during menstruation and subsiding slowly. Curiously the degree of pain does not appear to be related to the extent of the disease and the cause remains unknown.

The character of pain may vary as does its apparent origin. It may be generalised throughout the abdomen and like the pain of severe dysmenorrhoea, but localisations are frequent.

1. Pain in right iliac region like a 'grumbling appendix'.
2. Cramping pains, constipation, pain on defaecation may mimic obstruction and bowel malignancy, possibly in the pelvic colon or rectum. These symptoms occur in 10% of cases.
3. Deep dyspareunia suggests disease around the recto-vaginal septum and Pouch of Douglas.

B. **Menstrual Disturbance**. This is a frequent complaint. It may take the form of pre-menstrual 'spotting', menorrhagia or polymenorrhoea. Lesions in the wall of the bladder may result in 'menstrual haematuria'.

C. **Infertility**. Although infertility is a common complaint the relationship to endometriosis is not clear. Approximately 30% of endometriotic patients have the complaint. Various explanations have been suggested such as retroversion of the uterus, dyspareunia or altered ovarian function. Patients with retroversion of the uterus but no endometriosis are not commonly infertile. Dyspareunia could be a reason but if the infertility is due to endometriosis it is most likely the result of ovarian dysfunction caused by adhesions preventing normal ovulation.

It is claimed that deep nodular deposits in the recto-vaginal septum are associated with 71% incidence of infertility. These patients usually have severe dyspareunia.

ENDOMETRIOSIS

Physical Examination

Physical signs tend to be indefinite. There may be enlargement of the ovaries, retroversion of the uterus, evidence of tender nodules or adhesions but all of these are speculative not diagnostic. Nevertheless, endometriosis should always be kept in mind when patients have symptoms referable to the pelvic cavity. Examinations should be made at the time of menstruation when lesions will be at their largest and haemorrhage may be seen.

Laparoscopic examination is the only way of making a positive diagnosis. The lesions can be seen and their number and location estimated. Endometriosis of long-standing may be very difficult to diagnose due to obliteration of the pelvic cavity by adhesions. Histological confirmation must be obtained if feasible.

Non-invasive methods of Diagnosis

In recent times attempts have been made to devise antibody tests for diagnosis of endometriosis but, so far, the results have not proved reliable enough to be employed in clinical practice. The same may be said for imaging techniques such as ultrasound, computerised tomography and magnetic resonance imaging.

Differential Diagnosis

Due to the mixture of symptoms and the variation in appearance of the pelvic structures, conditions such as pelvic inflammatory disease and tumours of the ovary and bowel must be considered and eliminated.

Histogenesis

There are three theories.
1. Retrograde spill of menstrual debris through the tubes. This has been proved to take place in most women.
2. Metaplasia of embryonic cells. These are derived from the primitive coelom and may remain in and around the pelvis and differentiate into Müllerian duct tissue.
3. Emboli of endometrial tissue may travel by lymphatics or blood vessels and become established in various sites.

The first of these theories is most favoured.

Treatment
1. MEDICAL TREATMENT.

Any treatment must be aimed at eliminating pain and, if the patient desires, restoring fertility. Since ovarian hormones are responsible for growth and activity in endometrium the immediate objective of therapy must be to reduce their production or oppose their action.

A variety of steroids have been employed. In the beginning these were mainly used to induce pseudo-pregnancy, the idea being that the ectopic endometrium would undergo decidual change which ultimately would be destroyed by necrosis and heal by fibrosis. The contraceptive pill in high dosage and Provera (medroxy progesterone acetate) were reasonably successful in relieving pain but side effects such as weight gain, depression, mastalgia and irregular breakthrough bleeding made them unacceptable to some women.

ENDOMETRIOSIS

Treatment (*contd*)

2. DANAZOL

Danazol is an 'impeded androgen' i.e. a steroid hormone closely related to testosterone, which inhibits pituitary gonadotrophins, is anti-oestrogenic, anti-progestational, slightly anabolic, but has very little virilising activity.

A daily dose of about 400mg may abolish symptoms, and after about a year may produce complete regression and even allow pregnancy.

At that dose level, side effects include amenorrhoea, weight gain, acne and muscle cramps, none of them except amenorrhoea invariably present.

Increased dosage may result in hot flushes and loss of libido, and mild but reversible degrees of voice change and hirsutism.

Danazol impairs glucose tolerance and induces insulin resistance, and diabetic patients would require to increase their insulin intake. It also alters lipoprotein metabolism.

It is not clear how Danazol acts. Does it inhibit (a) the activity of hypothalamic releasing factors, (b) FSH or LH synthesis, (c) steroidogenic enzymes or (d) the action of steroid hormones on tissues?

Some patients do not tolerate Danazol.

3. GESTRINONE

This is a derivative of 19-nortestosterone. It has slight androgenic activity and is markedly anti-oestrogenic and anti-progestogenic. It interacts with the pituitary steroid receptors and decreases gonadotrophic secretion resulting in diminished follicular growth and anovulation.

A bi-weekly oral dose of 2.5 to 5.0mg for 6 months induces amenorrhoea, disappearance of pain and regression of the endometrial deposits.

Side effects include weight gain, acne, seborrhoea and mild hirsutism.

4. GONADOTROPHIC RELEASING HORMONE ANALOGUES

These substances are given continuously to desensitise the pituitary receptors for the hypothalamic releasing hormone (GnRH).

RH Analogue $\longrightarrow$ Pituitary receptors desensitised

↓

FSH and LH output reduced

↓

Ovarian function depressed

↓

Hypo-oestrogenism

↓

Regression of endometrioid deposits

This is the hoped for result of this form of therapy. Studies have been encouraging. The analogues can be given by injection or nasal spray. Symptoms are reduced. Adverse effects are the result of a pseudo-menopause condition – hot flushes, atrophy of the reproductive organs and bone loss which may be considerable even with the short six month course.

PAIN Both Danazol and gonadotrophin releasing hormone analogues are often successful in relieving pain but in both instances recurrence is not uncommon. A second course of therapy may be more effective.

INFERTILITY Unfortunately almost all studies of the effects of therapy on infertility have lacked proper controls and the position is still in dispute.

ENDOMETRIOSIS

Surgical Treatment

Where infertility is not a problem radical surgery to remove both ovaries is said to be a lasting cure for endometriosis, since it removes the oestrogenic stimulus to endometrial growth.

In many cases the patient wishes relief from pain but also desires to retain the possibility of future pregnancy. In these circumstances only conservative surgery can be employed.

The intentions in conservative surgery are:

1. To ablate as many endometrial deposits in the pelvic cavity as possible.
2. To restructure the pelvic anatomy by destroying adhesions which interfere with ovarian and tubal function.
3. To destroy endometrial deposits in the ovaries.
4. To deal with sensory nerve pathways.

In view of the many vital structures such as the bladder, rectum, colon and ureters in close proximity to each other conventional open surgery is not always feasible. Laser surgery under laparoscopy with its almost microscopic accuracy may be employed. Endometrial deposits and adhesions can be vaporised easily without damaging tissue outside a radius of a fraction of a millimetre from the target. Similarly the laster destruction of ovarian lesions can be carried out without destroying any of the functional tissue.

The question of dealing with sensory nerve pathways is difficult to answer. Severe pain is a feature of a number of gynaecological conditions especially those related to malignancy. Elsewhere in this book operative techniques are described which involve interfering with sensory conductivity centrally i.e. at the spinal cord level (see pages 235, 236). Recently a local operative procedure, paracervical uterine denervation, has been recommended. This consists of vaporising the utero-sacral ligaments by laser at their attachment to the posterior aspect of the cervix where the sensory fibres emerge from the uterus. Two difficulties are associated with this procedure. First, the ureters must be avoided and, secondly, veins lying lateral to the ligaments must not be injured. Unfortunately severe pain is often associated with severe endometriosis and adhesions may make the operation very difficult.

Reports in the literature record complete relief from pain in 50% of patients followed for more than a year and another 41% obtained moderate relief.

ENDOMETRIOSIS

Recommendations for treatment of Endometriosis

These are based on the extent of the condition, the local effects such as extensive adhesions affecting the ovary and recto-vaginal cul-de-sac, and the patient's desire for pregnancy.

Attempts have been made to stage the condition, although this is very difficult due to the extreme variability of both the anatomical changes and symptomatology.

Stage	Symptoms and Signs	Recommended Treatment
I and II mild	Pain. Small lesions with no scarring or adhesions.	Laparoscopic laser destruction of lesions. No hormones.
III moderate	Small scattered lesions. Scarring with peri-ovarian tubal adhesions. Severe pain.	Laser destruction of lesions. Hormones. Conservative surgery if no relief from hormones.
IV severe	Ovarian deposits greater than 2.5cm plus marked adhesions to other structures. Obliteration of recto-vaginal cul-de-sac. Severe pain.	Conservative surgery plus hormones. Hysterectomy and bilateral salpingo-oophorectomy if age or local lesions make these operations necessary.
V very severe	Lesions as in stage III plus involvement of bowel, bladder, ureter.	Barium meal and IVP should be carried out in case there is danger of fistulae. Otherwise, radical surgery is required followed by hormones if surgical removal has been incomplete.

Fertility

Claims of high pregnancy rates following laser treatment have been recorded, but as with medical treatment there has been lack of controls in these studies, especially untreated patients.

Recurrence

Apart from radical surgery all other forms of treatment are associated with significant rates of recurrence of symptoms. Nevertheless the recurrent symptoms seem to be less severe than in the original episode and hormonal treatment may control them.

DYSMENORRHOEA

Dysmenorrhoea implies pain during menstruation, and most women experience some degree of pain at least on the first day of the period when the loss is heaviest.

Many women will also describe varying sorts of discomfort before the period starts, but this symptom should be regarded as a manifestation of the Premenstrual Tension Syndrome (see p. 140).

The pain may be secondary to organic disease such as endometriosis or infection, but primary dysmenorrhoea, which is being discussed here, occurs in the presence of a normal genital tract.

Nature of the Pain

It is usually described as having two components: a continuous lower abdominal pain attributed to vascular congestion, which radiates through to the back and sometimes down the thighs; and an intermittent cramping pain.

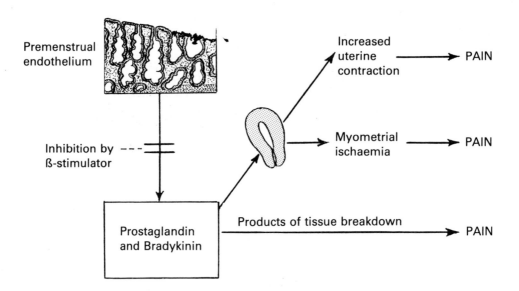

Aetiology

There is increased myometrial activity during the periods in women with dysmenorrhoea and uterine blood flow is reduced especially during intense contractions. It is thought that this hyperactivity is the result of excessive quantities of prostaglandins synthesised during the breakdown of the premenstrual endometrium.

Retrograde Menstruation has also been regarded as a cause. Recent work has shown that this phenomenon is much commoner in the presence of severe dysmenorrhoea.

DYSMENORRHOEA

Clinical Features of Primary Dysmenorrhoea

The patient is usually a nulliparous girl between 16 and 26 who is becoming increasingly disabled at the time of her periods, is incapable of work and often has to spend 1 or 2 days in bed. There is no characteristic personality or physique but the hysterical patient will make the most of her primary dysmenorrhoea as she will of any other gynaecological complaint. Childbirth does not abolish dysmenorrhoea but reduces its severity, perhaps because of the psychological changes of motherhood or the effects of childbirth on the uterine innervation.

Beta-stimulator drugs which inhibit prostaglandin synthesis have been proved experimentally to abolish uterine contraction and ischaemia and the pain which accompanies them.

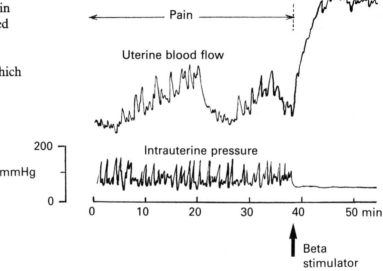

Management

Organic disease must be excluded, usually by examination under anaesthesia and by laparoscopy. Thereafter the problem is to find a suitable drug which will alleviate the pain sufficiently to allow a normal existence during the period time. It is fortunate that such patients tend to improve or at least complain less, as they grow older.

Women suffering from severe dysmenorrhoea need sympathy and support. A moralistic attitude should be avoided ('pain' comes from the Latin word poena, punishment) and the doctor should never imply that he believes the pain to be 'all in the mind'. If drug treatment is ineffective, which is very unlikely, some consideration may be given to the advisability of presacral neurectomy (p.139). In some cases the pain may be controlled by hypnosis.

DYSMENORRHOEA

Drug Treatment

1. **The Contraceptive Pill**. Dysmenorrhoea is very unlikely in the absence of ovulation, probably because of the pseudo-atrophy of the endometrium. The disadvantages of this efficacious treatment are the well known side-effects and perhaps the prevention of pregnancy.

2. **Analgesics**. If the prostaglandin theory is correct the most effective drugs will be those which inhibit the synthesis of prostaglandin, and this includes all the antipyretic analgesics.

   Aspirin and paracetamol are widely used.

   Mefenamic acid (Ponstan). This drug is said to prevent the action of prostaglandin on muscle as well as inhibit its production.

   Flufenemic acid (Arlef)
   Indomethacin (Indocid) } These drugs are usually prescribed for the relief of rheumatic pain but have been used with success in dysmenorrhoea. They tend to cause gastric bleeding.

3. **Beta-receptor Stimulators** (ritodrine, terbutaline, salbutamol). These drugs should in theory be most effective of all but, in practice, the dose required seems to carry too many side-effects.

MEMBRANOUS DYSMENORRHOEA

This is a rare condition in which the endometrium is cast off at menstruation in large strips or even as a whole piece called a 'cast'. The cause is unknown; and if the contraceptive pill (which will control the condition) is unacceptable, treatment with progesterone alone should be tried, say norethisterone 5mg daily from the 5th to the 25th day. Membranous dysmenorrhoea is said not to be a cause of infertility.

PRESACRAL NEURECTOMY

Division of the superior hypogastric plexus in order to interrupt afferent pain stimuli from the pelvis.

This operation might be offered as a last resort to a patient whose dysmenorrhoea was not relieved by any other means. Efferent pathways are also divided and there is transient atonicity of bowel and and bladder after the operation, and perhaps menorrhagia as a result of vasodilation. It is impossible to be certain of removing all the nerve trunks.

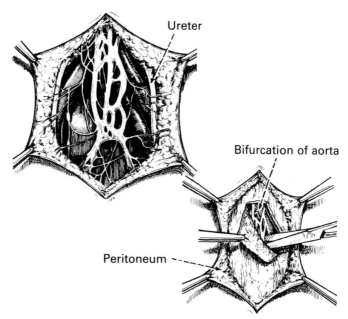

Ureter

Bifurcation of aorta

Peritoneum

SECONDARY CONGESTIVE DYSMENORRHOEA

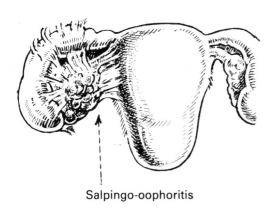

Salpingo-oophoritis

Generalised pelvic pain in menstruation due to some organic cause such as salpingo-oophoritis, endometriosis, pelvic venous congestion or even acute uterine retroversion. There may be no signs on palpation other than restricted mobility and tenderness, and laparoscopy is needed for diagnosis. The treatment is of the cause.

Mid-cycle pain (mittelschmerz) is associated with pelvic inflammation but may occur alone. It is sometimes accompanied by slight vaginal staining and is caused by changes in oestrogen level.

139

PRE-MENSTRUAL TENSION SYNDROME

The premenstrual tension syndrome (PMT) includes a large group of symptoms which appear regularly and predictably about 12 days before the onset of menstruation. The symptom pattern will vary with the individual, but 75% of women will acknowledge at least one of the symptoms listed below.

WATER RETENTION

Weight gain (up to 7 lb)
Painful breasts
Abdominal distension
Feeling of bloatedness

PAIN

Headache
Backache
Tiredness
Muscle stiffness

AUTONOMIC REACTIONS

Dizziness/faintness
Cold sweats
Nausea/vomiting
Hot flushes

MOOD CHANGES

Tension
Irritability
Depression
Crying spells

LOSS OF CONCENTRATION

Forgetfulness
Clumsiness
Difficulty in
   making decisions
Poor sleeping

MISCELLANEOUS

Feelings of suffocation
Chest pains
Heart pounding
Numbness, tingling

Clinical Features

The average age at presentation is 35 although symptoms may appear at puberty. Marriage and childbirth do not affect PMT but there is usually a preponderance of the more articulate patients, especially professional women who must appear before the public and cannot easily stay off work.

The most common complaints are abdominal distension, breast tenderness, irritability and a desire to avoid any activity, but any one symptom may dominate the others. A diagnosis of PMT requires that the symptoms must definitely be associated with the premenstrual phase of the cycle, they must not appear regularly at any other time and they must be quickly relieved when the period starts.

Pre-menstrual tension syndrome may occur in post-menopausal women on hormone replacement therapy during the combined oestrogen/progestogen phase.

PRE-MENSTRUAL TENSION SYNDROME

Aetiology

Several theories exist but none has been conclusively confirmed and most are based on conjecture rather than fact.

1. **Fluid retention** due to cyclical fluctuations in steroid hormones. Fluid retention is the commonest component and the most easily measured (weight fluctuation of more than 1.5kg from morning to evening or day to day) and emotional lability might be related to cerebral oedema.

2. **Endocrine aetiology**: Progesterone deficiency, oestrogen/progesterone imbalance, raised aldosterone level during luteal phase, raised prolactin and excessive ACTH production from pro-opio-melano-cortin, causing an endorphin deficiency have been postulated. In many cases the endocrine profile is normal.

3. **Evolutionary phenomenon**: PMT, by causing post-ovulation sexual hostility to the male, could reduce the likelihood of coitus in an infertile phase of the cycle. Confining coitus to a fertile phase would improve survival of the species.

4. **Neurotic personality**: Many severely neurotic women do not suffer from pre-menstrual tension syndrome; and pre-menstrual tension syndrome is not related to psychiatric illness.

Treatment is empirical. Many regimes are used and none is universally effective.

1. **Pyridoxine (vitamin B6)**
   This is based on disordered tryptophan metabolism in sufferers from endogenous depression. Pyridoxine corrects the reduced brain 5-hydroxytryptamine. 20 mg twice daily or more can give subjective relief.

2. **Progesterone**
   Progesterone itself is available as Cyclogest pessaries. Some women find these aesthetically displeasing, and oral progestogens such as dydrogesterone 10mg twice daily or norethisterone 5mg daily orally may be employed for the last three weeks of the cycle. The fact that pre-menstrual tension syndrome may be produced artificially in post-menopausal women during the oestrogen/progestogen phase of cyclical hormone replacement detracts from progesterone as a treatment.

3. **Bromocriptine (Parlodel)**
   The dose of 2.5mg twice daily orally requires to be achieved gradually to minimise nausea. Lassitude and dizziness may occur on Bromocriptine and it is best reserved for subjects who complain principally of breast pain and who have elevated or high normal serum prolactin (60 – 360mU/l normal range).

4. **Danazol**
   Danazol has been shown in double-blind crossover studies to relieve the symptoms of pre-menstrual syndrome in a significant number of women. 200mg daily continuously for several months is as effective as higher doses and produces fewer side effects. Side effects such as weight gain, nausea and acne may occur. Benefit to PMT is not dependent on producing amenorrhoea.

PRE-MENSTRUAL TENSION SYNDROME

Treatment (*contd*)

5. **Oestrogen**

   Cycle suppression using high-dose HRT has been recommended (J. Studd, London). Two Estraderm TTS 100 patches are used concurrently, adding 5mg Norethisterone orally for 7 days each month to avoid endometrial hyperplasia.

6. **Ovarian ablation**

   In rare cases where severe symptoms make normal existence impossible, the ovaries may be temporarily suppressed using an LHRH analogue and occasionally hysterectomy, bilateral oophorectomy and unopposed oestrogen hormone replacement therapy may be justified.

CHAPTER 7

GYNAECOLOGICAL INFECTIONS

INFLAMMATION IN THE LOWER GYNAECOLOGICAL TRACT

The vulva, vagina and ectocervix under normal conditions are the habitat of various types of infective agents, but they are only a threat if normal defence mechanisms are altered.

Defence mechanisms

1. **Vaginal acidity.**

   Glycogen is produced by vaginal epithelium by ovarian steroid activity. This is converted to lactic acid by Doderlein's bacillus (a type of B.acidophilus). This maintains the vaginal pH between 3 and 4 which inhibits most other organisms.

Normal vaginal flora

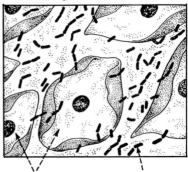

Desquamated cells   Organisms mostly lactobacilli
(Note absence of pus cells)

2. **Thick layer of vaginal squamous epithelium.**

   This is a considerable physical barrier to infection. Continual desquamation of the superficial kerato-hyalin layer and glycogen production, both dependent upon ovarian steroid action, prevent bacteria settling. In children and post-menopausal patients the epithelium lacking steroid stimulation is thin and easily traumatised.

3. **Closure of the introitus.**

   In children and virgin adults the vaginal canal is only a potential space kept closed by the surrounding muscles and provides another physical barrier. This, however, alters and becomes of little importance with sexual activity and pregnancy.

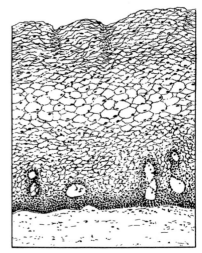

Functional vaginal epithelium: intermediate cells rich in glycogen.

4. **Glandular secretions** from the cervix and Bartholin's glands maintain an outward fluid current helping to clear the canal of debris. In addition, cervical secretion contains immunoglobulins, especially IgA, and there are varying numbers of polymorphs, lymphocytes and macrophages.

VULVAL INFLAMMATION

Vulval inflammation is not uncommon but is usually an extension of infection from the vagina. A mild reaction may arise due to physical and anatomical conditions in the area, such as (a) moistness and (b) proximity of urethra and anus.

The area is not only naturally moist but also warm. This is particularly so in obese patients. The folds of fat harbour moisture, and chafing occurs between them. The proliferation of bacteria is encouraged. Urinary incontinence and unsuspected glycosuria may add to this. It is important to test the urine for sugar in all patients.

Incidental factors may intensify any reaction resulting from these conditions e.g. the wearing of nylon underwear which is heat-retaining and non-absorptive. Associated with this may be chemical factors increasing the reaction such as washing underclothes with detergents, using toilet powders, perfumes and deodorants. The clinical result is irritation and itching leading to scratching. Continual itch-scratch-itch leads to maceration of the skin and may invite serious infection. Careful attention to personal hygiene is essential. Obese patients should be encouraged to lose weight and all of the incidental factors mentioned above should be avoided.

It must be remembered that itching may be a sign of a more serious disease such as impending liver failure or Hodgkin's disease.

Search for lice or scabies should be made where circumstances suggest the possibility.

One of the complications of vulvar inflammation is **obstruction of the duct of Bartholin's gland**. Cystic dilatation and abscess formation are apt to follow. The condition occurs during a woman's sexual life. Any organism, staphylococcal, coliform or gonococcal may be found.

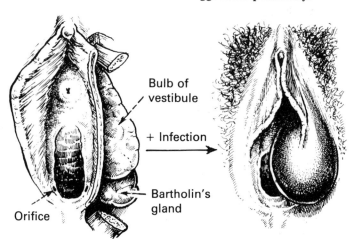

Bulb of vestibule

+ Infection

Bartholin's gland

Orifice

The gland lies partly behind the bulb of the vestibule and is covered by skin and bulbospongiosus muscle. The duct is 2cm long and opens into the vaginal orifice lateral to the hymen.

Treatment

Marsupialisation (Gk. marsipos, a bag)

The cyst or abscess is widely opened within the labium minus and drained, and its walls sutured to the skin leaving a large orifice which it is hoped will form a new duct orifice and allow conservation of the gland. A ribbon-gauze pack is inserted for 48 hours.

If the treatment is not successful, complete excision may be necessary.

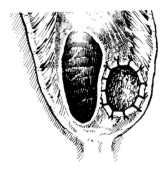

145

VAGINAL DISCHARGE AND INFECTION

A small amount of vaginal discharge is normal in adult life.

Composition
Tissue fluid, cell debris, carbohydrate, lactobacilli, lactic acid. The pH is about 4.5, a degree of acidity which inhibits the growth of organisms other than the lactobacilli.

Source of Vaginal Discharge
Vulva: Greater vestibular glands, glands of vulval skin.

Vagina: Mainly desquamated epithelial cells which liberate glycogen. The lactobacilli metabolise the glycogen to lactic acid.

Vaginal transudate (secretion from tissues and capillaries of the mature vagina) is often described: vaginal epithelium is certainly not water resistant (like transitional epithelium). There are no mucosal glands.

Cervix: Alkaline mucous secretion which becomes copious and watery during ovulation.

Uterine glands also discharge into the vagina.

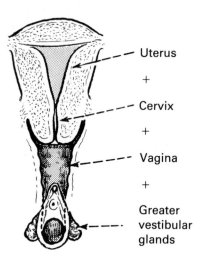

Uterus
+
Cervix
+
Vagina
+
Greater vestibular glands

Clinical Features

Volume: The need to wear a pad or tampon continuously suggests excessive discharge.

Onset: Sudden onset means infection. Onset can be associated with the end of a pregnancy, the contraceptive pill, a course of antibiotic, a sexual adventure.

Colour: Normal discharge is white but stains yellow or pale brown. A greenish-yellow colour suggests pyogenic infection, commonly accompanied by an unpleasant odour. A red or dark brown suggests blood.

Irritation: Any discharge can in time excoriate the vulva but only candida and trichomonas cause itching.

COMPLAINTS OF VAGINAL DISCHARGE

Women will complain if:
- (a) there appears to be an excessive amount of staining on the clothing.
- (b) they detect an offensive smell.
- (c) they suffer irritation.

There is often little correlation between symptoms and signs. Fastidious or neurotic women will complain of what is really normal; and gynaecologists regularly observe heavy and purulent discharge in women who deny any symptoms at all.

Examination
1. Vulva, perineum and thighs are inspected for signs of excoriation. The vestibular glands and urethral meatus are observed and palpated.
2. Vaginal walls and and cervix are examined through a speculum. Normal vaginal epithelium is pink, the rugae are well marked and the epithelial surface of the cervix smooth and moist. Normal discharge is like curdled milk and is white and odourless.
3. A bimanual examination should always be made.
4. Specimens of discharge are taken for microscopy and culture, and a cervical smear for cytology. Chlamydia must be excluded.

LEUCORRHOEA
This means an excessive amount of normal discharge – a very subjective assessment. The patient will complain of constantly having to change her clothes but there will be no irritation and appearance will be normal. The smell will be the normal vulval odour (from the action of commensal bacteria on the secretions of the apocrine sex glands), microscopy will reveal normal appearances and culture will grow only lactobacilli.

The patient should be reassured and given an explanation of normal physiology. No local treatment is necessary.

Almost 20% of all patients attending gynaecological clinics complain of vaginal discharge, indicating some form of infection. The infective agents form two groups:
1. In 90% of cases the inflammation is usually relatively mild and is due to one of three agents:
   - (a) Candida albicans
   - (b) Gardnerella vaginalis
   - (c) Trichomonas vaginalis.
2. The remaining 10% are more serious. They may cause painful sores, tumour-like lesions, spread into the pelvis or cause generalised infection.

VAGINAL DISCHARGE

CANDIDA ALBICANS

This is yeast and exists in two forms – slender branching hyphae or as a small globular spore which multiplies by budding.

Source of infection

This organism may exist as a normal commensal in the rectum and small numbers may be found in the vagina, the acid medium suiting their survival without symptoms arising. The patient's fingernails may harbour the yeast. Sexual transmission is also possible. Symptomatic infection is most likely to arise when there are predisposing conditions e.g.

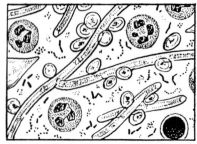

Mycelia and spores of C. albicans. Note the presence of leucocytes.

1. **Pregnancy**. The vagina provides a tropical micro-climate and the high concentration of sex steroids in the blood maintains an increased glycogen formation in the vaginal epithelium and may alter the local pH.
2. **Immunosuppressive Therapy**. This includes cytotoxic drugs and corticosteroids. There is also thought to be a natural degree of immunosuppression during pregnancy.
3. **Glycosuria**. This may be due to undiscovered diabetes, but again a mild degree of glycosuria may exist in a normal pregnancy due to lowering of the renal threshold for sugar.
4. **Antibiotic Therapy**. Systemic antibiotics destroy the normal bacteria thus reducing the competition for nutrients leaving the field clear for C.albicans.
5. **Chronic Anaemia**. Normal iron stores are needed to maintain an adequate immune reaction. This also entails adequate folic acid intake. The angular stomatitis of chronic anaemia is due to Candida infection.

Clinical features

The patient is usually between 20 and 40 when oestrogen support of the epithelial glycogen content is at its highest. The complaint is of irritant discharge and dyspareunia. Examination reveals an inflamed and tender vagina and vulva with white plaques resembling curdled milk adhering to the vaginal wall and vulva. Removal of the plaque reveals a red inflamed area. Pre-pubertal or post-menopausal infection is uncommon, but if it does occur after the menopause the symptoms tend to be severe.

Treatment

Nystatin pessaries each containing 100,000 units of the antibiotic are used for the vaginal infection, one pessary being inserted night and morning for 7 days followed by one nightly for a further 2 weeks. Smears should be taken to make sure the infection has been cured. Nystatin cream containing the same concentration is applied 3 or 4 times daily to the vulva. Other preparations used are amphotericin, clotrimazole, miconazole and oral fluconazole (for monilia).

Both partners require treatment. Boilable or disposable underwear should be worn and sheaths used during coitus.

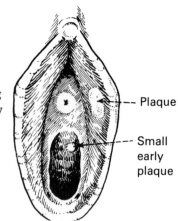

-- Plaque

--- Small early plaque

VAGINAL DISCHARGE

GARDNERELLA VAGINALIS

For a long time a large number of cases of vaginitis were labelled non-specific because of disagreement regarding the infective agent. These cases were characterised by a non-irritating, foul smelling discharge. Ultimately, careful bacteriological studies have established the fact that although the discharge contains a mixture of bacteria, the one constant feature in 90% of cases was the presence of a tiny gram-negative cocco-bacillus which was a facultative anaerobe – Gardnerella vaginalis.

Clinical features

The patient complains of a foul-smelling discharge, and examination confirms both the discharge and the odour. In appearance the discharge is thin, greyish and sometimes shows bubbles. A vaginal smear reveals the presence of 'clue' cells. Gram staining is usually negative but can be variable.

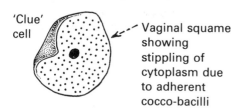

'Clue' cell

Vaginal squame showing stippling of cytoplasm due to adherent cocco-bacilli

Pus cells tend to be few in number. Doderlein's bacilli are also scanty but frequently many other bacteria are present. The pH of the fluid is raised. Although the main complaint is of malodorous discharge some patients will have pruritus, frequency, dysuria and dyspareunia.

Treatment

Oral Metronidazole 200mg t.i.d. for 7 days or a single dose of 2g appears to be effective. Male partners should also be treated.

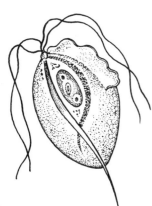

TRICHOMONAS VAGINALIS

Trichomonas vaginalis is a protozoan organism, pathogenic to man, which infests the vagina in the female and the urethra, prepuce and prostate in the male. It is a common cause of irritant vaginal discharge.

T.Vaginalis is a single-cell organism about 20μ x 10μ, with four flagellae and an undulating membrane which gives it a characteristic jerky movement. It is transmitted mainly during sexual intercourse but can be acquired from infected articles such as a contaminated speculum or even a lavatory seat. It multiplies by binary fission and feeds by osmosis and phagocytosis.

Pathology

Passing from host to host during coitus T.vaginalis attaches itself to the vaginal epithelium and multiplies rapidly, taking glycogen away from Doderlein's bacilli which disappear. The vaginal pH rises to about 5.5, allowing the increase of bacterial pathogens which aggravate the infection and resulting discharge.

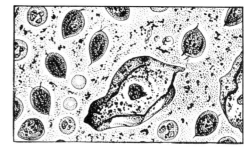

VAGINAL DISCHARGE

TRICHOMONAS VAGINALIS (*contd*)

Clinical features

In the acute phase the patient complains of severe vaginal tenderness and pain, and an irritant discharge. The vagina is seen to be inflamed, sometimes with a patchy strawberry vaginitis, and there is a copious offensive, frothy discharge. Frequently there is a burning sensation, pruritus, dysuria and dyspareunia. In the latent or dormant phases there are no symptoms although the presence of the organism can be demonstrated, often in a cervical smear.

Incidence

Perhaps 18% of the female population. T.vaginalis is commonly found in patients with gonorrhoea, and has an association with cervical dysplasia. No cause-and-effect relationship has been proved.

Diagnosis

Diagnosis is by observation of the motile organisms in a fresh smear diluted with saline and by laboratory culture.

Treatment

Always systemic and, if possible, including the patient's sexual partner.

Metronidazole (Flagyl) 200mg thrice daily for a week, or 2g orally once.

Nimorazole (Naxogin) 2gm as a single dose taken with food.

Short courses are useful with patients whose cooperation is uncertain, but are more likely to cause nausea and gastritis.

The post-treatment vaginal smear should be normal, but T.vaginalis can linger in the urethra, Skene's and Bartholin's glands, and reinfection of the vagina may call for further treatment.

The nitro-imidazoles are complex drugs and at least one of them, metronidazole, is active against anaerobic organisms and has also been used in alcoholism, Crohn's disease and rheumatoid arthritis. It is also effective as a potentiator of radiotherapy applied to hypoxic cancer cells, and a case of peripheral neuropathy has been reported after prolonged dosage. Care is necessary if the drug is being given to a pregnant woman, although no harmful effects on the fetus have been demonstrated.

VAGINITIS

ATROPHIC or SENILE VAGINITIS

This sometimes arises at times when ovarian activity ceases with the onset of the menopause, after surgical removal of the ovaries or following ablation by radiotherapy.

Clinical features

Symptoms may be mild, consisting of irritation with discharge. In other patients the changes may be severe. Pain can be the main feature and the discharge purulent. Examination of the vaginal mucosa reveals a rash of petechial haemorrhages and there may be ulceration. Smears show rounded epithelial cells, with no glycogen, many polymorphs and bacteria. In neglected cases intra-vaginal adhesions may develop. Trouble of this nature is more frequent and more acute after surgical removal or destruction of the ovaries than after normal menopause. Fortunately the condition is becoming increasingly uncommon with hormone replacement therapy. Oestrogen quickly reverses the changes.

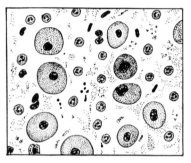

Vaginal smear of atrophic type, with numerous polymorphs, a mixed bacterial content and para-basal epithelial cells.

VULVO-VAGINITIS in CHILDREN

This is a rare condition and only arises in certain circumstances viz.
- (a) Sexual interference.
- (b) Insertion of foreign bodies by the child herself.
- In (a) the changes will be those of physical damage to the tissues. Infection will depend to some extent on whether the person guilty of the offence is a carrier of a specific agent.
- (b) In this case infection may arise from bowel commensals.

Many of the examples of vulvo-vaginitis may arise from the irritation caused by threadworms. Scratching will lead to maceration of the skin which in turn will encourage bacterial contamination.

Vaginitis due to foreign bodies is sometimes seen in adults. Tampons, contraceptive devices and supportive pessaries used for prolapse may be left, forgotten, in situ. These give rise to an offensive purulent discharge. Bacteriological investigation will give an indication of the type of infection and the appropriate treatment following removal of the offending body.

A secondary vaginitis may arise due to contamination of the vagina through fistulous openings (vesico-vaginal or recto-vaginal) following injury, surgical operations or tumour growth. Repeated attacks of infection may occur. Treatment is obviously repair of the fistula where this is possible.

In all cases of vaginal discharge the possibility of malignant disease in the tract must be considered.

VAGINAL DISCHARGE AND INFECTIONS

The second group, the 10% of infections which cause serious disease or present difficulties in diagnosis, are almost all sexually transmitted. In addition to being a serious threat to the individual they present a public health problem. If their presence is suspected or diagnosed it is better that they be dealt with by a specialised department experienced in their treatment and possessing the laboratory facilities for continuing assessment.

VIRAL DISEASES

HERPES

This is an important gynaecological problem. The virus may affect the lower genital tract or the mouth. It is highly infectious – 80% of women in contact with male carriers become infected. The symptoms are severe. There may be recurring attacks every 3 or 4 weeks and they represent a potential for wide dissemination to others in the immediate environment. There are two varieties of the virus – 1 and 2. The incubation period is short – 3 to 7 days.

Clinical findings

The disease affects the vulvo-vaginal and peri-anal regions but may be transmitted to the mouth. The patient complains of burning, itching and hyperaesthesia of the area and the skin shows evidence of acute inflammation – oedema and erythema. There is usually a vaginal discharge. If the peri-urethral area is involved there may be dysuria and retention of urine.

The specific lesions start as small indurated tender papules which become vesicles and quickly break down to form shallow ulcers, 5mm or more in diameter, with a yellowish grey slough in the base. These can be seen on the vulva and labia but in some cases they are confined to the vagina and cervix and there may be no external evidence of the disease. In these circumstances the ulcers may be large and could be mistaken for carcinoma of the cervix. The inguinal nodes are enlarged. The infection is accompanied by general symptoms of malaise, headache and neuralgia due to spread to the sacral ganglia. There is no intense dyspareunia.

The acute phase lasts for 4–5 days. The lesions heal over 8–10 days and then a latent period ensues during which the virus remains in the sacral ganglia. Further attacks may follow. The disease may occur during pregnancy, and infection of the baby may prove fatal.

Diagnosis

This is made from the appearance of the vesicles and ulcers and is confirmed by examining cervical and vaginal smears. These reveal large cells and sometimes multi-nucleated giant cells the nuclei of which contain eosinophilic inclusion bodies. The chromatin of these nuclei is compressed against the nuclear membrane. Some degree of immunity may be conferred during recurrent attacks and a search for antibodies will help to differentiate primary from second attacks.

Chromatin at nuclear membrane

Eosinophilic inclusion bodies

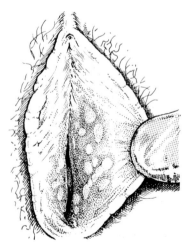

VAGINAL DISCHARGE AND INFECTIONS

HERPES (*contd*)

Treatment

The acute local symptoms can be alleviated by applying ice for 20–30 minutes. Similarly non steroidal soothing creams may be used. Analgesics such as 2% lignocaine can be employed. Repeated applications of Acyclovir, 3% as an ointment, provides effective treatment but only if started at the onset of signs or symptoms. Oral Acyclovir may be given in doses of 200mg 4 hourly for 5 days. It inhibits proliferation of viral DNA without damaging host cells. Silver nitrate 10% may be applied to the ulcers and Betadine can be used to control secondary infection. Care should be exercised with all preparations during pregnancy.

It has been claimed that the herpes virus may have some etiological activity in relation to cervical cancer.

CONDYLOMATA ACUMINATA

This disease is due to infection by the human papilloma virus of which there are 40 types. Two, numbers 6 and 11, are particularly associated with condylomata. The infection is transmitted sexually and more than 50% of contacts develop lesions. Infectivity is greatest just after appearance of a wart.

Clinical findings

It starts as a single warty growth which quickly spreads to form multiple growths showing a tendency to fuse. They are pinkish with dry surfaces unless macerated and are of softer consistency than the ordinary skin wart. The growths become luxuriant in moist areas and especially during pregnancy. They affect the labia, the peri-anal area, the perineum, the lower part of the vagina and may even spread on to the thighs. Secondary infection may give rise to purulent discharge.

Differential Diagnosis

There are 4 conditions which must be excluded when considering the diagnosis.

1. **Syphilitic condylomata**. These are more widespread and not confined to the genital area. They are also flatter and more rounded. Treponemes can be found in the tissue fluid. Serological tests will of course confirm the diagnosis.

2. **Benign papilloma**. This is commonly single and similar to ordinary skin warts.

3. **Verrucous carcinoma**. This is a locally malignant lesion but vulval carcinoma is rare in pre-menopausal patients. Biopsy will differentiate the two conditions.

4. Sometimes condylomata affect the cervix and can resemble carcinoma.

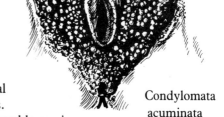

Condylomata acuminata

Histology

The warts have a central core of connective tissue covered by a thick layer of prickle cells. Chronic inflammatory changes are present in the dermis.

Treatment

An ointment containing 20% of Podophyllin is often used but it is not very effective and can be painful. It is also dangerous in large lesions. Systemic absorption has proved fatal. Electro-cautery or laser can be used. Surgical excision may be required.

VAGINAL DISCHARGE AND INFECTIONS

MOLLUSCUM CONTAGIOSUM

This is a highly infective pox virus, one of the largest known and can be seen under the microscope. It is commonly transmitted by sexual contact but towels and clothing can carry the infection. Whitish papules with dark umbilicated centres are produced. They are firm in consistency. Mostly they affect the genital region but can spread to other parts of the body. Spread is rapid. The disease is common in infants. Sometimes there is a cheesy discharge from the warts.

Histology

The epithelium undergoes hyperplasia extending deeply into the dermis.

The germinal layer of cells contains cytoplasmic inclusion bodies which push the nucleus aside. These cells desquamate when they reach the surface and spread the infection.

Treatment

This is a simple matter of killing the virus by local treatment to prevent spread of infection.

1. Phenol can be applied to the centre of a nodule.
2. Diathermy and cryosurgery are used in a similar fashion.

Normal epithelium

Desquamated cells

Germinal cells with dark inclusion bodies growing towards surface

New germinal layer

BACTERIAL INFECTIONS

CHLAMYDIA TRACHOMATIS This is a widespread gynaecological infection.

Clinical features

The initial symptoms in women are often mild. Discharge may be present, varying from watery to frankly purulent according to the severity of the reaction to the disease. In severe cases there is obvious cervicitis which looks like an infected erosion. Sometimes there is a punctate haemorrhagic inflammation with micro-abscesses. Occasionally there are few changes in the vagina and the first evidence of infection is the appearance of a salpingitis. It is an important cause of chronic pelvic inflammation. A gelatinous exudate is formed in the pouch of Douglas which proceeds to multiple adhesions and tubal occlusion. It is an important cause of infertility. Ophthalmia neonatorum is very common.

Reiter's syndrome may arise with urethritis, arthritis and conjunctivitis, but this is more common in the infected male. It is related to reactivity between chlamydia antigens and HLA antigens. There may be spread to cause perihepatitis with so-called violin string adhesions to the parietal peritoneum. This is accompanied by acute pain in the upper right quadrant. The condition may be mistaken for cholecystitis or pancreatitis. It has been suggested that chlamydia may be involved as an aetiological agent in carcinoma of the cervix.

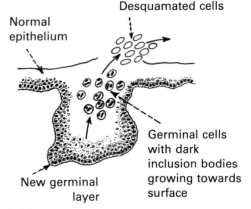

Chlamydia

154

VAGINAL DISCHARGE AND INFECTIONS

CHLAMYDIA TRACHOMATIS (*contd*)

Diagnosis

The organism can be seen under the microscope. It is intracellular. Staining by an immuno-fluorescence technique confirms the diagnosis. It multiplies like bacteria, but like viruses can only do so within cells. It contains both DNA and RNA.

Treatment: Tetracycline 500mg at 6 hourly intervals for 2 weeks. If the patient is pregnant erythromycin is preferable since there is a danger of hepatic damage with tetracycline therapy.

LYMPHOGRANULOMA VENEREUM (LGV)

This is a disease previously thought to be of viral origin but now attributed to a strain of chlamydia trachomatis. It is rare in the UK and is mainly seen in seaports of the Far East, Africa and South American tropical zones.

Clinical findings

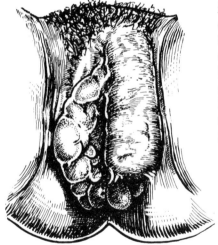

The primary lesion is a small painless ulcer with raised irregular borders which may involve the labia, clitoris or urethra. It appears 1 to 3 weeks after infection. Several weeks later the inguinal and iliac lymph nodes enlarge, become soft and fluctuant and this is followed by rupture creating discharging sinuses. The lesions eventually heal with the creation of large fibrous scars. In the process the urethra may be virtually destroyed and the rectum stenosed. Recto-vaginal fistulae may form and extensive surgical treatment may be required. The pelvic organs may be involved in the same way giving rise to intestinal obstruction and various fistulous communications. Histologically the reaction is of granulomatous type. Lymph channels are often obstructed giving rise to elephantiasis of the vulva. The picture shows an advanced case of LGV.

Treatment Tetracyclines or erythromycin are effective.

GRANULOMA INGUINALE

This is another ulcerative condition found in tropical areas. It is due to a Gram-negative organism found intra-cellularly as encapsulated rods, named Donovania granulomatis. The lesion begins as a painless nodule which breaks down to form an ulcer with a granular red base. It occurs in the genital, inguinal or peri-anal areas. It later invades the lymphatics and the local glands enlarge but do not break down. Large numbers of histiocytes packed with bacteria accumulate in the area. It may cause ulceration of the cervix and extend to the endometrium. If the patient is pregnant abortion often occurs and if the pregnancy goes to term there is very high fetal morbidity. The condition has to be differentiated from syphilis especially the secondary stage with condylomata lata. In some cases it may resemble carcinoma. Secondary infection is common.

Treatment The condition responds to tetracycline given for 2 or 3 weeks. Both of these diseases may be followed by squamous carcinoma.

VAGINAL DISCHARGE AND INFECTIONS

CHANCROID

This lesion is due to infection by Haemophilus Ducreyii. After a short incubation period a red macule appears which quickly changes to a pustule and then an ulcer. The ulcers are numerous and vary in size from millimetres to several centimetres. They are well defined with projecting margins but shallow with a greenish slough in the base. These ulcers are soft and painful. This, together with the short incubation period helps to differentiate them from syphilitic lesions. The labia majora, clitoris and peri-anal regions are affected. Two weeks later the local lymph nodes tend to enlarge and suppurate. There is usually secondary infection and the discharge is foul-smelling. Microscopically the lesions consist of granulation tissue infiltrated by lymphocytes and plasma cells. The bacillus can be demonstrated in scrapings from the ulcer stained by Giemsa.

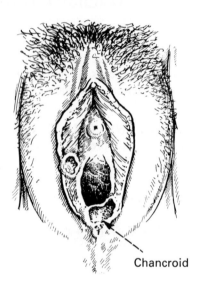

Chancroid

Treatment

Co-trimoxazole 960mg twice a day by mouth is usually effective. Tetracycline may also be used. If the lymph nodes suppurate they should be aspirated through adjacent healthy skin, but do not incise.

GONORRHOEA

Gonorrhoea in the female carries a high risk of salpingitis and sterility, but early diagnosis is difficult to achieve. Symptoms are often mild or absent, and since the incubation period is about 2 weeks (longer than in the male) very few women consider the possibility of such an infection.

Clinical features

The classical history is of urethritis, vaginal discharge, menstrual upset of sudden onset, but any infection in the genital area however it presents, may be gonococcal. After the acute phase vaginal discharge will persist, followed by signs of pelvic inflammatory disease (PID).

'Metastatic' signs – conjunctivitis, dermatitis, arthritis – are very rare in gynaecological practice.

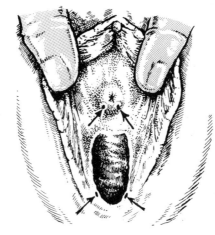

Examination

The labia are held apart, and the urethra, Skene's ducts and Bartholin's ducts examined for signs of infection. These ducts should be 'milked' for specimens of pus, if any, and swabs are taken from the cervix which is the main reservoir of infection.

Diagnosis is a laboratory procedure. Intracellular diplococci may be seen with Gram-staining, or the more time-consuming immunofluorescent method, but the evidence of positive culture is essential. Search should also be made for trichomonas, candida and chlamydia, and blood is sent for tests for syphilis.

Treatment

1.2 mega-units of procaine penicillin daily for 3 days. There is a need for 'single shot' treatments in venereal patients, and acceptable cure rates have been achieved with 1.2 mega-units of procaine penicillin along with 2g of probenecid (Benemid) to enhance blood levels and delay excretion. If the patient is sensitised to penicillin or the organism resistant, large oral doses of cephaloridine, tetracycline, and doxycycline are effective.

SYPHILIS

Syphilis is an uncommon disease in gynaecological practice, but any genital sore should come under suspicion.

PRIMARY SYPHILIS

The chancre (a corruption of 'cancer') has an incubation period of about a month and its appearance is often accompanied by pyrexia and malaise. The most common site is the vulva and then the cervix, but infection can occur anywhere. The chancre is the point at which the treponema enters the body.

The typical chancre is about 1cm in diameter and begins as a reddish papule which becomes ulcerated. It is painless and highly infective. The inguinal glands are markedly enlarged.

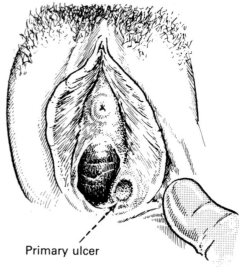

Primary ulcer

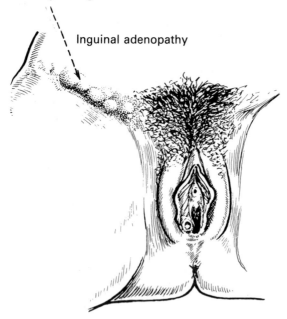

Inguinal adenopathy

Diagnosis requires the identification of T.pallidum in the exudate of the chancre or in material aspirated from an enlarged gland. Treponemata are not easily recognisable in stained preparations and the dark-ground illumination of fresh specimens is used. Light is reflected off the edges of the organisms, making them easy to perceive and they are recognised by their shape and movement. T.pallidum must be distinguished from other treponemata.

DIAGNOSIS OF SYPHILIS

Positive identification of T. pallidum is difficult for various reasons including the failure, so far, to grow the organism in vitro. The usual method of diagnosis is by serological tests which become positive 4–6 weeks after infection.

Reagin This is a non-specific antibody which appears in the tissues after infection with syphilis and many other bacteria and viruses. Its presence is detected by complement-fixation tests which are modifications of the original Wasserman reaction (WR) or by flocculation tests in which a reaction is observed under the microscope between infected serum and cardiolipin antigen.

False positives are usually weaker than a reaction due to syphilis, but if a positive result is obtained further tests are made. A false positive reaction may be obtained in the presence of latent yaws.

Principle of Fluorescent Tests (FTA)

1. Anti-human globulin is combined with fluorescein. } →

2. Dead treponeme is combined with test serum. If subject is infected, the treponeme acquires a coating of globulin antibody. } →

3. 1 and 2 are combined and the treponeme becomes fluorescent. } →

Reiter's Test is a complement-fixation test using a non-syphilitic treponeme as the antigen. A positive result means that the reagin is present because of a treponeme, and of course probably T. pallidum.

Treponemal Immobilisation Test (TPI). This is a specific for syphilis but is expensive. Live T. pallida are used (from a rabbit chancre) and are seen to be immobilised if combined with syphilitic serum.

Fluorescent Treponemal Antibody Tests are becoming very widely used for verification of the 'positive WR'.

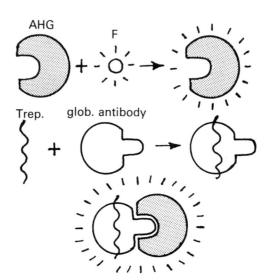

AHG

F

Trep.   glob. antibody

159

SYPHILIS

Signs and symptoms of the spread of T.pallidum throughout the whole body appear usually about 2 months after the primary stage, and the disease may present in this phase to the gynaecologist.

There is likely to be a mild pyrexia and malaise, but the dominating signs are a generalised lymphadenopathy and mucocutaneous lesions. 'Snail track' ulcers appear on mucosal surfaces, and the skin develops a very wide variety of macular and papular rashes. In warm moist areas such as the breast flexures and the vulva, the papules become hypertrophic and flattened and present as 'condylomata lata' which are highly infective.

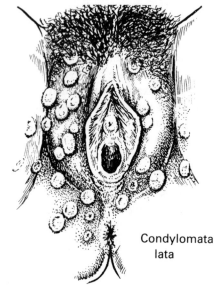

Condylomata lata

Diagnosis is by the demonstration of T.pallidum in the lesions and by serological tests.

Treatment of early contagious syphilis

T. pallidum is sensitive to many antibiotics, but reactions are common and care is required in treatment. Most patients receiving effective treatment for early syphilis with any antibiotic will display some degree of the Jarisch-Herxheimer reaction – rigors, sweating, headache, for about 24 hours. It can be modified by giving prednisolone 5mg 6-hourly.

Penicillin

This is the drug of choice, but the large doses required may induce some hypersensitive reaction, vaso-vagal, or even anaphylactoid.

The requirement is a blood level of 3μg per cent for about 2 weeks, and one mega-unit of procaine penicillin intramuscularly every day for 14 days is regarded as curative. The oral route is unreliable because of variable rates of absorption, and the uncertainty of patient cooperation.

Other Antibiotics

If the patient is sensitive to penicillin, many other drugs are available, including the tetracyclines, erythromycin, and doxycycline. These are given orally for 10–15 days, double the usual dosage, and Vitamin B and nystatin should be given concurrently because of the tendency to diarrhoea, pruritus ani, and candida infection.

If not treated in the early stages syphilis leads to a complex immune reaction with a chronic host-parasite relationship. The final stage involving cardiovascular and nervous lesions can appear months later.

TOXIC SHOCK SYNDROME

TOXIC SHOCK SYNDROME

This is an uncommon syndrome which can arise in women using tampons. It is due to the staphylococcus which may be carried by the woman herself in various sites such as the vagina, cervix, perineum or nasopharynx. It is extremely dangerous and may prove fatal. The infection becomes established in the vagina, usually aided by the presence of a tampon.

Clinical signs

There is a rapid onset of fever often with vomiting, diarrhoea, muscular aches, skin erythema. The blood pressure drops to very low levels and the patient becomes confused and stuporose. Swabs should be taken from the various sites where the organism may be carried and tests of function should be made so far as possible in relation to the kidney, liver, muscle, central nervous system and blood platelets.

Treatment

Crystalloid solutions and plasma should be given rapidly to reverse the hypotension. Methicillin or oxacillin 1–2g every 4 hours can be administered to subdue the infection. Check for a retained tampon.

Prophylaxis

Strict genital hygiene should be maintained with frequent baths. Tampons must be changed frequently – 3–4 times daily and an external pad worn at night – no internal tampon.

Following recovery, checks should be made to see if the patient is still carrying staphylococci.

Finally

In many cases of vaginal discharge the bacterial population is mixed and no specific cause for the symptoms can be discovered. Sometimes the complaint has begun as a specific infection e.g. trichomonas, but other contaminants have overgrown the initial organism. Good hygiene is necessary to clear up the general growth. Subsequent tests may reveal the offending organism.

MONITORING CVP

There is at present a general agreement that in the presence of acute peripheral circulatory failure, management is made easier by passing a catheter into a vein near the heart and monitoring the Central Venous Pressure (CVP).

CVP is technically the pressure in the right or left atrium, but for practical purposes it is taken as the pressure recorded in one of the great veins, preferably the superior vena cava.

CVP is an indicator of the amount of blood returning to the heart and continuous monitoring is necessary. Pressure at the right atrium varies between 0–15cm H_2O in the normal state and 2–15cm at the ante-cubital vein. In shock, if the pressure is persistently below say 5cm then rapid transfusion is required.

Technique

A special manometer set is used. A catheter is passed into a neck vein and the manometer adjusted so that the zero of H_2O is at the level of the right atrium.

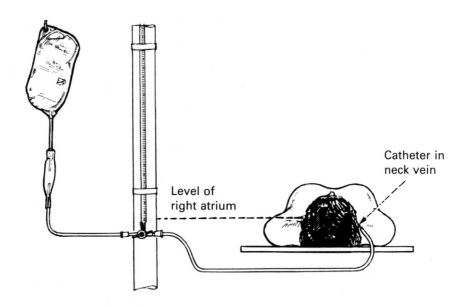

Level of
right atrium

Catheter in
neck vein

INFLAMMATION OF THE UPPER GYNAECOLOGICAL TRACT

This is the result of:
1. Spread from the lower tract of infections such as chlamydia, gonococcus or trichomonas and it begins in the cervix. It may not spread further but it remains a potential threat.

or 2. Diseases blood-borne from other parts of the body.

or 3. A few cases may be related to birth trauma or abortion.

CERVICAL ECTOPY

An overgrowth of columnar epithelium replacing the squamous epithelium round the cervical os. It has a raw appearance and a velvety feel. It is an ectopy of columnar epithelium and in modern terminology is so described. However the word 'erosion' is still widely used, but should be reserved for erosion by malignancy.

Aetiology:
1. Parturition:
2. Contraceptive pill.
3. Persistence of a condition which is normal in infancy.

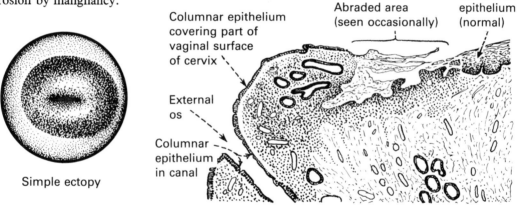

Simple ectopy

CERVICITIS

An infection of the cervical epithelium and stroma, usually following ectopy.

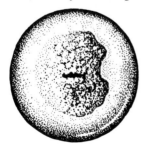

ECTROPION

An ectopy or infection in a gaping or lacerated cervix.

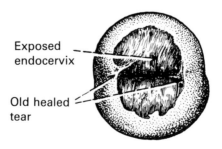

Symptoms

There may be no symptoms with any of these conditions which are observed at examination, but usually there is a complaint of discharge, and they are common causes of post-coital bleeding. Cervicitis has never been proved to have a special liability to malignant change.

163

CERVICAL ECTOPY AND CERVICITIS

CRYOSURGERY This has been developed as an alternative to cautery and diathermy and is useful as an outpatient procedure.

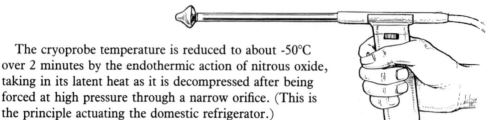

The cryoprobe temperature is reduced to about -50°C over 2 minutes by the endothermic action of nitrous oxide, taking in its latent heat as it is decompressed after being forced at high pressure through a narrow orifice. (This is the principle actuating the domestic refrigerator.)

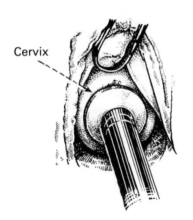

Cervix

Treatment takes about 2 minutes and is almost painless. Extreme cold causes adherence between tissues and metal and 30 seconds must be allowed for thawing before the probe is removed. The patient will have a watery discharge for 2 weeks, and coitus should be avoided for a fortnight.

DIATHERMY

More extensive lesions must be treated by surgical excision or by diathermy.

In diathermy the infected tissue is destroyed by the great heat generated where the diathermy probe or point touches the cervix and sends high frequency current through the body to the indifferent electrode strapped to the leg.

The burnt tissue sloughs off over 2 weeks and the raw area is gradually re-epithelialised. This method requires general anaesthesia, and the discharge is more offensive than that following cryosurgery.

TRACHELORRHAPHY

Sometimes the cervix is so torn and infected that surgical excision is the best treatment.

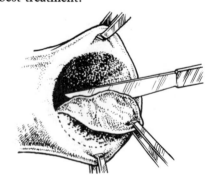

LASER

Laser therapy may be employed at a colposcopy clinic.

CERVICAL POLYPS

Cervical polyps are nodular or pedunculated growths arising from the endocervix, and associated with chronic cervicitis. A polypoid fibroid of the uterus may present as a cervical polyp.

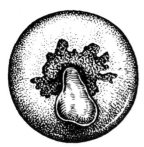

Cervical polyp
with cervicitis

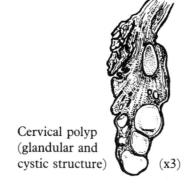

Cervical polyp
(glandular and
cystic structure)   (x3)

Polyps are common causes of irregular bleeding, especially after coitus, and should always be removed for examination, although malignancy is unlikely.

Polyps may be avulsed at an outpatient clinic by torsion using sponge forceps.

RARE CAUSES OF CERVICITIS

CHANCRE

Secondary infection is uncommon so the characteristic hard indurated base does not form. A chancre may be papular or ulcerative in which case it looks like an erosion. On palpation it may be mistaken for cancer.

A herpes simplex infection of the cervix may resemble a chancre.

TUBERCULOSIS

This is usually secondary to tubal and uterine infection and may be proliferative or ulcerative – in appearance not unlike ectopy.

It is usually found in association with chronic pelvic inflammation and infertility, and the diagnosis is histological.

If there is any doubt about the nature of a cervical lesion, a biopsy should always be taken before applying cryosurgery or diathermy.

INFECTION OF THE UTERUS

ENDOMETRITIS

Acute inflammation may develop in response to infection following childbirth or abortion, or the insertion of a contraceptive device; or as part of a gonorrhoeal infection. Actinomyces infection may be associated with neglected intra-uterine contraceptive devices and may be detected on a Papanicolaou smear.

Chronic Endometritis is a rare condition because of the frequency with which the endometrium is shed. The diagnosis is histological and there are no specific signs or symptoms, but the microscopic appearances are of infiltration mainly by plasma cells and lymphocytes. (For TB endometritis see p.170).

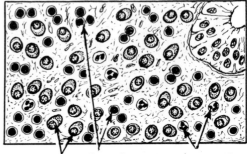

Plasma cells   Lymphocytes   Leucocytes

Senile Endometritis

Post-menopausal endometrium has little resistance to infection, and endometritis may arise from cervicitis or from tumour. If the cervix is stenosed by infection or tumour, the uterus becomes distended with pus and the condition is known as pyometra. Cervical dilatation will release the pus but curettage must be done to exclude malignancy and in such a situation it is very easy to perforate the uterus.

Metritis

Acute inflammation of the myometrium is a serious condition resulting from infection introduced during childbirth or abortion (see septic abortion p.407).

'Chronic Metritis'
'Fibrosis Uteri'
'Chronic Subinvolution'
'Myohyperplasia'

Many patients at gynaecological clinics are found to have an enlarged mobile 'flabby' uterus, often retroverted and sometimes associated with general pelvic inflammation. Menstrual irregularities and congestive discomfort or pain are complained of and the cause is not known. The histological appearances are normal unless there is other infection.

Treatment

If there is no organic cause, the menstrual irregularity may respond to sex steroid hormones. In the woman over 40 who wishes no more family, there is much to be said for simple hysterectomy.

PELVIC INFLAMMATORY DISEASE (PID)

Infection of the fallopian tubes usually involves the ovaries and peritoneum, and the combined infection is called pelvic inflammatory disease (PID).

ACUTE PID

The history is often of a prolonged period followed by the gradual onset of pelvic pain and irregular bleeding. The patient is fevered and on examination there is abdominal tenderness and guarding, and extreme tenderness of the vaginal fornices.

Acute PID may follow operations, but it is usually a result of ascending infection, and may be associated with the intrauterine device. It must be treated actively to avoid the development of a chronic infection.

Bacteriology

It is unusual to be able to isolate pathogens from the infected area, but their demonstration in the cervix points to the probable cause. N.gonorrhoea and Chlamydia trachomatis are said to be commonest, but anaerobic organisms are often found in pelvic abscesses.

Differential diagnosis

Appendicitis

Signs are mainly right sided, and the menstrual cycle is undisturbed.

Diverticulitis

This is a disease mainly of older women and signs are left sided.

Torsion of pedicle of a cyst

There may be a history of intermittent pain over several months. A cyst should be palpable.

Tubal pregnancy

The history may be helpful, but in young women in whom salpingitis and tubal pregnancy may co-exist the distinction can be very difficult. A ß-HCG pregancy test aids diagnosis.

Management

A laparoscopy is advisable if there is any doubt, especially as this nearly always makes it possible to exclude tubal pregnancy. An intrauterine device, if in the uterus, should be removed. After swabs have been taken from the vagina and cervix a broad spectrum antibiotic such as doxycycline or ampicillin should be given. If acute signs and symptoms persist, a laparotomy should be carried out to search for abscess formation. No surgical procedure beyond drainage should be performed.

PELVIC INFLAMMATORY DISEASE

CHRONIC PID

The patient complains of pelvic pain made worse during the periods which are irregular and heavy. Dyspareunia is common.

Examination Some swelling may be felt but often there is little to find except tenderness in the fornices. An exact diagnosis and estimate of the degree of PID cannot be made without laparoscopy.

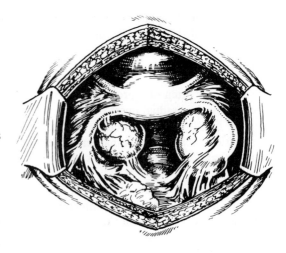

Pathology All degrees of inflammation are met with from salpingitis alone to a widespread inflammatory reaction involving all the pelvic tissues. It is rare to recover any organism in PID, other than in the case of tuberculosis. The ascending infection first attacks the tubes which are sealed off by oedema and adhesions. The tubes either swell up with watery exudate forming a hydrosalpinx or pyosalpinx; or they become very thickened and adherent to the ovary. The ovary may also be the seat of abscess formation, and the uterus and adnexa, normally mobile, become fixed by adhesions.

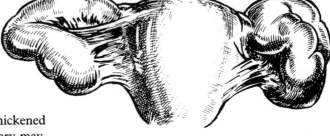

Blocked and distended tubes in PID

Treatment The course of chronic PID is not predictable, and mild degrees may resolve spontaneously. In such cases the patient should be treated by rest, and although the infective organism may not be identified, a broad spectrum antibiotic is usually given. Hydrosalpinx and any abscess formation must be relieved by laparotomy and drainage, and dyspareunia may be relieved by correcting the uterine retroversion with a sling operation (p.266). In advanced cases however the only effective treatment is operation to remove the uterus and tubes and perhaps the ovaries as well.

PELVIC CELLULITIS

Infection of the fibro-fatty connective tissue of the pelvis (the 'visceral layer') of the pelvic fascia – p.23).

Acute Cellulitis		Chronic Cellulitis
Primary Follows injury to vagina or cervix at childbirth or abortion. Follows pelvic surgery. Associated with radiotherapy for carcinoma of the cervix.	**Secondary** Simply an extension of pelvic inflammatory disease.	Mainly inflammatory thickening of the uterosacral and transverse ligaments of the uterus.

The classical identifying sign is a hard inflammatory mass somewhere in the pelvis.

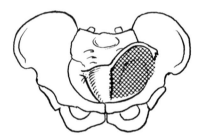

1. A lateral swelling in the tissues below the broad ligament. Note the displaced uterus.

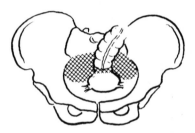

2. Posterior swelling in the tissues round the rectum (the 'horseshoe swelling').

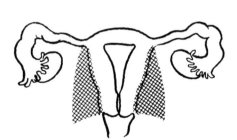

3. Bilateral swelling alongside the uterus.

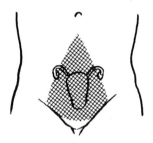

4. Anterior swelling in Scarpa's fascia of the abdominal wall.

Complications These are rare, as is the disease itself.
1. Suppuration.
2. Thrombosis of the pelvic and femoral veins with the risk of pulmonary embolism.
3. Development of chronic cellulitis.
4. A pelvic abscess may form and, if not drained surgically, will usually point below the inguinal ligament.

GENITAL TUBERCULOSIS

Tuberculosis is a rare disease in gynaecology. It attacks the fallopian tubes and the endometrium, and lesions elsewhere in the genital tract are uncommon. It is possible that infection may be acquired from a sexual partner.

Clinical Features

The patient is usually a young woman seeking treatment for primary infertility or complaining of irregular menstruation or perhaps abdominal pain.

Diagnosis

1. Histological evidence from curettings. This is the commonest method and it is assumed that the tubes are also infected.

2. Bacteriological evidence from guinea-pig inoculation or laboratory culture.

3. Biopsy from any suspicious ulcerated area in the vagina or vulva.

4. By laparoscopic inspection and biopsy.

Once evidence of genital infection is obtained, the respiratory and urinary tracts must also be investigated.

Pathology

This infection is blood borne, usually from a primary focus in the lung or kidney, and it infects the tubes, spreading thence to the endometrium.

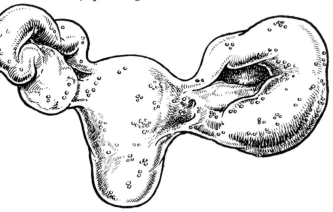

The tubes may appear normal (endosalpingitis) but usually display the distortion and swelling of chronic infection, and small pinhead tubercles appear on the serosa.

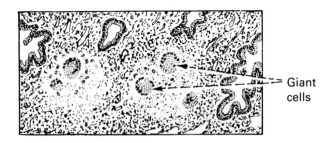

Giant cells

The endometrium also shows tuberculous follicles, best developed in the premenstrual phase. There may be debris in endometrial glands.

GENITAL TUBERCULOSIS

Treatment

Chemotherapy

A combination of rifampicin, isoniazid and ethambutol has been used effectively in recent years. Dosage is based on body weight and the first two drugs are given in combination for a year. The ethambutol is withdrawn after 90 days. Cure may be assumed if the endometrium shows no signs of tubercle, and the patient's menstrual cycle is normal.

Surgery

This means removal of uterus, tubes and ovaries, although conservation of one ovary would be permissible in a young woman. Surgery is indicated when chemotherapy has failed (about 5% of cases) or in combination with chemotherapy in the older woman. All infected tissue must be removed to avoid subsequent fistulous openings in bowel or bladder.

TUBERCULOSIS and INFERTILITY

Failure to conceive is probably the most important consequence of genital tuberculosis, and 90% of women presenting with the disease will never have had a pregnancy. Pregnancy after successful treatment may be looked for in about 10% of patients, but there is a considerable chance of ectopic gestation.

ACQUIRED IMMUNE DEFICIENCY SYNDROME – AIDS

AIDS is now the most serious of all gynaecological infections. It has reached pandemic proportions affecting almost all countries and regions. In some parts of the world such as the sub-Sahara region of Africa and in some sections of the public in western countries, e.g. drug addicts in the U.S.A., there are epidemics. It is due to the human immune deficiency virus (HIV) or, in scientific terms, retrovirus oncornavirus.

Transmission

There are several modes of infection and risk factors.

A. Sexual

1. Relationships with prostitutes. Multiplicity of sexual partners increases the risks. The same dangers exist with promiscuity.
2. Male homosexual activities. Again there are likely to be multiple partners.
3. Sexual contact with individuals of the same or opposite sex in southern parts of Africa.
4. Abrasions around the genital or anal regions increase the risk of infection.

It is said that circumcision provides some protection but this is scarcely reliable.

B. Non-sexual

1. Addicts using needles in common for intravenous drug injections. Although some authorities provide a free supply of sterile needles the very nature of drug-taking induces carelessness.
2. Injection of blood or blood products can be dangerous if proper precautions are not employed. For a time and in certain areas, Factor VIII treatment for haemophilia was associated with the occurrence of AIDS in a number of patients. This was due to using contaminated blood for Factor VIII preparations. The danger has been eliminated by heating all Factor VIII material to destroy the virus. The same potential danger exists in relation to blood or plasma for transfusion. Blood donors require rigorous testing for evidence of viral infection.

It is difficult to provide an adequate description of this disease. The symptomatology is such that almost every organ may appear to be affected at one time or another. There is a mixture of:

1. Constitutional disease with fever, sweating, etc.
2. Neurological symptoms and lesions.
3. Malignant tumours.
4. Liver or renal failure.
5. Secondary infections.

The course of the disease is erratic, associated with progressive loss of immune resistance. Death is almost inevitable but may be delayed for years. To understand the main features of the disease it is necessary to recall some of the mechanisms involved in the normal immune process.

NORMAL IMMUNE MECHANISM

This depends upon the activities of lymphocytes, of which there are two basic types, B and T.

B lymphocytes

These are so called because they were first discovered in the bursa of Fabricius in the bowel of chickens.

When the body is invaded by a foreign antigen, such as in an infection, B lymphocytes are transformed and become plasma cells capable of secreting specific antibodies into the tissues and blood causing destruction of the antigen. This reaction is very rapid, almost immediate, and results in humoral immunity.

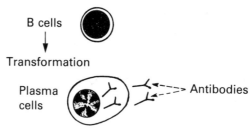

These B cells form 25% of the blood lymphocytes.

T lymphocytes are named thus because they are processed in the Thymus. They form 70% of blood lymphocytes.

T cells are also stimulated by foreign antigens and undergo transformation into several specific types whose function is to control and aid the B cells. There are 3 main types:

1. T cells which control the
   production of B cell antibodies.

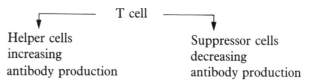

2. T cells which control the
   over-all production of lymphocytes.

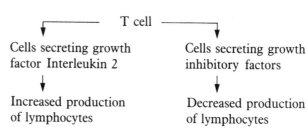

These changes in T cells follow the B cell phase and are therefore delayed. They produce cell mediated immunity. The various activities of the T cells make certain, in normal circumstances, that the immune reaction is tailored to the needs of the body at any particular phase of infection.

3. Killer cells. These kill other cells by direct contact if the latter have been infected.

HIV INFECTION AND THE IMMUNE SYSTEM

The Human Immunodeficiency Virus (HIV) and the B lymphocytes

The reaction is very slow and up to 6 months may elapse before antibodies appear in the blood. Usually, however, their appearance coincides with the eruption of symptoms. They seem to have little or no influence on the course of the disease and in the later stages they may disappear from the blood.

HIV and the T cells

Although B cells react and produce antibodies, initially it is the effect of HIV on the T cells which ultimately destroys the whole immune apparatus. The virus attacks T cells, especially those of the helper variety commonly called T4 lymphocytes which stimulate production of antibodies and increase the number of lymphocytes.

Curiously one of the antigens of these lymphocytes, the differentiation antigen CD4, has an affinity for the virus and acts as a receptor. On the other hand, although brain tissue and muscle may be infected by the virus, there is no CD4 antigen to act as a receptor in these regions.

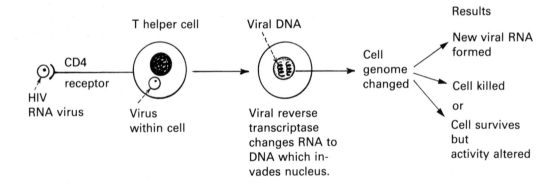

Ultimately there is a progressive lymphopenia affecting both B and T cells.

T cells also influence polymorphs and macrophages in much the same way as lymphocytes. Normally, in infection they increase chemotaxis and phagocytosis. With HIV infection these activities will diminish and this explains the ease with which secondary infections by organisms of very low pathogenicity can establish themselves, spread rapidly and cause septicaemia.

ACQUIRED IMMUNE DEFICIENCY SYNDROME – AIDS

The progress of the disease can be roughly divided into 4 phases, but these phases are ill-defined, variable in time of onset and duration.

Phase 1

Following infection there may be no symptoms but in a considerable proportion of infected individuals an acute illness resembling infectious mononucleosis appears with fever, night sweats, enlarged lymph nodes, diarrhoea and a blood lymphocytosis. Antibody formation occurs. In other individuals this feverish episode is delayed for varying periods.

Phase 2

A symptomless period usually ensues which may last for 7 years or more. Despite the lack of symptoms the virus goes on replicating within the body. During this period there is frequently enlargement of lymph nodes in various parts of the body. As a result the name 'Persistent generalised lymphadenopathy' is often applied to indicate a particular phase.

Phase 3

This is the turning point in the disease when the virus has replicated and is beginning to reduce the ability of the patient to mount an effective immune response to ordinary infections. Symptoms of the type observed in the initial phase may reappear. Further development means a change from mere infection by HIV to full-blown AIDS syndrome. Fifty per cent of infected individuals progress to phase 4 within 10 years. The phrase 'AIDS related complex' is used to indicate a particular stage in the disease but this phrase is not particularly useful because of the erratic behaviour of the infection.

Phase 4

The final phase is characterised by repeated attacks of intercurrent infection due to progressive immuno-deficiency. The core antigen increases. T4 helper lymphocytes progressively diminish. The viral DNA is integrated into the genome of infected cells producing more HIV.

Pneumonia due to pneumocystis carinii is one of the commonest complications but the list of secondary infections is very large and includes parasites, viruses, bacteria, fungi etc. They are almost entirely of the type which cause minor, localised lesions in normally immune individuals, but in AIDS patients they spread rapidly and can be fatal.

Three conditions are particularly characteristic of the immuno-deficiency state:
1. Kaposi sarcoma, usually an indolent growth in the skin, becomes aggressive.
2. Hairy leukoplakia of the tongue.
3. Lymphomas are common in AIDS patients and lymphoma of the brain is almost diagnostic.

ACQUIRED IMMUNE DEFICIENCY SYNDROME – AIDS

Intercurrent infections frequently found in AIDS patients

Minor infections and infestations which remain localised in normally immune persons and produce mild symptoms if any, spread rapidly and cause life-threatening clinical conditions in the AIDS patient whose immunity is seriously compromised.

Infective Agents	Clinical Results
Parasites	
Pneumocystis carinii	Pneumonia
Cryptosporidium	Severe diarrhoea
Strongyloides stercoralis	Severe diarrhoea
Toxoplasma gondii	Chorio-retinitis
Viruses	
Herpes	Pneumonia
J.C. virus	Leuco-encephalopathy
Bacteria	
Species usually causing minor lesions e.g. skin spots	Septicaemia
Fungi	
Cryptococcus neoformans	Pneumonia Meningitis

The final condition of the patient is pathetic due to these infections, wasting and possibly dementia.

Paediatric AIDS

Infection of the fetus or newborn from the mother can occur in two ways.

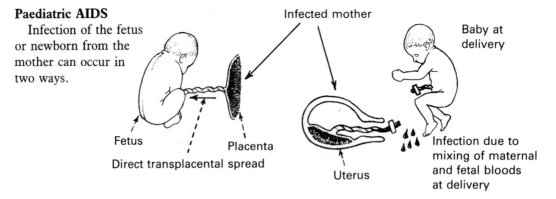

Infected mother

Baby at delivery

Fetus

Placenta

Direct transplacental spread

Uterus

Infection due to mixing of maternal and fetal bloods at delivery

Spread to the offspring occurs in one third of all AIDS patients. Symptoms are similar to those occurring in the adult but, in addition, lymphoid interstitial pneumonia and parotid gland enlargement occur in the infant.

Initial tests for antibody may be positive in the infant but if they become negative the child is not infected. If infection has occurred further tests at 15 months will be positive. In most cases of infection however, the child dies within 1 year.

Haemophilic children who were infected by contaminated Factor VIII show a slow progress of the syndrome with prolonged asymptomatic periods.

ACQUIRED IMMUNE DEFICIENCY SYNDROME – AIDS

Treatment

Earlier forms of treatment were aimed at preventing and treating secondary infection in the final phases of the disease. They were directed especially at pneumonia due to pneumocystis carinii which is common in these patients and, if untreated, causes death within 1 year.

Drugs have been used in a prophylactic manner to prevent secondary infection occurring. There are several preparations but some, such as nebulised pentamidine, while being effective against pneumocystis, are too specific and have no influence on other common infections such as toxoplasmosis. Oral drugs e.g. co-trimoxazole, sulpha-methoxazole-pyrimethamine, dapsone and dapsone-pyrimethamine, have a more general action.

Four methods of treating or preventing the viral infection itself are in various stages of development:

1. **Anti-viral drugs**

   These show some promise but whether they can produce a cure or merely modify the course of the disease is not yet clear. Zidovudine and didoxyinosine are two such. The latter has a disadvantage in that diabetes mellitus and Raynaud's syndrome have occurred during therapy.

2. **Gene therapy**

   An altered virus, a so-called mirror image of the AIDS virus has been constructed. The apparent idea is that the individual will be 'infected' with the artificial virus which will then occupy the viral receptors on T lymphocytes thus preventing entry of the AIDS virus and protecting the immune system.

3. **Vaccination**

   It is obviously impossible to use whole AIDS antigen for vaccination for fear of actually infecting the individual. Sub-units of the antigen have been used and there are indications of some success but, unfortunately, while treatment may protect against systemic infection there is no protection against the mucosal invasion during sexual activity. There is also evidence that the antigenic sub-units can vary and so also does the degree of immunity.

4. A new drug treatment with **benzodiazepine derivatives** is being tried.

   These drugs are known to interfere with reverse transcriptase reaction and would therefore stop the replication process.

A new viral disease similar to AIDS and named HIV2 has appeared in West Africa. It produces a milder symptomatic form of the disease but can end in the fully developed AIDS. Already it has spread to France, Portugal and West African communities in Britain, especially London.

ACQUIRED IMMUNE DEFICIENCY SYNDROME – AIDS

Management

With the rapid spread of HIV infection it is inevitable that general practitioners will be drawn into the treatment and management of cases. The practitioner should take all precautionary measures in the way of protective clothing including disposable gloves, and should arrange for some method of dealing with blood which may be spilled. In regard to the patient the following routine should be established.

1. Regular follow up every 3 months to determine progress.
2. Check weight.
3. Full blood count.
4. Erythrocyte sedimentation rate.
5. Examine especially for tumour growth e.g. Kaposi sarcoma, lymphoma.
6. Watch for opportunistic infection and treat immediately.
7. Arrange for expert psychological handling when necessary.
8. If possible leave HIV positive cases who require surgery to the end of a list so that special precautions can be observed.

Prevention of spread

1. Educate patients regarding risks of multiple sexual partners.
2. Indicate the use of barrier contraception.
3. Blood for transfusion must always be tested for HIV antibodies. If circumstances make this impossible, withdraw blood from the patient and store for future use.
4. In cases of infertility where donor semen is to be used for in vitro fertilisation, store it in cryo-preservation conditions for 3 months until certain that the donor is free of infection.
5. There are a large number of factors which can only be controlled by education and legislation. Some of these are:
   (a) Drug production, pushing and dealing.
   (b) Drug consumption.
   (c) All new drugs or other substances which may be habit forming.
   (d) Prostitution, both male and female.
   (e) The current fashion of casual sex. Television, newspapers and magazines must bear a great deal of blame for this.

Ethical considerations

Guidelines have been laid down by the General Medical Council and the British Medical Association. The main features are:

1. Confidentiality must be maintained at all times. The only exception to this rule is when the practitioner establishes that the health of another person is threatened. This must be explained to the parties concerned.
2. Tests must not be carried out without the consent of the patient.
3. Care must be exercised in dealing with the family and sexual partner of the patient. It is essential to establish a frank and open relationship with the patient so that both practitioner and patient can trust each other and all matters can be discussed freely.
4. Doctors who are themselves HIV positive must make every effort to protect patients, limiting their practice including treatment methods such as minor surgical procedures which carry a risk of transmitting the infection.

CHAPTER 8

DISEASES OF THE VULVA

VULVAL DERMATOSES (Syn: VULVAL DYSPLASIA: VULVAL DYSTROPHY)

The skin of the vulva appears to react differently from skin elsewhere. It is more easily irritated by friction and by local application of antiseptic, anaesthetic and antihistamine creams, and it has long been recognised that the treatment of vulval carcinoma by radiotherapy produces a much more intense inflammatory reaction in vulval skin than in other parts of the epidermis. Transepidermal water loss is higher in the vulva, and it more readily becomes dry and irritable.

Vulval dermatoses is the term applied to non-infective non-neoplastic diseases of the vulval skin. Their management is moving more and more into the province of the dermatologist, but the symptoms of itching, soreness and dyspareunia will usually take the patient in the first place to the gynaecologist.

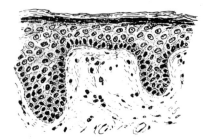

Normal vulva

Classification

There is at present no generally accepted classification, although attempts have been made to standardise terminology. Diagnosis is by biopsy which may show only non-specific histological changes, treatment is nearly always symptomatic, and there is continuing uncertainty about the association between dystrophy and malignancy.

The classification given here is based on a mixture of clinical and pathological descriptive terms, and is useful to the gynaecologist. There should always be cooperation with the pathologist and the dermatologist.

1. Dermatological conditions: Eczema, psoriasis.
2. Conditions displaying lichenification:
   (a) Lichen simplex (Neurodermatitis).
   (b) Lichen sclerosus et atrophicus.
   (c) Lichen planus.
   (Many skin conditions develop lichenification if traumatised.)
3. Kraurosis (atrophy due to oestrogen withdrawal). This is really a result of ageing. It may give rise to dyspareunia.

LICHENIFICATION

Repeated scratching produces a leathery condition called lichenification, and skin badly affected in this way eventually becomes whitish and rather shiny. Lichenification is common in vulval dermatoses and makes diagnosis difficult.

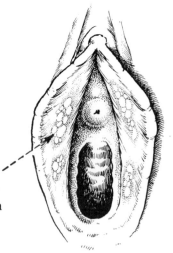

VULVAL DERMATOSES

LICHEN SIMPLEX (Neurodermatitis)

Lichen simplex is a common cause of severe vulvo-perineal pruritus. The vulva is reddened and inflamed, and marked by scratching and rubbing which leads to lichenification.

Normal

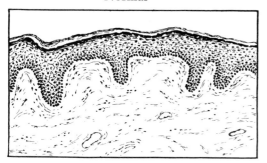

Lichen Simplex

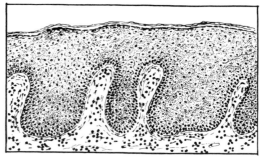

The normal vulva is covered in ordinary squamous epithelium except that on the labia minora there is no keratinisation, and no sweat or sebaceous glands. The epithelium is thin and flexible with well marked papillae.

The epidermis is much thickened and there is proliferation of the papillae. There is a retention of nucleated cells in the superficial epidermis (a characteristic of inflammation) and the dermis shows an invasion of leucocytes.

Management

1. Steroid Cream.   The condition responds rapidly to the thrice daily application of steroid creams such as 0.025% fluocinolone (Synalar), and in severe cases the 0.2% strength may be required initially. Steroid creams may themselves induce atrophy if their use is prolonged.

2. If there is much infection the application of a local antibiotic is indicated.

3. A search is made for any causal factors such as contact sensitivity.

4. A vaginal swab is examined for the presence of candida.

5. The urine is tested for sugar.

6. Biopsy. Once the condition has resolved, a biopsy should be carried out (preferably under general anaesthesia to avoid the use of local anaesthetic) to exclude any underlying condition. In the case of vulval dystrophies, diagnosis by clinical appearance only is not easy.

VULVAL DERMATOSES

LICHEN SCLEROSUS ET ATROPHICUS (LSA)

This is a form of atrophy associated with scleroderma – a progressive fibrosis and loss of mobility of the skin.

Aetiology is unknown, and although the disease can affect both sexes at all ages in any area of skin, it is most commonly seen in the vulvo-perineal skin of middle-aged women.

Appearance

The disease starts as a flat pinkish-white macula. Further patches appear and coalesce, and the vulva becomes moist and reddened. There is gradual sclerosis and contraction of the tissues, and scratching may induce lichenification.

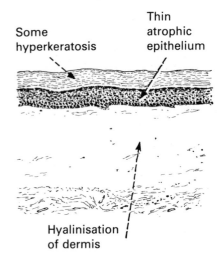

Some hyperkeratosis

Thin atrophic epithelium

Hyalinisation of dermis

Histology

There is atrophic thinning of the epidermis with some hyalinisation of the dermis. The keratinised layer is thickened, giving a whitened appearance ('leukoplakia').

Management

Pruritus responds to bland creams such as zinc and castor oil, or to low concentration steroid creams which must be used with caution in case they increase the atrophic change. Because of the sclerosis, dyspareunia tends to be marked and is difficult to treat. Oestrogen creams are of no use, and testosterone creams which are used to induce a thickening of the atrophic skin may induce virilising symptoms.

Malignant Associations

The atrophy in LSA is held to have some association with subsequent malignancy, and once the diagnosis has been confirmed by biopsy, the patient must be kept under observation.

VULVAL DERMATOSES

LICHEN PLANUS (LP)

This is a rare type of lichenification, and presents as flat-topped papules in areas of skin trauma, such as the insides of wrists, the neck and the vulva. The histological appearance is characterised by a curious 'saw-tooth' acanthosis.

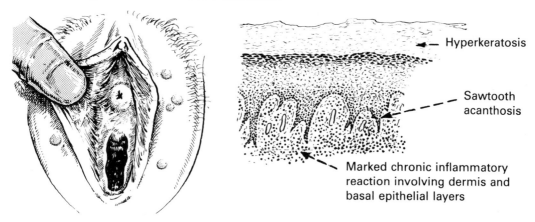

- Hyperkeratosis

Sawtooth acanthosis

Marked chronic inflammatory reaction involving dermis and basal epithelial layers

Management

LP may be an autoimmune disease and treatment is difficult. The itching is severe and does not respond as well as other dystrophies to steroid creams, and bland preparations should be tried. The disease tends to remit, but may be pre-malignant.

KRAUROSIS

The term means dry or brittle, and the condition is an exaggeration of the normal physiological atrophy. It requires no treatment unless the patient complains of dyspareunia, in which case a plastic operation to enlarge the orifice is necessary, and even then the atrophic shrinkage will continue. A dystrophic condition may of course be superimposed on kraurosis, and biopsy is then necessary.

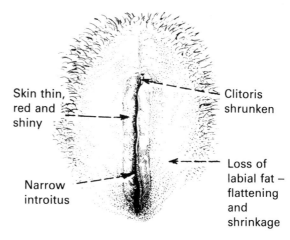

Skin thin, red and shiny

Clitoris shrunken

Narrow introitus

Loss of labial fat – flattening and shrinkage

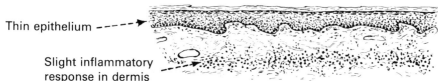

Thin epithelium

Slight inflammatory response in dermis

SIMPLE TUMOURS OF THE VULVA

The complaint is usually a of a 'lump' or 'swelling' at the vaginal introitus. (In many cases the patient may mistake prolapse of various types or hernia for tumour growth.)

The tumours can be divided into two groups: (a) Non-neoplastic and (b) Neoplastic swellings.

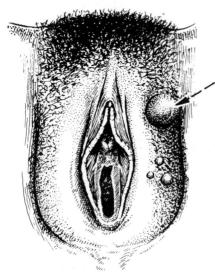

NON-NEOPLASTIC SWELLINGS

These are the result of blockage of ducts of glands, congenital malformations or due to trauma.

Sebaceous cyst of the vulva occurs in the hairy region of the labium majus. The cyst may become infected and cause pain. On examination, multiple cysts are usually found, mostly small. If painful they can be removed. The cyst contains whitish, cheesy sebaceous material.

Inclusion cysts are sometimes found in the perineum.

Cyst of Bartholin's gland This is the commonest simple tumour of the vulva. Caused by obstruction of the duct, the cyst almost always becomes infected and requires surgical treatment (see p.145).

A **cyst or hydrocele of the canal of Nuck** (an embryonic remnant of a peritoneal pouch which extends along the round ligament).

If causing discomfort the cyst is excised.

An inguinal swelling may cause the patient to believe she has a vulval swelling.

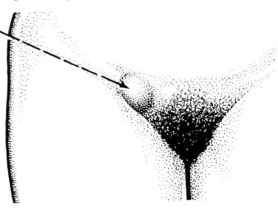

Vulval varicosities may produce tumour-like swellings. Treatment is by excision or injection of sclerosing agents.

Vulval haematoma is a result of direct violence or wounding (it is most commonly found with childbirth). The haematoma spreads widely because of the loose tissue structure. Treatment is by incision, evacuation and drainage.

Endometriosis is uncommon in the labia majora or other parts of the vulva. It enlarges and becomes tender during menstruation. Treatment is by excision.

It is difficult to categorise endometriosis. Its behaviour varies very much and many suggestions as to its origin have been made – e.g. congenital lesion, metaplastic change, embolic origin from uterus, true neoplastic growth.

SIMPLE TUMOURS OF THE VULVA

NEOPLASTIC SWELLINGS

Lipoma is found rarely. It arises from the subcutaneous tissues of the vulva and usually becomes pedunculated and dependent with growth. Treatment is by excision.

Fibroma is also uncommon but presents as a pedunculated tumour like a lipoma but is firmer. It arises from the fibrous tissue of the round ligament and the vulvar connective tissue. Treatment is by excision. Very rarely it is found to be a myoma. These tumours on occasion become sarcomatous.

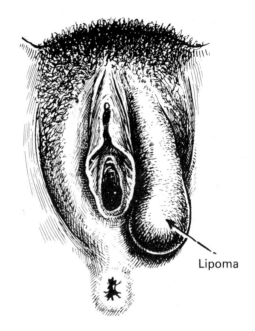

Lipoma

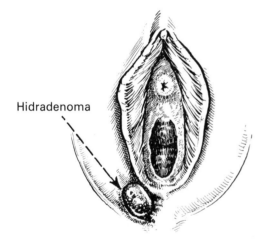

Hidradenoma

Hidradenoma is a rare tumour of sweat gland origin. It appears as a small nodule on the labium or in the interlabial sulcus. The overlying skin tends to ulcerate and bleed, giving a fungating appearance. The tumour is excised and shows a cystadenomatous structure. It also shows a typical two layer epithelium with some mucous secretion. Intracystic papillary protrusions occur. It may undergo malignant change.

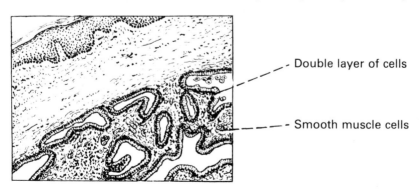

Double layer of cells

Smooth muscle cells

Condylomata acuminata, due to viral infection, form a moist mass of small warty growths. The lesion is often included in the list of simple tumours (see p.153).

Urethral caruncle is dealt with on page 193.

SIMPLE TUMOURS OF THE VULVA

PIGMENTED MOLE

These are very common on and around the vulva. They vary in colour from yellowish to black and may be flat, macular lesions or warty. Some are hairy, others smooth. Hairy moles rarely become malignant. All junctional non-hairy growths should be removed since these are the type most likely to undergo malignant transformation.

During fetal life melanin-pigment-forming neuroectodermal cells migrate to the skin and are found in small numbers in the basal layer of the skin.

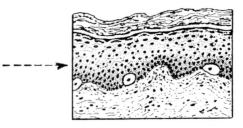

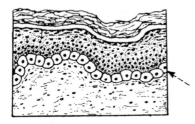

The common congenital pigmented mole or lentigo is the result of an abnormality of migration, proliferation and maturation of these neuroectodermal cells. A continuous layer of pigmented cells is found adjacent to the basal epidermal cells.

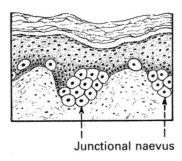

Junctional naevus

In this case proliferation is local and confined to the dermoepidermal junction.

ACCESSORY NIPPLES

Small areolae may be found on the pubis or labia majora and resemble naevi.

VULVAL DYSTROPHY

VULVAR INTRA-EPITHELIAL NEOPLASIA (VIN)

In all cases of marked 'dermatosis' the possibility of early malignant change should be considered. It is helpful to apply acetic acid to the area. Areas of hyperplasia show up as white spots (VIN BLANC). These can then be biopsied and studied microscopically.

NON-INVASIVE CARCINOMA of VULVA
(Bowen's Disease of the Vulva)

This rare disease presents as scaling, erythematous patches rather like psoriasis. Histology shows the thickened and disorganised epidermis with nucleated cells at all levels, and characteristic Bowen's cells – large epithelial cells (keratinocytes) with large nuclei containing mitotic figures. This is thought to be an indication of vulvar intra-epithelial neoplasia (VIN).

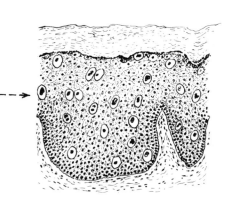

Treatment is by local excision, but the opinion of a dermatologist must be sought.

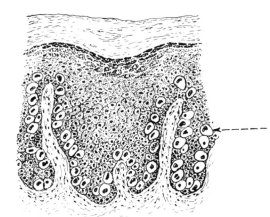

PAGET's DISEASE of the VULVA
(Extra-mammary Paget's Disease)

This malignant disease starts as an erythematous, irritant plaque which becomes eczematous (oedema and exudate) and spreads. Histology shows the characteristic Paget's cells – large round, clear-staining cells with large nuclei, often mitotic. These represent metastases from an underlying carcinoma which must be looked for, and a more extensive biopsy may be required. The breasts should always be examined, and the treatment is as described for vulval carcinoma.

CARCINOMA OF THE VULVA

(SQUAMOUS EPITHELIOMA: INVASIVE CARCINOMA)

The most common site is the labium majus followed by the clitoris, but it may arise anywhere including the vestibule when it will involve the urethra. Two or more growths are occasionally seen.

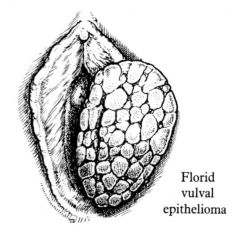

Florid
vulval
epithelioma

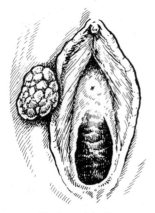

Early epithelioma

Histology. It is usually a squamous cell carcinoma (p.216). However any tissue contributing to the vulva may give rise to malignant change. Rare tumours are melanoma, basal cell carcinoma and sarcoma.

Spread. The tumour will spread locally if neglected, to involve the whole vulva and will invade the vagina. Metastatic spread is along the lymphatic system.

Clinical Features. This is a disease of old women and the average age is over 60. The patient may have had a pruritus of long standing but quite often the tumour is symptomless except for being palpable, until it ulcerates. The appearance is often uncharacteristic, and the old descriptive terms ('cauliflower, ulcerated, indurated') are not relevant to diagnosis. *Any lump on the vulva must be histologically examined.*

The inguinal glands will often be enlarged, but absence of enlargement does not guarantee absence of lymphatic spread.

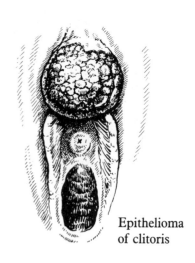

Epithelioma
of clitoris

CARCINOMA OF THE VULVA

LYMPHATIC SPREAD

1. To the superficial inguinal glands which lie along the inguinal ligament and the saphenous vein (vertical group). These nodes lie between the layers of the superficial fascia in relation to numerous superficial vessels.

   Drainage may be contralateral i.e. cells from a tumour on the right labium might drain via the left inguinal glands.

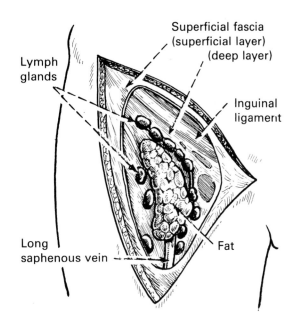

2. Thence to the deep femoral nodes accompanying the femoral vessels, and from there to the external iliac, common iliac and para-aortic glands.

3. This path is not invariably followed. The superficial nodes are occasionally bypassed and a tumour near the midline might drain via the vesical lymph channels direct to the internal iliac group.

4. Some tumours spread along the lymphatic system more quickly than others and there is no reliable correlation between the size of the tumour and the likelihood of gland involvement.

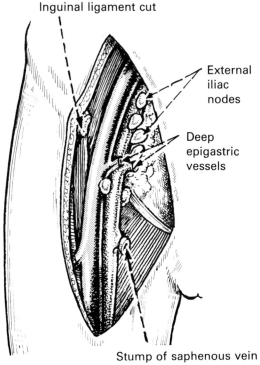

CARCINOMA OF THE VULVA

Treatment

A radical vulvectomy with dissection of the superficial and deep inguinal glands and the external iliac glands is accepted as the ideal treatment, but in the case of a frail patient the deep glands might be left untouched. Radical vulvectomy is an uncommon operation, better performed in centres which specialise in such work.

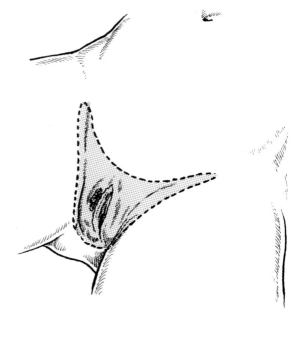

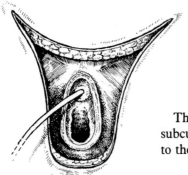

The whole vulva, skin and subcutaneous tissue are excised down to the periosteum.

The wound should be closed completely if possible, undercutting and mobilising skin if necessary. In this picture closure is incomplete, but the small raw area should heal in a few weeks. Drains are shown which remain in place for the first few days.

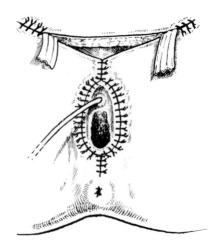

CARCINOMA OF THE VULVA

DISSECTION of DEEP INGUINAL and EXTERNAL ILIAC NODES

The picture shows the extent of the dissection required to make a thorough clearance of the nodes which may be involved.

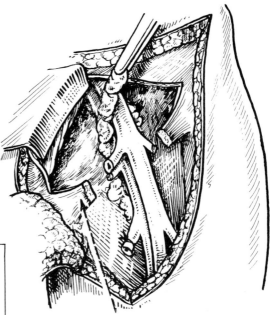

Inguinal ligament cut

To achieve this exposure the inferior epigastric vessels must be divided and inconstant vessels may be a cause of haemorrhage.

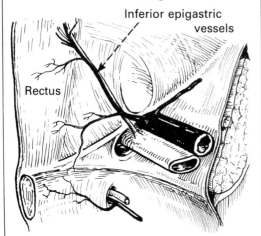

The anterior abdominal wall from inside, showing epigastric vessels.

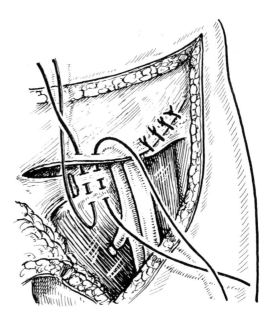

The inguinal ligament is not easily reconstituted and the aponeurosis must be sutured to pectineus muscle and its fascia. Hernia is sometimes a sequel of this operation.

CARCINOMA OF THE VULVA

COMPLICATIONS OF RADICAL VULVECTOMY

Immediate

1. **Shock**   If the operation is long and the patient old, this may contribute to the operative mortality.

2. **Thrombosis and pulmonary embolism**
   These well-recognised risks of pelvic surgery are increased in elderly patients.

Later

1. Chronic oedema is likely if there has been any thrombosis.

2. Coitus should be possible after this operation, but removal of the clitoris and the erectile tissue round the ostium vaginae puts an end to all erotic sensation in that area. This consequence of radical vulvectomy should be explained beforehand to patients who are sexually active.

PROGNOSIS AFTER RADICAL VULVECTOMY

This depends on three factors:

1. **Histology**. The more differentiated the tumour the better.

2. **Lymphatic spread**. Lymph node metastases occur in about 50% of patients, and the lateral pelvic nodes are involved in about 15%.

3. **The duration of tumour symptoms**. Elderly women may not immediately recognise a 'small wart' for what it is, or may lack the courage to consult their doctor.

RESULTS

If the nodes are not involved, a 70% 5-year cure rate may be looked for in the best hands. This falls to 40% when the superficial nodes are involved; and below 20% if the disease has reached the pelvic nodes.

RADIOTHERAPY in the TREATMENT of CARCINOMA of the VULVA

This is not a treatment of choice. Squamous carcinoma is a relatively resistant tumour, and the lethal dose required produces a severe reaction in the vulval skin which is peculiarly sensitive to irradiation. The inflammatory changes which follow treatment cause much discomfort and distress and may take a year or more to subside. Nevertheless radiotherapy has a place in the treatment of very old and frail patients. Such patients, perhaps in their fifties, might be offered radiotherapy as an alternative to a mutilating and sexually crippling operation.

DISEASES OF THE URETHRA

CARUNCLE

A small tumour arising from the posterior part of the lower end of the urethra. It is composed of a very vascular stroma, almost a haemangioma, usually infected and covered with squamous or transitional epithelium.

Clinical Features Caruncles are red in colour because of their vascularity, and extremely sensitive. The patient is usually an elderly woman complaining of dysuria and bleeding.

Treatment Caruncles should be excised and sent for histological examination although malignant change is rare. The base of the tumour on the urethral mucosa should be cauterised.

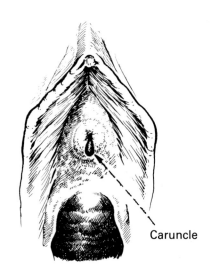

Caruncle

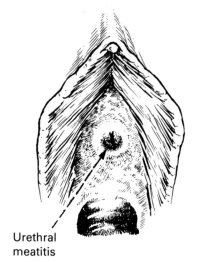

Urethral meatitis

URETHRAL MEATITIS
(Granulomatous Caruncle)

Chronic infection of the peri-urethral tissues. It is often called a caruncle but is not neoplastic and is often symptomless. 'Granulomatous' caruncle is often seen, while the true caruncle is uncommon. Treatment if needed is by cautery and there is a tendency to recurrence. Infection in this area must involve the paraurethral gland network and complete cure is difficult. A search should be made for a vaginal or bladder source of the infection.

DISEASES OF THE URETHRA

PROLAPSE of the URETHRAL MUCOSA

This forms a symmetrical swelling round the meatus and at first sight looks like a caruncle. If it causes symptoms the cautery should be applied. Larger prolapses must be excised.

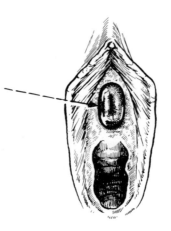

CYST of SKENE'S DUCT
(Paraurethral gland)

A firm cyst is palpated in the posterior wall of the urethra. It may be mistaken for a urethrocele, but it cannot be reduced by pressure. When it is being dissected out care must be taken not to create a urethral fistula.

URETHROCELE

This is a descent of the urethra from its position under the pubic arch. It is sometimes a cause of stress incontinence and may exist by itself or in company with a cystocele. Treatment is described in the section on prolapse.

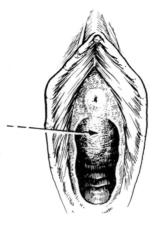

DISEASES OF THE URETHRA

CARCINOMA

This is a rare condition seen in elderly women. The tumour is a transitional or squamous cell epithelioma, and may arise in any part of the urethra.

Clinical Features   The patient complains of local pain, bleeding, dysuria. Inspection will reveal a tumour mass at the meatus, or if the growth is in the proximal urethra, a hard swelling in the vaginal wall. The inguinal glands may be enlarged by infection or metastases, but absence of swelling does not mean absence of spread since the urethra shares the lymphatic drainage of both vulva and bladder and the deep pelvic nodes may be the first affected.

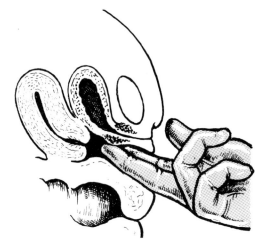

Always palpate
the whole urethra

Treatment

1. The disease is rare and experience of the results of different treatments is restricted.

2. The wide lymphatic drainage means that radical surgery should include removal of vulva, lymph nodes, bladder, uterus and vagina. Such mutilation is difficult to justify when it by no means guarantees a cure.

3. The tumour is not particularly radiosensitive, and large doses of irradiation are needed, which cause an unpleasant local reaction.

Probably the treatment of choice would be the insertion of radium needles round the urethra. This can be preceded by local excision (it is said that half the urethra may be removed without causing stress incontinence) and perhaps followed by lymphadenectomy.

Prognosis is poorer than for carcinoma of the vulva and depends very much on the stage of the disease and whether lymphatic spread has occurred.

OPERATIONS ON THE PERINEUM

1. Repair of Deficient Perineum

This condition is due to repeated stretching at parturition and repair is often done to complete an operation for prolapse. The perineal floor is only secondarily responsible for maintaining uterine position, and operation is really only necessary if the patient complains of discomfort or of unsatisfactory coitus.

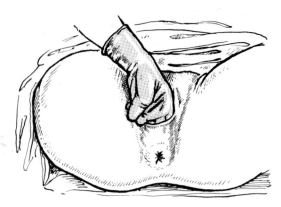

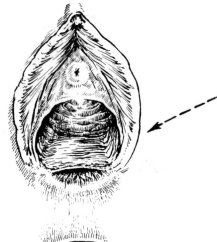

2. Repair of Complete Tear

The perineal body including anal sphincter and perhaps some rectal wall is completely torn through at parturition. The complaint is usually of faecal incontinence although the patient may be able to prevent this by using her levator ani muscles. Complete tears seen in gynaecological practice are usually the result of breakdown of a primary repair following delivery.

3. Enlargement of Vaginal Orifice

This is done by dividing the muscles of the perineal body, and it is required when the orifice is too small to allow intromission of the penis. The usual cause is stenosis following a perineal repair, but sometimes the patient may be an older woman with senile shrinkage or, very rarely, a young woman with a congenitally small orifice (see p.199).

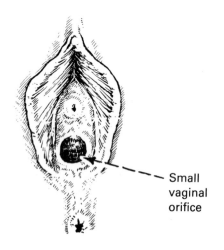

Small vaginal orifice

REPAIR OF DEFICIENT PERINEUM

The principle is mobilisation and removal of excess vaginal tissue and apposition of levator muscles adjacent to the perineal body.

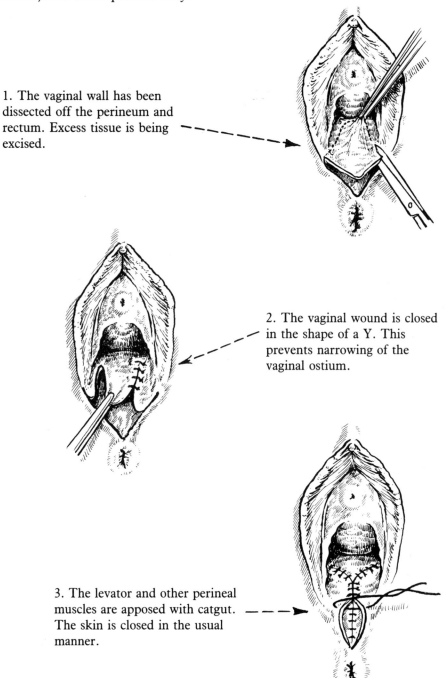

1. The vaginal wall has been dissected off the perineum and rectum. Excess tissue is being excised.

2. The vaginal wound is closed in the shape of a Y. This prevents narrowing of the vaginal ostium.

3. The levator and other perineal muscles are apposed with catgut. The skin is closed in the usual manner.

REPAIR OF COMPLETE TEAR

A complete tear of the perineum may occur at childbirth and the name implies that the anal sphincter has been completely disrupted. Such tears are normally repaired immediately, but if the primary repair breaks down 3 months should be allowed to elapse before attempting a secondary repair. If there has also been extensive damage to the recto-vaginal septum, and much infection, it may even be necessary to fashion a temporary colostomy to divert the faecal flow for a period to allow good healing.

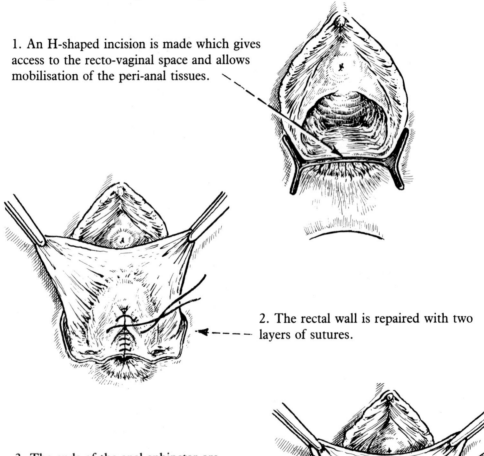

1. An H-shaped incision is made which gives access to the recto-vaginal space and allows mobilisation of the peri-anal tissues.

2. The rectal wall is repaired with two layers of sutures.

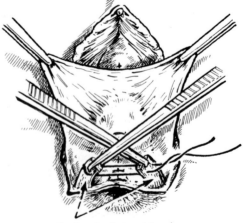

3. The ends of the anal sphincter are sutured together. (These are often difficult to identify.) The perineum is then repaired in the usual manner. After the operation the patient's bowels are confined for 4 days and then laxatives are given.

This sort of reconstituted perineal body looks well on completion but the late results are often disappointing especially in elderly women with atrophic muscles.

Ends of anal sphincter

OPERATION FOR ENLARGING THE VAGINAL OUTLET

PERINEOPLASTY

The principle is to divide all the fibres of the perineal body except the anal sphincter.

1. Making the longitudinal incision through skin and muscle. The finger in the rectum allows the surgeon to know how near his knife is to the rectal wall.

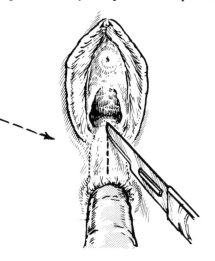

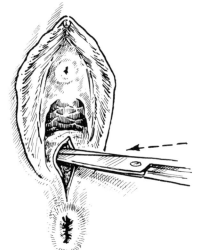

2. The cut muscles retract laterally, and the vaginal wall is further mobilised to allow closure without tension.

3. The longitudinal wound is then closed transversely with interrupted sutures.
   Vaginal dilators are used once the sutures are removed and continued with for several weeks until all tenderness is gone and coitus can be resumed.

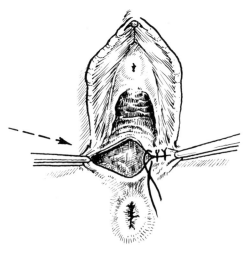

CHAPTER 9

DISEASES OF THE VAGINA

CYSTS OF THE VAGINA

Vaginal cysts are relatively common but rarely large. They are found in the anterior or lateral walls of the lower third of the vagina and in the posterior wall of the upper third, seldom larger than a walnut, sometimes multiple, and may be mistaken for a cystocele. These cysts are occasionally a cause of dyspareunia but usually cause no symptoms at all.

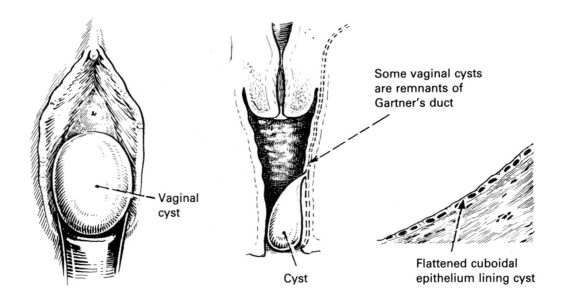

Vaginal cyst

Some vaginal cysts are remnants of Gartner's duct

Cyst

Flattened cuboidal epithelium lining cyst

Treatment is by excision or marsupialisation.

TRAUMATIC EPITHELIAL CYSTS (inclusion cysts) are found usually in the lower vagina, and are caused by infolding of epithelium at repair operations. If they cause symptoms they should be excised or marsupialised.

VAGINAL INFECTIONS

Vaginal infections are common and are dealt with in Chapter 7, 'GYNAECOLOGICAL INFECTIONS' (pages 144–161).

CARCINOMA OF THE VAGINA

Primary growths of the vagina are rare and the average gynaecologist will see only one such tumour for 30 of the cervix. Secondary growths are more common, especially extension from cervical cancer, and metastatic deposits may appear from disease elsewhere in the body.

Clinical Features

The patient is usually menopausal and complains of bleeding and discharge. If the bladder is involved, she will experience pain and dysuria.

The tumour is not at first painful and unless it appears in a woman who is still sexually active, it is not likely to present until it has penetrated the vaginal wall and caused bleeding. Old women often believe or affect to believe that all bleeding is from haemorrhoids.

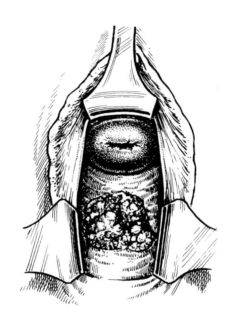

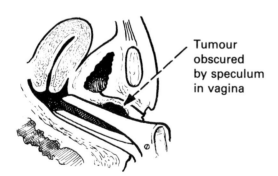

Tumour obscured by speculum in vagina

An early tumour can easily be missed if it is obscured by the blade of the speculum. The whole vagina should always be inspected, and cytological smears taken from any lesion at all unusual.

Histology

Eighty-five per cent are squamous carcinomas, occurring in women over 60. The remainder include melanoma, sarcoma, adenocarcinoma and clear cell carcinoma, all of which tend to be associated with middle-aged or even young women.

CARCINOMA OF THE VAGINA

Site and Spread

Tumours of the lower third have a much poorer prognosis than those of the upper and middle thirds, partly because spread to the inguinal nodes is quicker and because of the danger to the bladder.

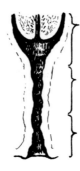

Upper third: approximately same drainage as cervix.

Middle third: any pelvic lymphatic channel may be involved.

Lower third: approximately same drainage as vulva.

Clinical Staging		Five Year Survival Rates
Stage 0	Intraepithelial carcinoma.	Should be curable with the use of colposcopy.
Stage I	Confined to the vaginal wall.	70–80%
Stage II	Invading subvaginal tissues.	30–40%
Stage III	Extension to the pelvic wall.	20–40%
Stage IV	Extension to other viscera.	0–30%

Prognosis depends on the stage, which depends on when the patient goes to her doctor, and on the position in the vagina. The lower third with its much quicker lymphatic spread is the least favourable.

Treatment   In stage 0 growths, good results have been obtained with local application of 5-fluorouracil cream, but for stage I onwards, radiotherapy is the usual treatment.
1. It can be applied at any stage.
2. It is more readily available than skilled radical surgery.
3. The patients are often elderly and poor surgical risks.

Radical surgery (radical hysterectomy, vaginectomy, lymphadenectomy) is claimed to give good results in experienced hands, and a cure rate of over 80% has been achieved for stage I. In stage IV where radiotherapy is only palliative, surgery which includes some form of exenteration is the better treatment if the patient is fit and the gynaecologist has the necessary experience.

In the past, stilboestrol was administered in pregnancy to women with a history of recurrent abortion. Female children of these pregnancies had an increased risk of developing vaginal adenosis and vaginal carcinoma in adolescence and early adult life.

PLASTIC SURGERY OF THE VAGINA

This is required when the patient is prevented from coitus by congenital absence of the vagina or by distortion and contractures due to injury. Such a situation is rare; but various operations have been devised.

The McIndoe-Bannister Operation – using a free skin graft from the thigh.

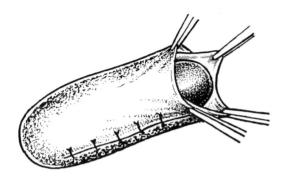

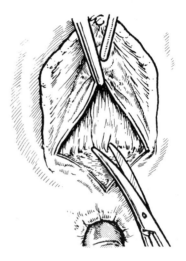

1. A plastic mould is covered with skin from the thigh. (This is done by a plastic surgeon.)

2. The space between urethra/bladder and rectum is opened up. The finger in the anus helps the surgeon to avoid damaging the rectum.

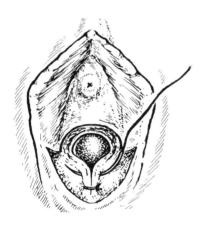

3. Mould and graft are inserted and kept in place by suturing the split ends of the labia minora. (The vaginal orifice may need enlarging later on.)

The mould must be kept in situ for several months and once it is removed the patient should have regular and frequent coitus to prevent contraction of the new vagina.

The main complications to be avoided are graft failure due to venous oozing or sepsis; and pressure necrosis of bladder or rectal wall from too large a mould.

PLASTIC SURGERY OF THE VAGINA

Williams' Operation

The formation of a cul-de-sac by suturing the labia majora in two layers. This means that the anterior wall of the new 'vagina' is the vulva. It is a simple operation which seems to provide a satisfying coitus for both parties.

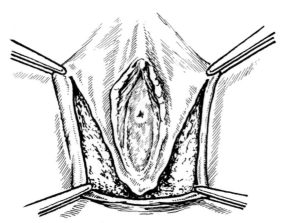

1. The labia majora are split down to the perineal muscles. Bleeding is free.

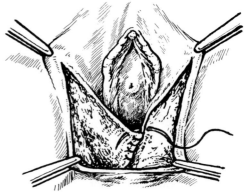

2. The inner margins of the labia are sutured together.

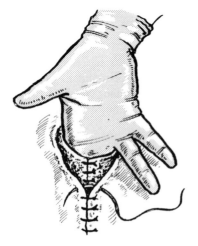

3. The outer margins are sutured. The resulting cavity should accommodate two fingers.

Other methods include the use of pedicle grafts from the labia, and encouraging natural epithelialisation of the dissected cavity without any grafting. There is sometimes a rudimentary vaginal depression already developed which can be enlarged to a functional size by using a pessary to maintain prolonged upward pressure.

CHAPTER 10

DISEASES OF THE CERVIX

CARCINOMA OF THE CERVIX

EPITHELIAL CHANGES

The cervix constitutes the lower third of the uterus.

It is in two parts: endocervical and vaginal or ectocervical. The dividing line is quite sharp and is determined by the character of the lining epithelium, which is clearly seen in the nulliparous patient around puberty.

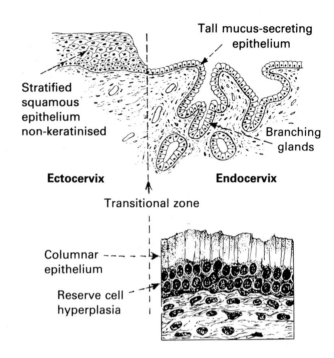

Stratified squamous epithelium non-keratinised

Tall mucus-secreting epithelium

Branching glands

Ectocervix   **Endocervix**

Transitional zone

Following puberty and with the beginning of sexual activity changes in the epithelium of the transitional zone appear. To begin with these are very mild, consisting of hyperplasia of reserve cells of the transitional zone. This may be a change induced by mild inflammatory reactions in the zone causing shedding of the columnar cells.

Columnar epithelium

Reserve cell hyperplasia

DYSPLASIA

This means a distinctive change in the type of epithelium. Initially the columnar mucus secreting epithelium of the transitional zone disappears and is replaced by squamous epithelium. This is a metaplastic change as distinct from true dysplasia. Metaplasia is a simple condition.

Benign squamous metaplasia
Stratification well defined with:

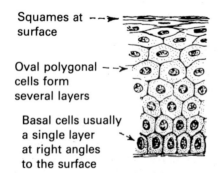

Squames at surface

Oval polygonal cells form several layers

Basal cells usually a single layer at right angles to the surface

In some cases the squamous epithelium shows a degree of proliferative activity with some cellular atypia. This is DYSPLASIA. It is regarded as the first of a series of changes which may lead to **cervical intra-epithelial neoplasia (CIN)** and subsequently to invasive carcinoma.

CIN 1 ≡ mild dysplasia

Upper two thirds stratified squames i.e. normal

Cells of basal third have high nucleocytoplasmic ratio; pleomorphic nuclei in layers at this level

CARCINOMA OF THE CERVIX

DYSPLASIA (cont)

The dysplastic change has been divided into 3 stages indicating increasing degrees of abnormality and nuclear activity, but in practice it is impossible to provide strict rules which will give a guide to classification of individual cases. All degrees of change are seen and the stages merge one into the other. Grading must lie with the individual pathologist.

CIN 2 ≡ moderate dysplasia

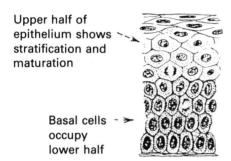

Upper half of epithelium shows stratification and maturation

Basal cells occupy lower half

From a diagnostic and prognostic point of view the position is made very difficult by the fact that the dysplastic change is not inevitably progressive. It is reckoned that 50% of dysplastic lesions disappear without treatment. However it is impossible to differentiate those which will do this from those which are destined to progress and therefore all dysplastic lesions require treatment.

CIN 3 ≡ severe dysplasia or CIN

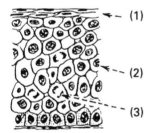

(1) There may be one or two layers of stratified epithelium on surface.

(2) Remainder is immature with large nuclei.

(3) Mitoses are common.

No attempt is made to differentiate between CIN 3 and carcinoma in situ (i.e. carcinoma which is contained within the superficial epithelial layer and shows no sign of invasion of the underlying stroma).

The changes creep over the cervical surface.

Classical CIN

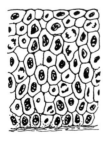

(1) Almost complete loss of stratification.
(2) Loss of polarity of the cells, the majority being at right angles to the surface; the remainder irregularly arranged.
(3) Variation in nuclear size with increase in nuclear/cytoplasmic ratio.
(4) Cells lose their squamous appearance.
(5) Mitotic figures found at all levels.

This is the final stage of the intra-epithelial lesion prior to invasion of the subjacent tissue. It is reckoned that only 10% of dysplastic lesions reach this phase but it is impossible to say which are the 10%. 2% of the total number of dysplasias progress beyond this intra-epithelial carcinoma to frank invasive cancer. The time scale appears to be long. It takes 10 years for the first signs of dysplasia to be converted into carcinoma in situ.

CARCINOMA OF THE CERVIX

Diagnosis of CIN

This is made in the first instance by examining smears of cells from the surface of the ectocervix. Care must be taken in making these smears. The abnormal epithelium, especially in CIN 3, is loosely attached to the underlying stroma and may be removed by over-vigorous preliminary swabbing, leading to misdiagnosis.

Most cases of advanced dysplasia are discovered in women around the age of 40 but the span extends from age 30 to 70 plus. This may be a true change in epidemiology or partly a result of the campaign to encourage all women to have a smear test.

The **CERVICAL SMEAR** is an out-patient procedure. The most consistent results are obtained by using an Ayre's spatula.

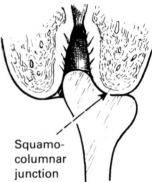

Place a speculum in the vagina to make the cervix visible. Put the larger rounded projection of the spatula in the cervical canal and rotate in a circle scraping the squamo-columnar junction.

The material obtained is smeared on slides, fixed in equal parts of 95% ethyl alcohol and ether, and stained by Papanicolou's method. The stains are (1) haematoxylin, to stain nuclei, (2) orange G and (3) a mixture of Bismark-brown, eosin yellowish and light green. Stains 2 and 3 are cytoplasmic stains. Mature cells take up orange G and eosin, immature cells the light green.

Squamo-columnar junction

When to take a cervical smear: The arguments on which cervical smear screening is based include two assumptions which are almost facts.
1.   An invasive cancer can be detected in its early precancerous stage, and destroyed by excision.
2.   The length of the precancerous stage extends to more than 10 years.

When to begin taking cervical smears: There is at present no agreed pattern of screening.

YES carcinoma of the cervix is related to sexual intercourse and screening should begin at the same time as sexual activity. At the present day this means about 18.

–   BUT there is nothing to be gained by treating positive smears early, especially as spontaneous regression to normal may occur in young women. The greatest number of changes from normal to CIN are detected in the age group 25–29.

Young women need to be accustomed to the idea of screening, and this is best done when they seek advice for some gynaecological condition, contraception or pregnancy. Women at present dying of cervical cancer are still, in the main, those who have never had a cervical smear.

–   BUT invasive cancer is a disease of the middle years, and intensive routine screening should be concentrated in the years 25–35.

When to stop taking cervical smears: The death rate from cervical cancer continues into old age, and there is no clinical reason why screening should ever stop until the patient no longer wants the service. A first smear should always be taken from any sexually active woman however young or old she may be.

How often to take a smear: For women who have previously been found normal, an interval of about 3 years is probably adequate. In the age group 35–45 a one year interval is advisable, to guard against false-negative smears.

CERVICAL SMEARS

INTERPRETATION of CERVICAL SMEARS Smears are reported in 3 categories:

1. **Negative** No signs of CIN

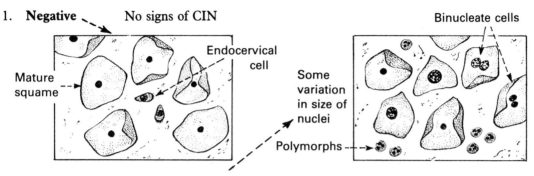

2. **Suspicious**: (doubtful, atypical, dyskaryotic). This means that some degree of cellular atypia is present (CIN 1), which may revert to normal.

3. **Positive**: Grossly abnormal cells are present, indicating the likelihood of a malignant process (CIN 2 or CIN 3).

In CIN 2 the smear shows a mixture of normal and dyskaryotic (abnormal nuclei) cells.

In CIN 3 the cells are almost all abnormal and show larger nuclei with coarse chromatin.

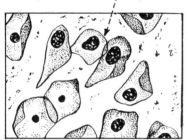

It is generally impossible to differentiate between CIN 2 and CIN 3 in smears, and histological examination of a biopsy is required.

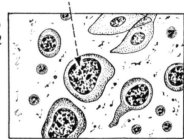

Repeat smears are required if appearances are obscured by inflammatory changes or if the results are inconclusive. It is also advisable in one particular instance: if there is evidence of infection by human papilloma virus. This virus (HPV) induces a distinctive change in the epithelial cells.

The cells are termed koilocytes. Often binucleate they have a large perinuclear halo and the cytoplasm is condensed at the periphery.

The smear should be repeated after 4 months even if these koilocytes show no evidence of dyskaryosis.

The average results in any smear test clinic are likely to be:

Normal 90%	HPV or CIN1 . . . . 3–5%
Inflammatory or unsatisfactory 3–5%	CIN2 or CIN3 . . . . 1–3%

It must be emphasised that dysplastic changes in the cervical epithelium do not of themselves produce any clinical signs or symptoms.

If dyskaryosis exists, further help can be obtained by the use of the colposcope.

COLPOSCOPY

Colposcopy means binocular inspection of the cervix with a magnification of up to 20 times.

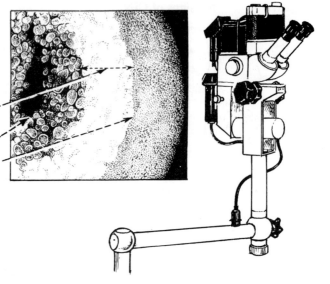

The colposcopist recognises two kinds of epithelium, the 'native' which may be squamous or columnar; and the metaplastic squamous epithelium which arises in the physiological transformation zone.

The transformation zone lies between the cervical canal and the squamo-columnar junction.

At birth it is covered by columnar epithelium, and at three stages, coinciding with maximum oestrogen stimulation – the perinatal period, the menarche, and the first pregnancy – it is particularly liable to squamous metaplasia, which may proceed to dysplasia.

Atypical epithelium

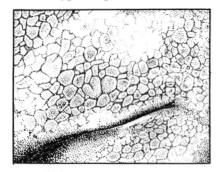

Mosaic appearance

Prior to examination with the colposcope the cervix is swabbed with acetic acid. Any focus of increased cellularity becomes white in colour indicating the areas requiring close attention.

Atypical epithelium may have a mosaic or tiled appearance because of the arrangement of the epithelial capillaries.

An experienced colposcopist can detect suspicious areas with great accuracy and take multiple punch biopsies without trauma.

TREATMENT OF CIN

Conservative treatment is indicated in younger women and in CIN 1.

CRYOSURGERY

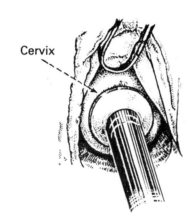

Cervix

This allows destruction of affected tissue to a depth of 3mm. It is quick and sufficiently painless to be used in the conscious patient.

DIATHERMY

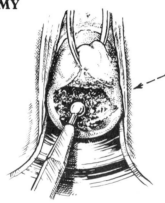

Diathermy under general anaesthesia will destroy tissue to a depth of 7–8mm.

CO$_2$ LASER

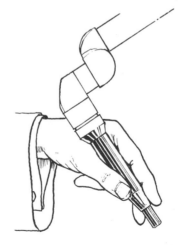

This instrument emits very powerful electromagnetic radiations which vaporise tissue to a depth of 7–9 mm. It can be used with great precision and causes very little trauma. The diameter of the laser beam at its focal point is 1.8 mm.

CONE BIOPSY by itself will deal adequately with about 90% of CIN lesions, but patients so treated must have a cytological follow-up for life.

HYSTERECTOMY is indicated for the woman over 40 who has persistently positive smears in spite of conservative treatment, and when the colposcope cannot reliably inspect the whole of the dysplastic area.

It should be remembered that if smears are positive after ablation of the lesion there is a 25-fold increase in the risk of developing invasive cancer.

CONE BIOPSY OF THE CERVIX

This means removal of a cone of cervical tissue along with most of the cervical canal. It is required when a cervical smear repeatedly shows malignant or dyskaryotic cells and when colposcopically directed biopsy is unsatisfactory. (Minor degrees of dysplasia can revert to normal.)

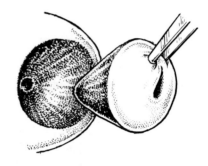

Advantages

1. It allows histological differentiation between invasive, micro-invasive and intra-epithelial disease.

2. In 90% of cases it is curative, removing all the affected tissue.

Disadvantages

1. A fairly high rate of immediate complications – haemorrhage, infection, cervical stenosis.

2. A tendency to spontaneous abortion in subsequent pregnancies.

A preliminary colposcopic inspection is preferable. The colposcopist identifies the limits of the lesion, and the subsequent biopsy tends to be smaller and less traumatic.

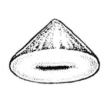

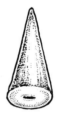

Cryo-cautery may be employed after cone biopsy to arrest bleeding.

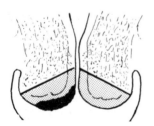

Childbearing age.

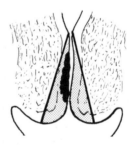

Post childbearing.

If colposcopy is not available, the considerations affecting the size of the biopsy may be modified by age and future childbearing intentions of the patient.

MICRO-INVASIVE CARCINOMA

Stage 1a

This is the stage between CIN 3 and clinical invasive carcinoma. It is characterised by the spread of malignant cells through the basement membrane to a depth of 3mm.

Degree of Malignancy

This depends on three histological factors:-
1. Depth of invasion below the basement membrane, and the width of the 'front' along which the carcinoma is advancing.
2. Invasion of lymphatic and capillary channels (capillary-like or CL involvement).
3. A staghorn pattern of advancing growth.

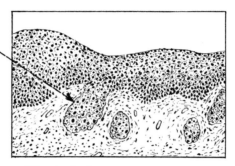

Histological assessment requires a good deal of experience. The diagnosis is entirely histological but colposcopists claim to be able to identify likely areas of micro-invasiveness with considerable accuracy.

Treatment

Most gynaecologists regard simple hysterectomy with a 1cm cuff of vagina as adequate, but more radical treatment may be required if the degree of invasion is more than minimal. It must be remembered that micro- or not, it is invading.

CIN DURING PREGNANCY

When persistently abnormal smears are obtained during pregnancy further investigation is hindered by the danger of severe haemorrhage associated with cone biopsy during pregnancy, and indeed such an operation should probably never be done. The bleeding is such that hysterectomy has, on occasion, been necessary, and there is a considerable risk of abortion.

Colposcopy is now regarded as a reliable method of screening. Difficulty arises when micro-invasion is suspected, and in such cases a wedge biopsy may be required.

CIN 3 is not affected by the pregnancy and further investigation and treatment may be delayed. If micro-invasive carcinoma is diagnosed, abortion should be advised.

CARCINOMA OF THE UTERINE CERVIX

This is said to be the most common malignant tumour of the female genital tract, but the incidence varies from country to country and appears to be significantly reduced where there is a vigorous campaign for early diagnosis and eradication of carcinoma in situ.

The growth is a squamous cell carcinoma in 95% of cases, the remaining 5% being adenocarcinomas. The site of the growth has no relationship to the histological type. It usually arises at the squamo-columnar junction. 20% of squamous carcinomas are found within the cervical canal, and occasionally an adenocarcinoma originates in the glands near the external os.

The cervix becomes very indurated; necrosis and ulceration commonly follow quickly.

Later, a large fungating mass is produced. Sloughing may leave an excavated crater.

The tumour may form a proliferating growth which pro-trudes into the vagina – a 'cauliflower', 'exophytic', 'everting' growth. This type bleeds easily and soon becomes ulcerated.

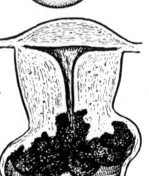

Sometimes the spread is in the substance of the cervix – 'excavating', 'endophytic', 'inverting' growth. The cervix becomes stony hard and enlarged – the 'barrel-shaped' cervix.

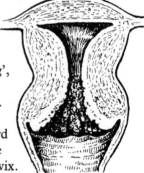

Histology of Squamous cell carcinoma

The appearances are typical, but cell nests are absent and keratinisation is rarely seen.

As stated above, the growth is almost always a squamous celled carcinoma but the cell morphology varies. Three main types of cell are described.

1. Plate-like with distinct cell borders resembling adult squames.

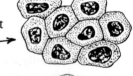

Central cells ovoid and obviously of squamous type

Peripheral cells cuboidal

2. Transitional cells. Similar to 1 but smaller.

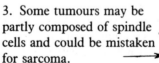

3. Some tumours may be partly composed of spindle cells and could be mistaken for sarcoma.

CARCINOMA OF THE CERVIX

ADENOCARCINOMA

This uncommon form of cervical malignancy usually arises from the columnar epithelium of the endocervix but in some cases it apparently takes origin from the ectocervix. While the latter may occasionally be true it must be remembered that most cases of cervical carcinoma are discovered when the disease is fairly advanced and sites of origin are questionable.

The most important point is that the histological type of lesion does not appear to alter the behaviour or spread of the tumour. With advances in chemotherapy and immunotherapy differences in tumour reaction related to histological types may become apparent.

The appearances in this form are typical of adenocarcinoma in other organs.

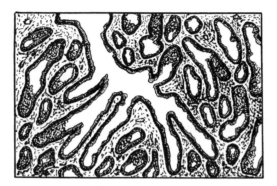

Low power. Tubular processes spread out from the lumina of the glands. The characteristic pattern is an aggressive adenomatous formation with very little fibrous stroma.

Many indeterminate patterns are seen on microscopic examination. Sometimes both glandular and squamous malignant cells appear together – adenocanthoma – and squamous metaplasia is common.

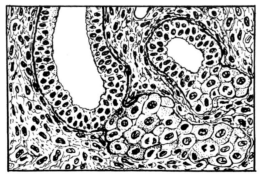

High power appearance of squamous epithelium which appears to originate by metaplasia from columnar epithelium.

CARCINOMA OF THE CERVIX

Aetiology

Two facts related to this disease have been recognised for a very long time.

1. Age at first coitus. The younger the individual the more likely is cancer to develop.
2. Multiplicity of sexual partners. The disease is common among prostitutes. It rarely if ever occurs in virgins e.g. nuns.

From these observations arose the idea that cancer of the cervix might be due to some factor or factors transmitted from male to female during the sexual act.

Recently, attention has been focused on viruses, two varieties in particular, Human papilloma virus (HPV) types 16, 18 and 31, and Herpes simplex virus (HS) type 2. Both of these viruses are extremely common in the female genital tract. Epithelial cells infected with HPV viruses, koilocytes, are easily recognised (see page 211) and are found in 80% of cases of dysplasia. Antibodies to both of these viruses are found in the sera of cancer patients, the concentration being 10 times that in control patients. Cells of all types of severe dysplasia and invasive cancer show integration of viral genomes into the cellular DNA. One of the effects of this is the inactivation of a cellular protein which controls cell proliferation. Experimental infection of animal cells grown in vitro with these viruses induces permanent transformation of the cells so that when re-introduced into the host animal tumour growth results.

All of these observations are strong evidence that these viruses are implicated in the development of cervical cancer.

There are however some facts which seem to indicate that this is not the whole story. The time span appears excessive – 10 years to reach carcinoma in situ and a further number of years before invasion occurs during which time many of the lesions disappear. Secondly, the incidence of viral infection in a population is so great that by comparison the occurrence of cancer of the cervix is a rare event. These two aspects of the disease tend to suggest the possible existence of a co-carcinogen. This may be an intrinsic factor such as alteration of immune reactions, or some mechanism which determines whether the viruses are allowed to express their activities fully. These and other possible co-factors still require investigation.

CARCINOMA OF THE CERVIX

Spread

Direct spread into adjacent tissues usually occurs first. Involvement of the corpus uteri may cause pyometra. Further spread to the parametrium induces the same signs and symptoms as chronic pelvic inflammation.

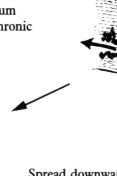

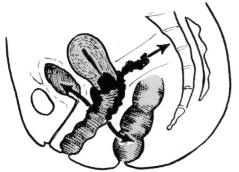

Spread downwards into the vaginal wall inevitably involves bladder or rectum causing fistulae. Backwards spread along the uterosacral ligaments leads to involvement of the sacral plexus causing intractable sciatic pain.

Lymphatic spread usually follows but may precede direct spread.

From the cervical lymphatics the spread is usually along the paracervical lymph tract to the external iliac nodes. Occasionally the extension is backwards to the internal iliac group.

Blood borne spread is exceptional.

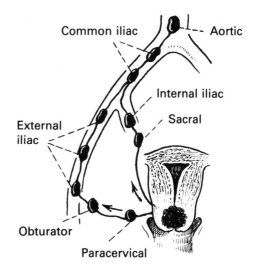

Symptoms

1. Irregular bleeding is one of the first complaints, either post-menopausal or post-coital. It is not often due to carcinoma but the possibility must be kept in mind.
2. Infection. The growth is soon infected from the vagina and a foul discharge is common.
3. Pain. This is due to spread of the growth to the pelvic cavity and is a late sign.
4. Cachexia occurs in advanced cases due to prolonged infection. There is mild but persistent fever, weight loss and anaemia.

219

CARCINOMA OF THE CERVIX

Signs

Inspection and Bimanual Examination

Early Stage

In this phase malignancy is not obvious and for a considerable time the tumour may feel and look like a simple ectropion even when moderately developed.

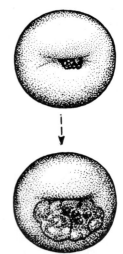

Moderately developed

It may still resemble an advanced inflammatory ectropion.

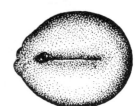

Even less conspicuous is an endocervical growth which in the early stages may be neither seen nor felt. Later, as it infiltrates, the cervix becomes barrel-shaped but the external os may still appear normal.

Later stages

The cervix becomes stony hard. It is fixed by the infiltration of the vaginal fornices. The surface of the growth is friable and bleeds on touch.

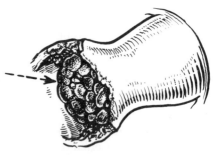

DIFFERENTIAL DIAGNOSIS OF CERVICAL CARCINOMA

Biopsy is necessary for histological confirmation, but in very few cases is there any doubt. If the growth is early, some normal tissue should be removed as well, and a diagram provided to show the pathologist where the biopsy was taken. It should be no bigger than necessary and cone biopsy is not done in the presence of naked eye evidence of malignant growth. Curettage should also be done if the external os is accessible.

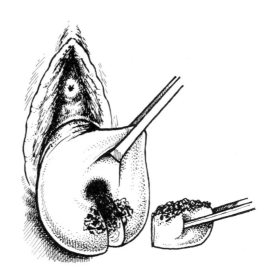

Very occasionally what appears to be a definitely malignant lesion turns out to be benign.

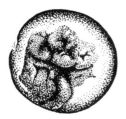

Cervicitis with ectopy is the commonest cervical lesion and if florid can be most misleading.

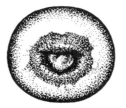

Mucous cervical polyps when infected can present a very suspicious appearance. (But all polyps require examination.)

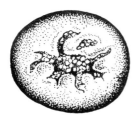

Tuberculosis is rare in the cervix. There is nearly always a history of genital tuberculosis.

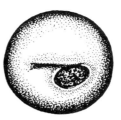

A **primary chancre** can appear in the cervix: ulcerated hard and indurated. In the United Kingdom it is rare.

221

CLINICAL STAGING OF CERVICAL CARCINOMA

Each growth is allocated to a stage according to the extent of spread.

Stage O   CIN 3
(Carcinoma-in-situ)

Stage Ia
Micro-invasive carcinoma not extending more than 3mm beyond the basement membrane and not invading capillary or lymphatic channels.

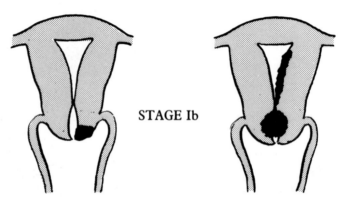

STAGE Ib

Stage 1b The growth is confined to the cervix or uterus. (This includes 'histological finds' not detected clinically.)

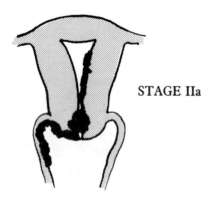

STAGE IIa

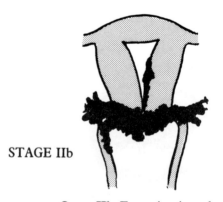

STAGE IIb

Stage IIa Extension to the vagina not beyond the upper two thirds.

Stage IIb Extension into the parametrium but not as far as the pelvic walls.

CLINICAL STAGING OF CERVICAL CARCINOMA

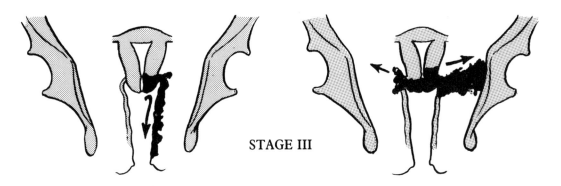

STAGE III

Stage III Extension to lower third of vagina or to pelvic wall.

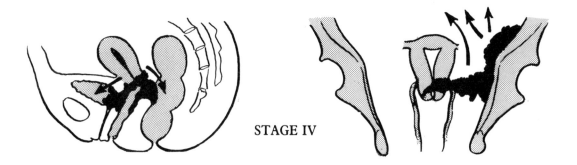

STAGE IV

Stage IV Extension through vagina into bladder or outside pelvis.

Classification is made after vaginal and rectal examination followed by cystoscopy and sigmoidoscopy when indicated, and doubtful cases are placed in the less advanced stage. There are two serious sources of error:

1. It is impossible to distinguish between malignant and inflammatory thickening in an indurated parametrium.

2. Pelvic lymph nodes can be invaded without being enlarged. The incidence of this is put at:

       Stage I, 15%   Stage II, 30%   Stage III, 45%

Surgeons who practise radical surgical treatment also classify their cases according to the 'percentage operability' of the total number of patients seen.

TREATMENT OF EARLY CERVICAL CARCINOMA

There is a high success rate in the treatment of the disease but survival depends mainly on three factors:

1. Early diagnosis.
2. Non-involvement of the lymphatics and lymph nodes.
3. Treatment should only be undertaken in oncology centres staffed by persons with extensive experience of malignant conditions and equipped to the highest standards. There is no place for a casual one-off approach.

Unfortunately, diagnosis at what appears to be an early phase i.e. clinical stages Ib and IIa cannot always be guaranteed. Lymphatic spread may have already occurred but been undiscovered due to an unusual route taken by the growth.

The choice of treatment lies between surgery i.e. hysterectomy and radiotherapy. Statistics show that in early stages, Ib and IIa, the results are equally favourable whichever mode of treatment is employed. In the United Kingdom radiotherapy is the more favoured but each has its advantages and disadvantages.

Before attempting treatment there are commonly pre-existing complications which must be treated – anaemia and sepsis. If surgery is contemplated anaemia could lead to shock since bleeding may be a problem during the operation. In the case of radiotherapy, the anaemia may cause the growth to be relatively anoxic. This results in radioresistance. The dose of radiation has to be increased, leading to possible damage to the normal tissues with post-radiation complications.

Sepsis is commonly present in the malignant cervix and difficult to eradicate. If it cannot be eliminated locally, antibiotic cover must be provided to prevent post-traumatic spread.

RADIOTHERAPY

Various machines, substances and techniques are employed according to circumstances: X-rays in accelerated form for external radiation using a Betatron, radium and artificial isotopes such as Cobalt 60, Caesium 137 and others for internal application to the growth. Techniques are constantly being improved. The bowel is very sensitive to irradiation and rectal necrosis and fistula used to be notorious complications but are now rare. The incidence of fistula is now no more than 1% and is almost entirely confined to Clinical Stages III and IV.

PREPARATION FOR RADIOTHERAPY

Physical

1. Anaemia must be corrected. A low haemoglobin level increases the anoxia of the growth and renders it less radiosensitive.

2. Local infection must be treated and a pyosalpinx may have to be removed surgically.

3. Renal function must be assessed, and intravenous pyelography is required to exclude involvement of the ureter.

4. X-ray scanning of the bony pelvis is carried out to exclude metastases, although these are rare in early cervical carcinoma.

Survival Rates (all stages)	
5 yrs	41%
10 yrs	28%
15 yrs	18%
20 yrs	11%

Compare the above results with those for Stages Ib and IIa

5 year survival rate	
Stage Ib	>80%
Stage IIa	>60%

Psychological

'Cancer' is still a fearful word; but the patient receiving radiotherapy is very likely to learn that cancer is her disease, and she should be prepared for this revelation.

The two routes of radiation should be described, and the patient told that she has a growth well within the curative power of modern radiotherapy. She should know what side effects may occur during treatment, and how long she will be in hospital. The patient who is sexually active, whatever her age, will have to be assured that coitus will still be feasible, and that although there will be no more periods she will be given hormone replacement therapy which will save her from the other effects of the loss of ovarian function.

Although radiotherapy will be in the hands of the expert oncological therapist, the gynaecologist should take part in the discussions regarding the therapy and should also be present when explanations to the patient are required. The first will inform the gynaecologist who may be called upon to deal with the after-effects of treatment. The second will give the patient added confidence in the presence of one who is already familiar to her.

COMPLICATIONS OF RADIOTHERAPY

EARLY

1. **Difficulties during insertion of radium or caesium**

Sometimes the cervical canal is not accessible or the fornices are so distorted by tumour that the proper vaginal application cannot be made. Technique must be adapted to the individual.

2. **Pyrexia**

Septic areas in a large growth can never be completely eradicated before treatment, and antibiotic cover must be given. If symptoms and signs of peritonitis appear, treatment must be suspended.

3. **Vagina**

A whitish membrane is seen to cover the vagina for a few weeks.

4. **Bladder**

Some irritation of the bladder base is inevitable and frequency and dysuria will be complained of.

5. **Rectum**

Proctitis – diarrhoea, tenesmus, sometimes bleeding is common and may take several months to disappear. Treatment is symptomatic by chalk and opium mixtures and steroid pessaries.

The intestines are equally sensitive and their reaction is manifested by nausea and perhaps diarrhoea.

LATE

1. **Genital Tract**

Ovarian function is destroyed and hormone therapy may be needed. The uterus becomes fibrotic and pyometra may develop. Some degree of vaginal atrophy is usual, although often slight, and subsequent sexual activity really depends on the age of the patient.

2. **Urinary Tract**

The incidence of vesico-vaginal fistula is less than 1% and fistula if it is going to develop will do so within 2 years.

3. **Alimentary Tract**

Intestino-vaginal fistula may occur especially if previous surgery has left adhesions between bowel and Pouch of Douglas. Rectal damage – ulceration, stenosis, fistula – is as rare as urinary fistula.

4. **Pelvic Skeleton**

The risk of avascular necrosis and spontaneous fracture of the neck of the femur has become very small with the development of modern megavoltage apparatus. A patient with this complication is likely to have had her treatment at least 25 years before.

5. **Skin Reactions**

Sometimes a degree of subcutaneous fibrosis may be observed a year or so after treatment.

INDICATIONS FOR SURGERY

Because of the availability and relative efficacy of radiotherapy with its very low risk, it has become necessary to justify recourse to surgery. It can be offered as the sole treatment or as an attempt to improve the results of radiotherapy, but whatever the basis the following conditions should prevail.

1. The gynaecologist must be particularly skilled and experienced in radical surgery and be working in a hospital which supplies high standards of clinical and laboratory support.
2. The patient must be a 'suitable subject' – in good general health, not too fat, not too old.
3. The growth must be 'operable' – not fixed to the pelvic wall. Operability is finally assessed by the surgeon once the abdomen is opened. This is a personal judgement and is not necessarily the same as the radiotherapist's staging.
4. The patient should be provided with enough information to allow her to choose between surgery and radiation. If she is sexually active she should know that radical surgery includes excision of the vagina.

For some patients, an operation of some sort must be done. These are (a) those in whom the growth has been proved to be radioresistant: and (b) those in whom the growth has invaded the bladder or rectum.

COMBINED RADIOTHERAPY AND SURGERY

There is no completely reliable method of extirpating cancer cells which have passed into the pelvic lymphatics and there is therefore a theoretical advantage to be gained in following radiotherapy with surgery, either a radical hysterectomy and lymphadenectomy, or a lymphadenectomy alone. Some very successful results have been reported; but the survival rates achieved are not so evidently superior as to place combined treatment beyond controversy.

1. The early case does very well with either treatment, and it may be difficult for the gynaecologist to convince both himself and his patient that a mutilating and dangerous operation is going to make more than a statistically marginal difference to her chance of survival.
2. It is known that pelvic nodes removed after irradiation often contain apparently unaffected cancer cells; although the primary should be destroyed. A regional lymphadenectomy without hysterectomy does seem a sensible supplementary treatment; but the operation has its risks of haemorrhage and thrombosis and is performed unnecessarily if the nodes turn out to be unaffected.
3. Radiotherapy requires a good blood supply to the tumour and tumour bed if it is to have its maximum effect, so the irradiation should be given first. This creates more difficulty for the surgeon who must operate on more fibrotic and avascular tissue with an inevitably greater chance of producing a ureteric fistula. It is usual in the United Kingdom, if combined treatment is being given, to omit the external radiation and operate about 4 weeks after the radium treatment when the increased vascularity has regressed and fibrosis is still minimal.

SCHEME OF TREATMENT OF CERVICAL CARCINOMA

1. It is now accepted that the best results will be obtained if all patients are treated in centres which specialise in the work and are staffed by radiotherapists and gynaecologists working in close co-operation.

2. Since both forms of treatment give equal results in favourable cases, adherence to one or other form becomes a matter of preference or prejudice. In the United Kingdom the average radiologist is more experienced in irradiation techniques than is the average gynaecologist in radical surgery.

Stage I   Radiotherapy.

Stage II   Radiotherapy alone or followed by surgery. (The nodes are more likely to be involved.)

Stage III   Radiotherapy alone or followed by surgery.

Stage IV   Radiotherapy alone if distant metastases are present. Pelvic exenteration if bladder or rectum is invaded.

CARCINOMA OF THE CERVICAL STUMP

Cervical carcinoma appearing after subtotal hysterectomy is called 'stump carcinoma' and is now a rare occurrence. Its treatment was formerly a subject of controversy; the absent corpus reduced the possible dosage of intracavity radium, and radical surgery was made more difficult by the pelvic fibrosis and adhesions between bladder, cervical stump and rectum. It is now recognised that treatment by modern radiotherapy offers much the same chance of cure as when the uterus is intact.

TREATMENT OF CERVICAL CANCER

ADVANTAGES OF RADIOTHERAPY
1. It eliminates the need for surgical procedures which are always alarming to the patient.
2. Residual after-effects tend to be less than those following surgical treatment.
3. Radiotherapy reduces the size of a large tumour, making surgery possible.
4. There is no mortality directly attributable to radiotherapeutic treatment.
5. Although ovarian function is inevitably destroyed by radiotherapy, coital function is preserved.

ADVANTAGES OF SURGICAL TREATMENT
1. Ovarian and coital function can in many cases be preserved.
2. Surgical treatment exposes the whole lesion allowing accurate staging of the disease including lymphatic spread.
3. If major complications follow radiotherapy they are difficult to treat because of the effects of radiation on the tissues.

ADVANCED STAGES OF CERVICAL CANCER
In Stages III and IV neither surgery nor radiotherapy offers real hope of cure. Only 30% of Stage III patients survive beyond 5 years and in Stage IV the percentage drops to 8%. Routine has no place in the treatment of these patients. Each is approached on an individual basis and treatment tailored to the circumstances. In a proportion of these patients the advance of the disease is related to radioresistance. Techniques have been tried to overcome this difficulty.

1. **Fractionation of Radiation Dosage**
   After the first dose of radiation the tumour begins to shrink, demand for oxygen is reduced and the flow and distribution of blood improves. The previously hypoxic cells then become sensitive to the next dose of radiation.

2. **Hyperbaric Oxygen**
   A multicentre randomised trial has shown a slight but definite advantage. Oxygen tents or pressure chambers mean that patients must spend longer periods under treatment. There are also side-effects such as earache, sinus pain, oxygen convulsions and claustrophobia.

3. **Chemical Sensitisers**
   These drugs mimic the sensitising effect of oxygen. Many compounds are successful in vitro, including nitrofurantoin (Furadantin), metronidazole (Flagyl) and the more active misonidazole which is neurotoxic. These chemicals are still the subject of clinical trial.

4. **Neutron Therapy**
   The effect of radiation depends on the energy of the bombarding wave or particle and that in turn is a reflection of their speed. Even if accelerated greatly they produce only a low degree of ionisation in the tissues. More recently it was found that neutrons, previously ignored as useless, could be accelerated and used clinically. The interaction was such that radioresistance no longer existed. Fast neutron therapy has caused disappearance of tumours hitherto regarded as untreatable.

The aims in advanced cancer must be to prolong life and, even more importantly, to prevent suffering. The wishes of the patient should be considered very much and nursing care is extremely important.

OPERATIONS FOR CERVICAL CARCINOMA

The best known consists of removal of the uterus and adnexa, most of the vagina and the fatty-fibrous tissue which 'pads' the pelvis and contains the lymph glands. This is known as the 'Wertheim hysterectomy' (although the original operation of Wertheim (1900) was less extensive).

The broad ligament is opened up and the ureter dissected off uterus and cervix. This is usually made difficult by the presence of inflammation.

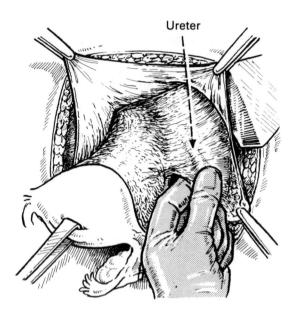

The ureter is being identified by palpation.

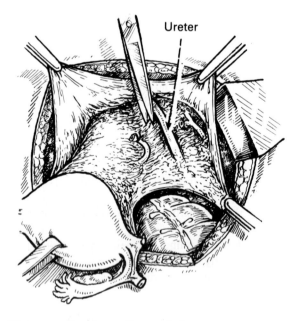

The ureter has been dissected clear down to the bladder and the uterine vessels divided.

The ureter can always be identified in the false pelvis and followed downwards, but dissection in the parametrium is difficult especially if the growth has infiltrated (stage II growth). The ureter has to be mobilised to protect it, but the more thorough the surgeon is, the greater the possibility of damage to the ureter's blood supply and development of fistula due to avascular necrosis.

RADICAL HYSTERECTOMY

After removal of the uterus the vaginal stump is usually closed, but sometimes a drain is required because of oozing.

In this description the hysterectomy is shown first, to be followed by the lymphadenectomy; but many surgeons carry out a 'block dissection' removing pelvic nodes and fat and then the uterus and vagina all in one piece. The essential end-result is to clear the pelvis down to the muscle fascia, leaving only vessels, nerves and the rectum and bladder.

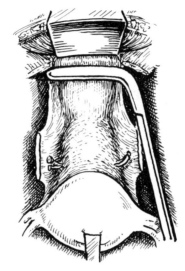

The vagina is severed below the special Wertheim clamp.

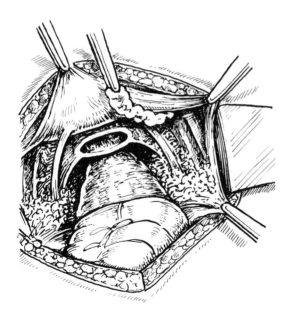

Dissecting out the fatty tissue and glands from the obturator fossa.

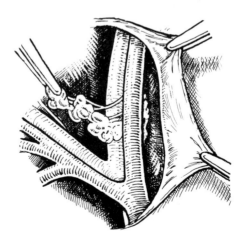

Dissecting out the external iliac glands. (Other accessible groups of nodes are also removed.)

231

RADICAL VAGINAL HYSTERECTOMY

An extended vaginal hysterectomy can also be done. It is known as Schauta's operation; and because of its technical difficulties and the impossibility of gland dissection by the vaginal route, it is little practised in this country. Those few surgeons who have experience of it report good results, although not better than abdominal surgery or radiotherapy.

SCHAUTA'S OPERATION

The object is to remove ovaries, tubes, uterus and vagina through the vulva.

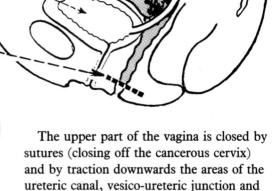

The vagina is circumcised, i.e. a circular incision is made right round the vaginal wall.

The upper part of the vagina is closed by sutures (closing off the cancerous cervix) and by traction downwards the areas of the ureteric canal, vesico-ureteric junction and posteriorly, the uterosacral ligaments become available for dissection. This is a difficult surgical exercise and may be accompanied by troublesome haemorrhage.

Site of dissection of ureter

Site of dissection of rectum and uterosacral ligament

Upper cuff of vagina closed and suture used as retractor

When the vagina with its contained cervix has been mobilised from bowel, bladder and ureter, the vesico-uterine pouch is opened and the uterine fundus pulled down to expose the adnexal ligaments for division. This allows removal of the whole genital tract other than the lower third of the vagina, and the operation area can now be closed.

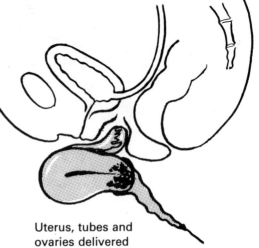

Uterus, tubes and ovaries delivered

PELVIC EXENTERATION

If the bladder or rectum or both are invaded by the growth, these organs can be removed along with the genital tract and pelvic lymph glands.

Anterior Exenteration

The bladder is more often invaded than the rectum. Cystectomy relieves the surgeon of the need for meticulous dissection of the ureters; but the urinary tract must be diverted.

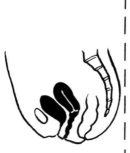

Organs removed

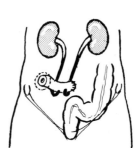

Uretero-colic implantation

Ileal bladder

Posterior Exenteration

This is the most acceptable to the patient involving only a colostomy, but it is the least often indicated.

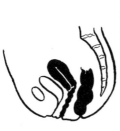

Organs removed

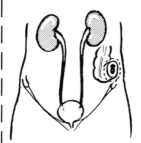

Colostomy

Total Exenteration

This leaves the patient with a colostomy and a urinary tract diversion and is a formidable operation.

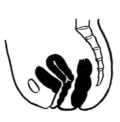

Organs removed

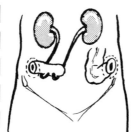

Ileal bladder and colostomy

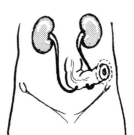

Wet colostomy (undesirable)

COMPLICATIONS OF RADICAL SURGERY

OPERATIVE

1. Haemorrhage
There is continual oozing throughout a long dissection, and a large vein may suddenly tear. Pelvic blood vessels are often abnormally distributed.

2. Shock
This results from a long operation, with continual blood loss, fluctuating blood volume, and acidosis. A high standard of anaesthesia is required.

3. Damage to adjacent organs
The presence of malignant or inflamed tissue makes it easy to tear the bladder or rectum when separating them from the vagina. The ureter can be damaged at any point in the pelvis but is at greatest risk near the infundibulopelvic ligament and adjacent to the cervix and vagina. Dissection is extremely difficult if there has been lateral spread of the tumour.

4. Assessment of operability
Sometimes remote or peritoneal metastases are found as soon as the abdomen is opened. On occasion the surgeon will find as the operation progresses that a full clearance is impossible or too dangerous for the patient.

POST OPERATIVE

1. Ureteric fistula

2. Complications of urinary diversion

3. Urinary Retention
The bladder falls down into pelvis allowing stasis and infection to develop. Also bladder tone is inhibited at least for several days. Pyelograms done several months later very often show a still atonic bladder with narrowing of lower ureter from fibrosis and dilatation and hydronephrosis above.

4. Ileus is not uncommon.

5. Obstruction
This is encouraged by the displacement of viscera and the introduction of a colostomy.

6. Sepsis
This gives rise to thrombosis and anaemia.

7. Thrombosis and embolism
These risks are always present with pelvic surgery. Very rarely there may occur thrombosis of a large pelvic artery.

8. Lymphocyst formation
Cystic collections of lymphatic exudate occasionally form in the pelvis, sometimes reaching the size of a 20 week pregnancy and falsely suggesting recurrence. Such collections should be investigated and removed.

It will be noted that most of these complications arise with more advanced disease – Clinical Stages III and IV.

PAIN IN ADVANCED CANCER

Pelvic cancer spreads mostly by local invasion to the lateral walls of the pelvis, and up the lymphatic chains in the lumbosacral gutter.

Local invasion involves the sacral plexus and pelvic viscera; lumbar spread involves the lumbar plexus lying in the fibres of the psoas, and the lumbosacral trunk.

By the time the growth has extended to the nerve trunks there is usually lymphoedema and ureteric obstruction as well. Death from renal failure will be near and analgesic drugs the kindest treatment.

The occasion does arise however when some interference with pain fibres is necessary, and the help of a neurosurgeon is sought.

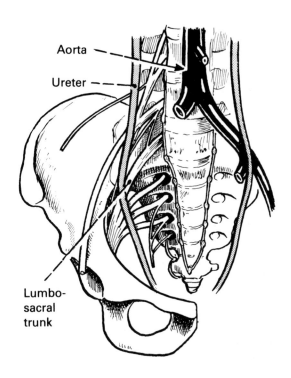

Aorta

Ureter

Lumbo-sacral trunk

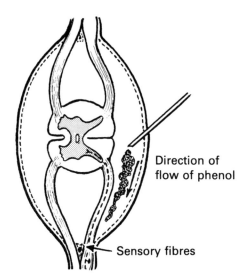

Direction of flow of phenol

Sensory fibres

Intrathecal Injection of Phenol

This is a technique requiring the special skill of the neurologist. The principle is to inject 1–2ml of phenol in glycerine into the cerebrospinal space with the patient lying on her side in such a position that the phenol gravitates to the posterior roots through which the pain fibres enter the cord. About 3–6 months of relief is obtained. Phenol must be kept away from the sacral nerves supplying the sphincters; and this technique is not suitable for the relief of perineal pain.

PAIN IN ADVANCED CANCER

Antero-lateral Cordotomy

This is the treatment of choice if the pain to be abolished is unilateral.

Fibres entering the cord from the sensory roots cross over within 3 or 4 segments of entering, and dissociation into well-defined tracts occupies at least 5 segments in the thoracic region. Division of antero-lateral fibres at the level T2 will permanently interrupt pain and temperature fibres above the level of spinal integration.

There is usually some residual muscle weakness and the patient has a slight limp. There is also constipation and temporary difficulty in starting micturition. This operation does not affect the functioning of a colostomy but it is not suitable for patients in whom the ureters have been transplanted.

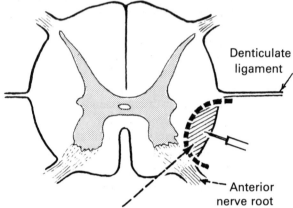

Denticulate ligament

Anterior nerve root

The anterolateral tract is destroyed by a needle electrode.

Bilateral Cordotomy

This is necessary for bilateral pain but carries much more disability. Permanent bladder and bowel dysfunction is the rule and the leg weakness is much more noticeable.

Posterior Rhizotomy (Section of a posterior root)

Three or four roots have to be severed because of overlap, and complete relief of pain is obtained at the expense of function. When proprioception and touch are lost the leg is useless. Paraesthesiae are troublesome and there is a tendency to ulceration, especially if the patient is bedridden.

TERMINAL CARE

Six thousand deaths from gynaecological cancer, half of them ovarian, take place each year in the United Kingdom. Terminal care may be said to begin once it has been accepted that palliative measures cannot or should no longer delay the natural course of a mortal disease.

PSYCHOLOGICAL SUPPORT

This should come from relatives, friends and clergymen as well as nurses and doctors. Dying patients may be affected by the fear of death, by anxiety about their dependents and by depression. The attitude to be taken and the amount of information to be given depends wholly on what is felt to be the kindest approach in each situation. It is cruel to destroy all hope before the patient has become philosophically prepared.

PHYSICAL SUPPORT

Pain must be relieved by adequate dosage of analgesic drugs, given routinely and not simply 'on demand'. Most analgesics cause drowsiness at first but this wears off after a few days. Nausea can be reduced by a phenothiazine such as prochlorperazine (Stemetil).

NORMAL NURSING CARE This

includes measures such as the prevention or treatment of bedsores, correction of constipation, sleeplessness, etc.

USEFUL ANALGESIC DRUGS (in alphabetical order)

Antiprostaglandin group (INDOMETHACIN, FLURBIPROFEN, etc.)	About 100mg tablet	6 hrs	Effective for pain of bone metastases.
DEXTROMORAMIDE (Palfium)	5 or 10mg tablet or suppository	2 hrs	Stronger than morphine but shorter acting.
DIAMORPHINE	40–100mg/24 hrs via syringe driver. Nursing staff can alter delivery as required.		
KETOROLAC	20mg tablet (SERVEDOL) 30mg i.m. injection (TORADOL)		
METHADONE (Physeptone)	5mg tablet	Up to 12 hrs	Weaker than morphine but longer acting.
MORPHINE	1. Up to 64mg in chloroform water 2. MST CONTINUS sustained release tablets	4 hrs 4 hrs	Best strong analgesic. Use with phenothiazine. 10 or 30mg tablet dosage. Use up to 100mg.
OXYCODONE (Proladone)	30mg suppository	8 hrs	Equal to morphine.
PHENAZOCINE (Narphen)	5mg tablet	8 hrs	Stronger than morphine.

CHAPTER 11

DISEASES OF THE UTERUS

UTERINE POLYPS

ADENOMATOUS or MUCOUS POLYP

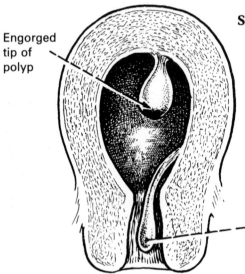

Engorged tip of polyp

Symptoms

Heavier but regular periods. Post-menopausal bleeding. Irregular bleeding on HRT.

Cramping pain – usually mild – as uterus tries to expel polyp.

Intermenstrual staining – usually due to congestion or necrosis, but malignant change must always be considered.

The polyp may be visible in the external os and there may be more than one. Endometrial polyps may be visualised by hysteroscopy.

PLACENTAL POLYP

This is due to the survival of chorionic tissue from a recent pregnancy. The tissue remains adherent to the uterine wall and enlarges with the accretion of fibrin and fibrous tissue.

Symptoms Menorrhagia and intermenstrual bleeding which may present some time after the pregnancy has terminated or aborted. Examination will reveal an enlarged uterus.

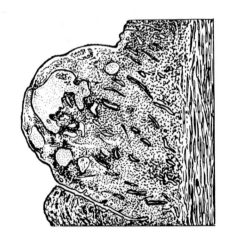

Treatment

All polyps must be removed, either by curettage or avulsion.

FIBROIDS

FIBROIDS (FIBROMYOMATA)

Fibroid is the gynaecological term for a leiomyoma of the uterus.

It is a circumscribed tumour of non-striped muscle with supporting fibrous tissue.

Fibroids develop in the myometrium and are not encapsulated, but they develop a false capsule of compressed myometrial tissue.

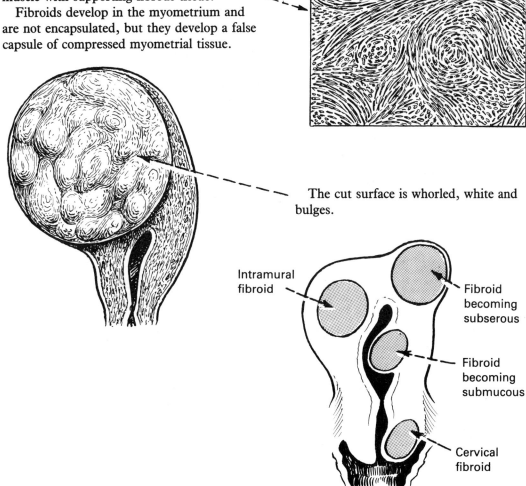

The cut surface is whorled, white and bulges.

Intramural fibroid

Fibroid becoming subserous

Fibroid becoming submucous

Cervical fibroid

Location of the fibroid describes the type.

They are sometimes conglomerate and multiple and vary in size from tiny (millet seed) to several centimetres in diameter.

Some fibroids develop a long pedicle and present as polyps.

Not uncommonly, hard faecal masses in gut are mistaken for uterine fibroids on bimanual examination.

FIBROIDS

The fibroid is the commonest tumour found in women (present in 15 to 20%) especially after 35 years of age.

They make the uterus bulky and irregular and enlarge the cavity so that there is a greater area of endometrium to be shed at menstruation. Menstruation tends to be heavy but the cycle is usually regular. Fibroids are associated with infertility and nulliparity.

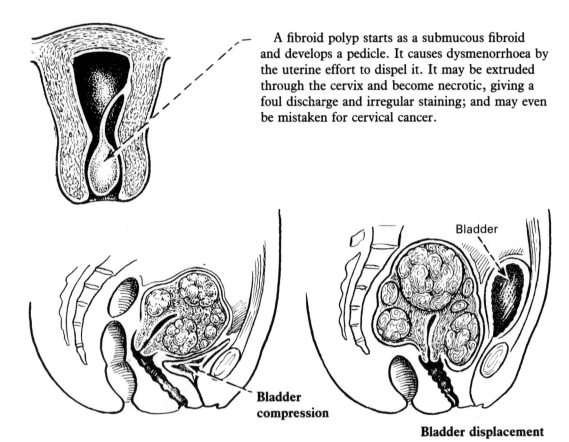

A fibroid polyp starts as a submucous fibroid and develops a pedicle. It causes dysmenorrhoea by the uterine effort to dispel it. It may be extruded through the cervix and become necrotic, giving a foul discharge and irregular staining; and may even be mistaken for cervical cancer.

Bladder compression

Bladder

Bladder displacement

FREQUENCY

The bulk of fibroids in the uterus gives
- A palpable abdominal tumour
- Urinary frequency
- A growth filling the pelvis leading to bladder displacement, retention and overflow and bowel difficulty.

FIBROIDS

DIAGNOSIS

1. This is suggested by a history of increasing menstrual blood loss in a woman commonly in her forties.

2. When the mass is large it will be palpable per abdomen, but in less advanced cases a pelvic examination will reveal an irregularly enlarged uterus.

3. **Examination** under anaesthesia and curettage will allow a more accurate assessment and the exclusion of endometrial carcinoma.

4. If a doubt as to the nature of the mass remains, ultrasound scanning will make a distinction between fibroids and an ovarian cyst.

5. The **diagnosis** may be made at laparoscopy.

COMPLICATIONS

1. **Sarcomatous change**. This is rare but occurs, and even asymptomatic fibroids must be kept under observation.

2. **Degeneration**. Fibroids tend to outgrow their blood supply and are subject to various forms of degeneration.
   Necrobiosis ('red degeneration') occurs in pregnancy and is a cause of pain. Usually this remits and no treatment is needed.
   Hyaline, mucoid, cystic degeneration. These changes may produce soft or hard fibroids, confusing the diagnosis.

3. **Torsion of the pedicle**. This can arise in the case of a polypoid subserous fibroid and gives rise to acute abdominal symptoms. If the torsion is subacute and the blood supply gradually reduced, the fibroid may develop a new vascularity through adhesions (paraditic tumour).

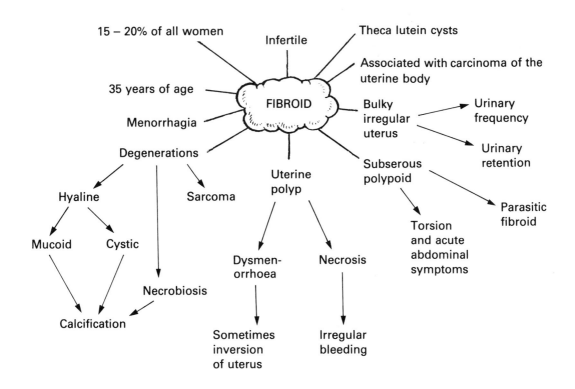

FIBROIDS

Treatment

Small fibroids found without symptoms should be ignored. Larger fibroids and those causing symptoms can be dealt with in two ways:-

    1.   Remove the fibroids and leave the uterus (myomectomy). This is indicated when the patient wishes to keep her uterus.

    2.   Remove the uterus with the fibroids (hysterectomy).

MYOMECTOMY

The approach to the tumour is made through the uterine wall, and the fibroid is shelled out by scissors and finger dissection. The false capsule may make the plane of dissection difficult to identify.

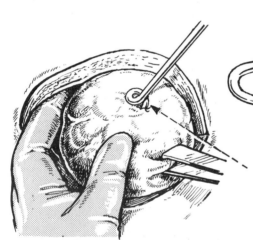

Myoma screw can be used to steady fibroid

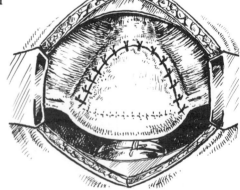

The resultant cavity is obliterated by buried sutures and the uterine wall flapped over to bring the suture line as low on the uterine wall as possible to reduce the risk of adhesions to bowel.

The disadvantages of myomectomy are possible haematoma formation and recurrence of fibroids. Hysterectomy is the treatment of choice unless the patient wishes to become pregnant.

HYPERPLASTIC CONDITIONS OF THE ENDOMETRIUM

The term endometrial hyperplasia is a much abused and confusing term. This is due to the various terminologies used and lack of agreement in defining histopathological appearances. It is also related to the fact that, unlike cervical carcinoma, it is extremely difficult to obtain repeated samples of material for examination from individual patients. Nevertheless it presents an important problem. Any hyperplastic condition must raise the question of development of cancer and it is essential to devise some form of criteria in order to assess the degree of danger of this happening. There have been many reports of the simultaneous existence of hyperplasia and carcinoma.

Various classifications of endometrial hyperplasia have been suggested. The simplest approach is probably the best – mild, moderate and severe. The differentiation of these grades is based on the microscopic architecture of the endometrium, evidence of cytological growth activity and cellular atypia.

Clinical Findings

Almost all patients are in the 3rd and 4th decades of life, but hyperplasia is not confined to these age groups. Occasionally it is found in young individuals and is not uncommon in post-menopausal patients. Haemorrhage is the presenting symptom but the severity or frequency is not related to the degree of pathological change.

Mild Hyperplasia

This is the most common type. Previously known as metropathia haemorrhagica, the endometrium has a characteristic appearance, often termed 'Swiss cheese' or cystic glandular hyperplasia.

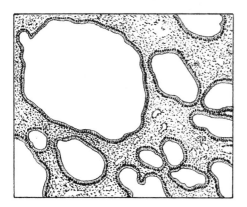

At low power magnification the pattern is a mixture of glands of varying sizes, a significant proportion of them being cystic. There is no crowding of the glands which are lined by cubical or columnar epithelium. Mitotic figures are present in small numbers. A similar gross picture may be seen in atrophic endometria but mitotic activity is absent.

HYPERPLASTIC CONDITIONS OF THE ENDOMETRIUM

Moderate Hyperplasia

In this grade of hyperplasia the most striking feature is the evidence of quite obvious hyperplasia – crowding of glands so that they are back-to-back, the epithelium is stratified and mitoses are relatively frequent. There is, however, no epithelial atypia.

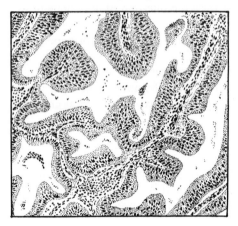
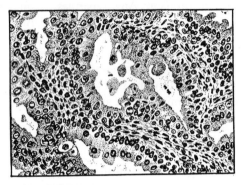

Severe Hyperplasia

At this stage cellular atypia is prominent, glands are distorted by intra-glandular polypoid formations. Mitoses are quite frequent.

These grades of epithelial change seem to form a graded series. Evidence of proof of this is difficult to find however. Some of the conclusions drawn from studies must be viewed with caution from an intellectual point of view, but in practice it must be accepted that any hyperplastic condition must be regarded with suspicion and treatment should be anticipatory.

Many cases have a history of profuse menstruation and some present clinical features which are said to be stigmata of the type of patient apt to develop endometrial carcinoma such as obesity, abnormal glucose tolerance curve and hypertension.

In some cases of localised adenocarcinoma of the endometrium, the surrounding endometrium shows evidence of hyperplasia, giving credence to the view that one condition develops out of the other. In addition, there are cases where it is microscopically difficult to state that the endometrial changes are hyperplastic but not malignant. This occurs with severe grades of hyperplasia and names such as adenoma malignum or Grade O in the histological classification of adenocarcinoma have been used.

Claims are made for the likelihood of adenocarcinoma developing according to the grade of hyperplasia. Mild – 1%, moderate – 5%, severe – 30%, and the time taken for malignancy to appear, milder – 10 years, severe – 4 years.

Treatment

This should be based on 4 main factors:
1. The age of the patient.
2. The desire of the patient to retain her fertility.
3. The severity of the hyperplasia.
4. The ability to control possible sources of oestrogen production.

In young patients wishing pregnancy, with mild hyperplasia, conservative hormonal treatment may be sufficient. In severe cases progestogens can be tried initially but, if results are not satisfactory in 6–8 weeks, hysterectomy is recommended.

CARCINOMA OF THE ENDOMETRIUM

This is one of the commonest gynaecological cancers. It is usually found in post-menopausal women (75%) most frequently between the ages of 55 and 65 years and the majority, (60%), in the latter part of that span. In the USA it is said to be the most common form of gynaecological malignancy, 1 in 1000 post-menopausal women developing it every year. This is in contrast to the UK where carcinoma of the cervix is the commonest cancer and 70 % are diagnosed before the age of 60.

It has been observed that patients suffering from this disease tend to show a number of characteristics in common:
1. A high proportion are married.
2. Of those who are married a large percentage are infertile.
3. If parous they are apt to have had repeated abortions.
4. Many have a late menopause, have a history of profuse menstruation, are obese, hypertensive, and have glycosuria or frank diabetes.

Symptomatology

The usual complaint is of a blood-stained watery discharge which, due to infection, quickly becomes foul smelling. If infection is marked the cervical canal may become blocked and pyometra develop.

Diagnosis is made by curettage and histological examination, ideally prededed by hysteroscopy.

Fractional curettage

This is a technique designed to detect early cervical involvement. Its value is doubtful and it is not really feasible except in the earliest stages of the disease.

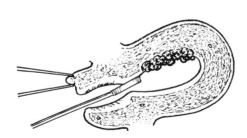 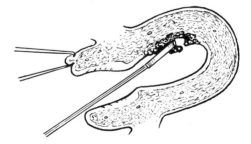

1. A cervical smear is taken, the canal is dilated a little, and curettings taken from the region of the internal os.

2. Dilatation is continued and a larger curette is used to obtain a biopsy from the cavity.

3. Curette the lower uterine cavity.

4. Curette the upper cavity.

5. Use sponge forceps to remove any polypi.

Each specimen is placed in a separate container of fixative and sent for histological study.

CARCINOMA OF THE ENDOMETRIUM

Typical early polypoidal fundal growth

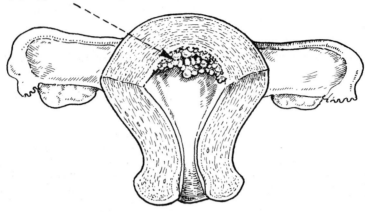

Histology

The majority of tumours (60%) are pure adenocarcinomata. They can be divided into 3 groups according to the degree of glandular differentiation.

Grade 1 – well differentiated. Gland forms are conspicuous. Mitotic figures are moderately numerous. - - - - →

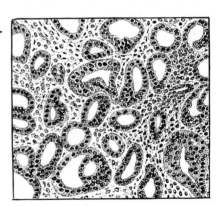

Grade 2 – patchy differentiation. Gland forms are much less prominent and many deposits consist of infiltrating single cell columns or solid masses.

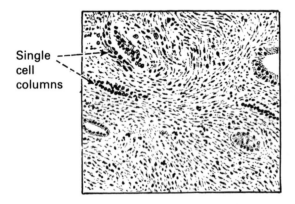

Single cell columns

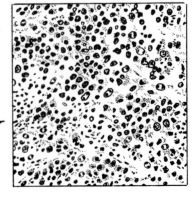

Grade 3. This type consists of solid masses of malignant cells of varying sizes and shapes with little or no stroma. Mitoses are numerous.

CARCINOMA OF THE ENDOMETRIUM

Further groups have been described.

Adeno-squamoid group

This has been divided into two groups:

1.   If the squamous cells are well differentiated the tumour is termed adeno-acanthoma (Histological Grade 1).

2.   Poorly differentiated squamous cells merit the name adeno-squamous carcinoma (Grade 2).

Adeno-acanthoma

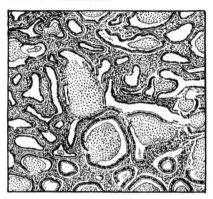

Adeno-squamous carcinoma

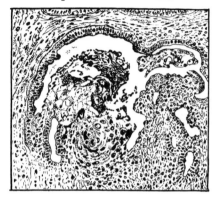

One other histological type is recognised and is apparently of prognostic significance.

Clear celled carcinoma

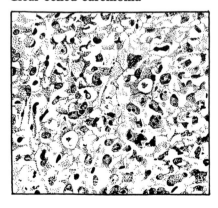

This tumour has a poor prognosis and is included with the Grade 3 adenocarcinomata. It occurs mainly in the elderly.

STAGING OF ENDOMETRIAL CARCINOMA

The classification given below is that of the Federation of Gynaecology and Obstetrics (FIGO) 1961.

Stage O   The histological appearances are suggestive of cancer but not conclusive.

Stage I   Growth confined to corpus.
  Ia   Cavity 8cm or less.
  Ib   Cavity over 8 cm.
Stage I growths are also graded according to histology (see pp.245–249).

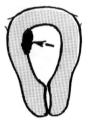

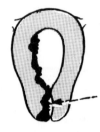

Stage II
  The growth has extended to the cervix.

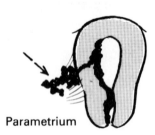

Parametrium

Stage III
  The growth has extended beyond the uterus but not outside the pelvis and not into the bladder or rectum.

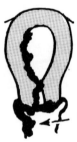

Vagina

Stage IV
  The growth has invaded the rectum or bladder or structures beyond the pelvis.

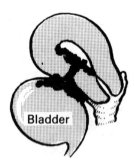

Bladder

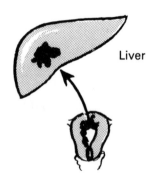

Liver

SPREAD OF ENDOMETRIAL CARCINOMA

In general this cancer is slow to spread from the uterine cavity, probably because the endometrium lacks lymphatics.

Local Spread
Slow invasion of the myometrium is the commonest spread. It may produce considerable uterine enlargement; or spread may involve the vaginal vault.

Venous Spread
This pathway might account for the occasional appearance of a low vaginal metastasis; but venous spread is not a common feature of uterine cancer.

Lymphatic Spread
The incidence of this (it is much debated) seems to be somewhere between 10 and 30%. All pelvic nodes, including the internal iliacs, the parametrium, the ovaries, and the vagina may be involved, probably with equal frequency. Lymphatic spread is more likely to occur when the tumour is anaplastic and the uterine wall is deeply invaded.

Tubal Spread
Malignant cells can pass along the tube in the same way that peritoneal spill may occur during menstruation. This may account for isolated ovarian metastases.

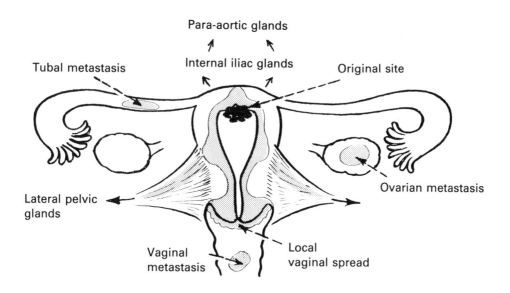

Distant metastases do occur in advanced cases. Pulmonary deposits are the most common. Most metastases are confined to adjacent structures and the peritoneum. Occasionally the liver, vertebrae or other bones may be affected.

AETIOLOGICAL FACTORS IN ENDOMETRIAL CARCINOMA

The actual cause of this cancer is unknown. Argument has centred around the undoubted association between this tumour and oestrogen. Increased incidences have been reported in women given oestrogen alone as post-menopausal hormone replacement therapy, in fat, diabetic, hypertensive women who commonly have a high plasma oestradiol even post-menopausally and in patients who develop oestrogen secreting tumours of the ovary.

The central position of oestrogen in the aetiology of endometrial cancer is strengthened by the fact that the addition of progestogen to the oestrogen in hormone replacement therapy appears to abolish the increased incidence of endometrial cancer. There can be no doubt that oestrogen can alter the behaviour of this tumour but there is still a question about oestrogen as a primary causal agent. Every normal woman is subject to the influence of unopposed oestrogen for 2 weeks out of every 4 for a matter of 30 years or more. There is also the fact that 75% of cases of endometrial cancer occur in the post-menopausal period when oestrogen values are low. Only a proportion of fat, diabetic and hypertensive women develop endometrial cancer and similarly only a proportion of women with endometrial cancer are fat, diabetic or hypertensive. The question remains whether oestrogen is a causal agent, or is acting in its normal capacity as a growth factor and is really to be regarded as a co-carcinogen. It may be that the lack of progestational activity alters the reaction to oestrogen.

PROGNOSIS OF ENDOMETRIAL CARCINOMA

While clinical staging is important in assessing the likely outcome of this disease it should be realised that staging can be difficult and a matter of opinion. Fortunately in most instances the growth is slow in developing and 75% or more are in Stage 1 at operation. Nevertheless it is customary to take the histological grade of the tumour as well as the clinical stage into consideration. A tumour of histological Grade 3 with its obvious capacity for rapid proliferation must affect the outlook and so it proves.

Various figures are quoted but the following are an example of the 5-year survival rates according to clinical staging.

Stage	Percentage survival
IA } IB }	80
II	50
III	30
IV	10

Assessing 5-year survival rates according to Federation International Gynaecology Obstetrics (FIGO) histological grading is reported as follows:

Grading	Appearance	Percentage survival
G1	Highly differentiated	100
G2	Differentiated part solid	66
G3	Mainly solid	57

Using both methods on similar cases we find that the 5-year survival rates for Stage 1 are the only ones altered significantly:

Stage and Histology	5-year survival Rates
I, G1 and 2	80%
I, G3	60%

Prognosis is also altered by individual findings. For instance, if the tumour has penetrated more than half-way through the myometrial thickness the prognosis is bad. In addition, the recurrence rate, up to 15%, is directly proportional to the histological grade.

TREATMENT OF ENDOMETRIAL CARCINOMA

This is by a combination of surgery and radiotherapy, sometimes with the added support of progestogens (pages 252, 255).

Conservative Surgery

This may be followed by a course of radiotherapy when the tumour has invaded more than 5mm into the uterine wall. Many clinicians give a course of progestogen prior to carrying out simple hysterectomy and salpingo-oophorectomy. This treatment tends to reduce the tumour before operation. 200mg medroxyprogesterone acetate (Provera) are given daily till operation (oral medication), or 100mg intramuscularly (Depo-provera) weekly, but no statistically significant improvement in cure rate has been demonstrated, possibly because the results are already so good.

Radical Surgery

A modified course of intracavitary radiation may be given, followed by a radical hysterectomy with removal of as much of the parametrial and vaginal tissue as possible, and also the pelvic lymph nodes.

There is no incontrovertible evidence that radical surgery will improve the result, and the morbidity, especially the risk of subsequent ischaemic necrosis of a ureter, is not so easily overcome in the older patient; the grandmother rather than the mother.

The trend is now for a more flexible approach. If the growth has extended beyond the uterus, or is anaplastic, megavoltage irradiation is given as well as intracavitary, or surgery more extensive than a simple hysterectomy is carried out (a 2cm 'cuff' of vagina is often removed). If the growth involves the cervix, the treatment is that of carcinoma of the cervix. If the patient is not suitable for surgery, radiotherapy and progestogen therapy alone are given. Progestogen therapy may have a useful palliative effect on advanced metastatic disease.

Results of Treatment

Stage I ——————— 80%
Stage II ——————— 50%
Stages III and IV ——————— very poor

The overall results are better than for carcinoma of the cervix, not because it is a less malignant tumour, but because treatment is usually given earlier. Post-menopausal bleeding is much more difficult to ignore than the irregular bleeding of the younger woman.

RECURRENCE OF ENDOMETRIAL CARCINOMA

The incidence of recurrence within 5 years is in the region of 30% and is accepted along with the 5-year survival rate as a measure of the effectiveness of the various systems of treatment.

Sites

Local recurrence is the commonest especially in the pelvic walls and vaginal vault; but endometrial carcinoma also recurs outside the pelvis in the para-aortic glands, the lungs, the skeleton and the lower vagina.

Prophylaxis

Pre-operative vaginal irradiation will very much reduce the chance of vaginal recurrence, and some radiotherapists advise pelvic megavoltage treatment as well. The basis of radical surgery is an attempt to clear the pelvis of lymphatic tissue which is not possible; and there is no agreement on whether lymphadenectomy, if technically feasible, is worth doing except on principle.

Treatment

Modern radiotherapy permits an attempt at cure, especially if the recurrence is restricted to the accessible vagina.

PROGESTERONE

Many endometrial carcinomata are hormone dependent and progestogens have been used as part of a combined primary treatment as well as for recurrent or metastatic growths.

The response is dose dependent. Small doses actually increase the rate of growth. High dosage reduces mitotic activity and the number of malignant cells and encourages differentiation and return to normal architecture.

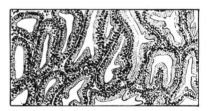

After progesterone

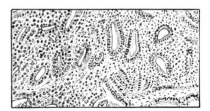

Before progesterone

Drugs used include: Medroxyprogesterone acetate (Provera) 100mg, twice daily.
Gestronol hexanoate (Depostat) 200mg i.m. for 12 weeks.

40% of patients with inoperable carcinoma or recurrence have objective improvement in 6–8 weeks.

MALIGNANT TUMOURS OF ENDOMETRIUM OF MIXED EPITHELIAL-STROMAL HISTOLOGY

These are rare tumours and show varying degrees of malignancy of either the glandular or stromal elements or both.

1. **Endometrial stromatosis** (also called endolymphatic stromal myosis or endometrial stromal nodule).

   This forms a nodular growth of stromal cells extending in an expansile fashion rather than by infiltration. It may however appear to invade the local lymphatics, but does not form metastases and is essentially non-malignant.

2. **Endometrial stromal sarcomas.**

   These are tumours of endometrial stromal cells. They vary in degree of malignancy and form 2 groups:

   (a) **Low grade malignancy.**

   Cure may follow local removal but they sometimes recur years later in the pelvis. Occasionally they may form pulmonary metastases. The patient has a prolonged survival and may be cured after radiation therapy.

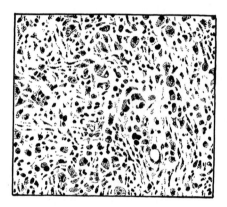

   (b) **High grade malignancy.**

   This type of stromal tumour shows numerous mitoses and is infiltrative from the start. There is early recurrence and widespread metastases occur even if there has been little local invasion of the myometrium. The prognosis is poor.

3. **Adeno-sarcoma.**

   This forms a polypoid mass in the uterine cavity consisting of a mixture of gland and stromal elements. The glandular tissue appears to be benign but the stroma shows the usual signs of malignancy – cellular atypia and mitotic activity. In 25% heterologous elements are found such as striated muscle and cartilage. Recurrences are confined to the pelvis. Distant metastases are rare.

4. **Carcino-sarcoma.**

   In this variant both epithelial and stromal elements are malignant. It forms a soft polypoid mass, usually haemorrhagic. Microscopically most of the growth is sarcomatous but there are foci of carcinoma – adeno, squamoid, undifferentiated or various mixtures of these. The sarcomatous parts show marked cellular atypia such as giant cells and other bizarre forms. The prognosis is poor. Treatment is surgical plus radiotherapy for recurrences and metastatic deposits.

MALIGNANT TUMOURS OF ENDOMETRIUM OF MIXED EPITHELIAL-STROMAL HISTOLOGY

5. **Mixed mesodermal tumours**.

These are often confused with carcino-sarcoma. They may be found in the vagina or cervix in children, but the uterine variety occurs in post-menopausal women. The growth in children has a grape-like appearance – botryoid sarcoma.

Bulky mixed mesodermal tumour showing haemorrhagic appearance.

Microscopic appearance of mixed mesodermal tumour.

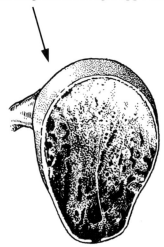

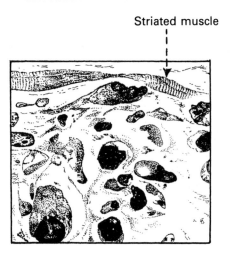

Striated muscle

In the uterus it presents as a large white polypoid mass, semi-necrotic with areas of haemorrhage. Microscopically the tumour is pleomorphic with areas of myxomatous, cartilagenous and bony tissue. Growth is very rapid and it invades adjacent organs quickly. The prognosis is extremely poor, the 5-year survival rate being 20% at most. Blood borne metastases are common.

SARCOMA OF THE UTERUS

Histological Appearances

The tissues of origin are the connective tissue and muscle of the myometrium or leiomyoma; or the endometrial stroma. These are composed of undifferentiated round- or spindle-celled masses. A special group of sarcomatous growths, the mixed mesodermal tumours, sometimes occur. In children, striated muscle is often a feature and a characteristic polypoidal growth occurs – sarcoma botryoides. Later in life carcinoma, sarcoma and various mesodermal tissues such as cartilage may be found.

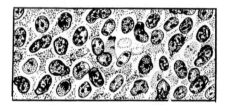

High power appearance of round cell sarcoma.

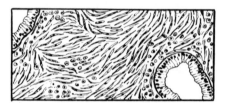

Low power view of spindle-cell sarcoma.

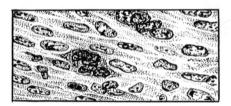

High power view of smooth muscle sarcoma.

Treatment

Sarcoma spreads by the blood stream and surgery should be limited to removal of the uterus and ovaries. If there are no remote metastases the patient should then be sent for external radiation.

Prognosis

This depends on the degree of spread and the histological differentiation and is generally poor. Circumscribed and pedunculated growths have a better prognosis than infiltrating ones, and the most hopeful outlook is in the case of a 'histological find' in a fibromyoma thought at operation to be benign.

SARCOMA OF THE UTERUS

A malignant tumour arising from the connective tissue or muscle of the uterus. This is a rare disease in contrast to the common benign tumour of connective tissue and muscle, the leiomyoma or fibroid. Sarcomatous change may occur in between 0.1% and 1% of fibroids.

Clinical Features

The patient is usually over 50 and presents with a complaint of fairly heavy bleeding of recent origin, accompanied by pain. Pelvic examination reveals a large intra-uterine mass with friable tissue palpable through the os. The tumour may originate from the vagina in the younger woman and from the cervix in the child; but these are very rare conditions indeed.

Pathology

Tumour tissue may infiltrate the whole myometrium and fill the uterine cavity (diffuse, infiltrating) or arise from a pedicle (circumscribed type). This type often presents as a cervical or vaginal polyp. If the malignant change originates in a fibromyoma (which is very rare) the sarcomatous area has a yellowish fleshy appearance with areas of necrosis.

Differential Diagnosis

The growth is obviously malignant as a rule, but biopsy is required to distinguish sarcoma from the more common adenocarcinoma.

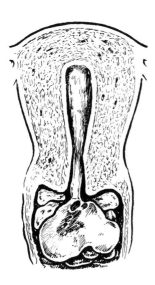

Pelvic examination in this case would suggest a cervical origin.

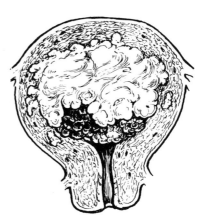

A diffuse infiltrating sarcoma.

CHAPTER 12

DISPLACEMENTS OF THE UTERUS

BACKWARD DISPLACEMENTS OF THE UTERUS

An alteration from the usual anteverted position of the uterus often with a change in the curve of the uterine axis. Most of the so-called displacements are merely variations of the normal and are of little clinical significance.

Anteverted Uterus

The uterus is approximately at right angles to the vagina and has a slight forward curve. This position has long been regarded as offering the best access to sperms at insemination.

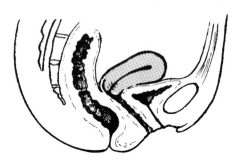

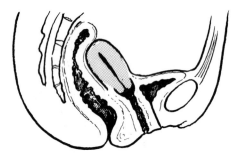

Retroversion

The long axis of the uterus is directed backwards.

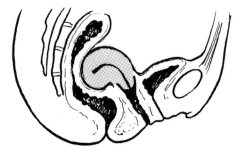

Retroflexion

The uterus is curved backwards. The cervix may remain in the normal position but is usually positioned as in retroversion.

Retroposition

The uterus is displaced backwards but the direction of its axis remains the same.

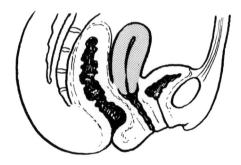

BACKWARD DISPLACEMENTS OF THE UTERUS

Causes of Displacement
'Complicated' displacement is
due to the presence of some other
condition such as a cyst or fibroid
or endometriosis. 'Uncomplicated'
displacement, where there is no
other abnormality, is of unknown
aetiology; the uterus in some women
appears to take up retro-displacement
spontaneously.

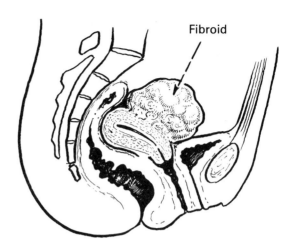

Fibroid

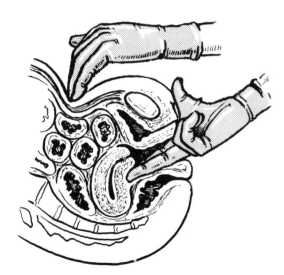

Diagnosis is by bimanual palpation.
The vaginal hand palpates a mass
in the Pouch of Douglas, the
abdominal hand detects the absence
of a uterine corpus in the expected
place. The possibility of tumours
and inflammatory masses must be
considered; and in fat women the
diagnosis can only be made with
confidence after an examination under
anaesthesia and the careful passage of
a sound to determine the direction in
which the uterine cavity lies.

SYMPTOMS OF DISPLACEMENT

Consequences of Uncomplicated Displacement

1. Very often none at all. The manifestations of hysteria were classically attributed to movements of the womb round the abdomen; a retroverted uterus is an attractive focusing point for a variety of functional complaints. If a symptomless retroversion is discovered, it should not be mentioned to the patient.

2. If the uterus is not mobile, coitus may be unbearable if the penis thrusts against the retroflexed uterus lying with prolapsed ovaries in the Pouch of Douglas (the 'ovarian entrapment syndrome'). If such pain occurs it can easily be reproduced by pressing with the examining fingers. It is quite possible for the patient to present with a complaint of dyspareunia and to have a retroverted uterus which has nothing to do with her complaint.

3. **Backache**
   Dysmenorrhoea
   Menorrhagia

   All these complaints are often difficult to explain and if a retroversion is found on examination, it is tempting to claim it as the cause. Very often the three complaints co-exist with a 'flabby' slightly enlarged parous retroverted uterus, a sequel to many pregnancies perhaps with some pelvic infection. In such a situation a 'pessary test' (vide infra) could be tried.

4. **Infertility**

   The retroverted cervix, pointing away from the posterior fornix is said to be at a disadvantage during insemination, but experience with mechanical and barrier methods of contraception suggests that the spermatozoa in a normal ejaculate are capable of overcoming such an obstacle. Many women with retroverted uteri fall pregnant. Some women with otherwise unexplained infertility conceive after surgical correction of retroversion.

TREATMENT OF DISPLACEMENT

This should only be offered if the patient has symptoms.

1. **Basculation**: This means manual correction of the displacement (Fr. bascule, a cradle). The technique can only be acquired by experience and often an anaesthetic is required. This manipulation might be performed after diagnosis by examination under anaesthetic or laparoscopy.

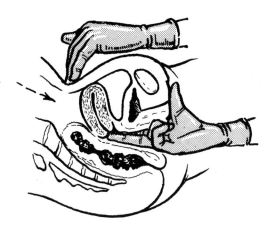

2. **Insertion of Hodge Pessary:**

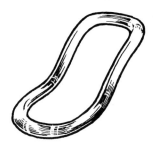

This is a rigid plastic pessary, oblong in shape, which was designed for insertion into the vagina in such a way as to maintain a uterus in the anteverted position once the retroversion had been manually corrected. It is now becoming obsolete but is still occasionally used in the 'pessary test'.

Pessary Test:
This is applied to patients in whom a chronic retroversion is suspected of causing dyspareunia. The pessary is placed as shown and will certainly maintain the anteversion. If properly fitted it does not interfere in any way with coitus, and if it abolishes the dyspareunia it is removed. The retroversion and its symptoms may not recur but, if they do, a sling operation should be considered.

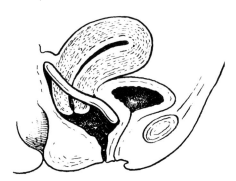

SLING OPERATION ON UTERUS

This is seldom required and indicated only after at least one positive pessary test. Two operations are described both of them making use of the round ligaments to hold the uterus forward. These ligaments have a considerable capacity for stretching and a permanent correction can never be guaranteed.

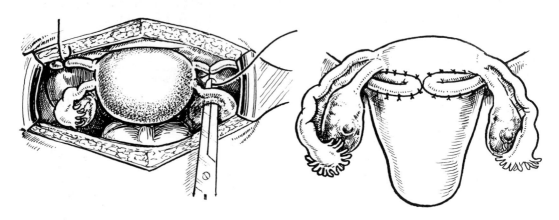

Baldy-Webster Sling Operation (now rarely, if ever, performed)

Silk sutures are attached to the round ligaments and pulled back under the fallopian tubes so that the ligaments may be attached to the back of the uterus.

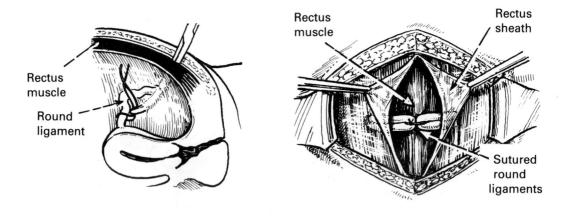

Gilliam's Ventrosuspension Operation

The sutures are attached as before and the loops of round ligament are pulled up through peritoneum and rectus muscle fibres, to be sutured to each other across the recti. This operation can also be performed under laparoscopic visualisation. The round ligaments are picked up with forceps and sutured to the rectus sheath through two small incisions, and there is no need for formal laparotomy. Synthetic absorbable sutures may be preferable as silk can cause abscess formation.

CHRONIC INVERSION OF THE UTERUS

The uterus is turned inside out through the cervix. This is a very uncommon condition.

Causes of Chronic Inversion
(Acute inversion causing severe shock is an obstetrical problem.)

1. Unnoticed partial inversion after labour progresses to chronic inversion. This is caused by too much fundal pressure and cord traction in an effort to expel the placenta.

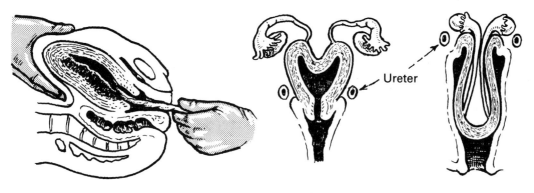

Expelling the placenta.   A few days later.   A few months later.

2. Attempts of the uterus to expel an intracavitary tumour. The tumour is usually a fibromyoma and if the pedicle will not stretch, or if there is no pedicle, inversion develops.

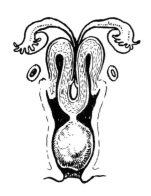

Note the short thick pedicle.

If the cervix is also inverted, the vagina will follow, bringing the bladder with it. Note the position of the ureters.

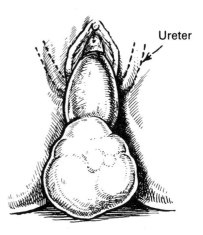

267

CHRONIC INVERSION

Clinical Features

The patient complains of irregular
bleeding, and of 'something coming down'.
Examination reveals a mass usually infected,
distending the vagina. Bimanual examination
will, if the patient is not too fat, confirm the
base of a uterus in the usual place.

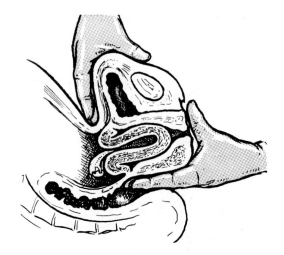

Differential Diagnosis

This includes a fibroid polyp and cervical
neoplasm, but inversion must always be
thought of. To attempt 'avulsion of a polyp'
in a case of inverted uterus would produce
extreme and perhaps fatal shock.

Surgical Treatment

Operative correction is best done by the abdominal route (Haultain's operation).

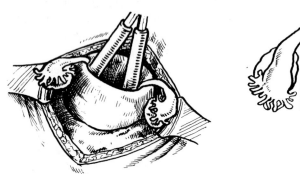
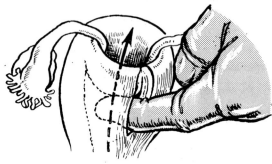

This operation may be made very difficult by the presence of adhesions or a large tumour, and
the 'upside down' anatomy makes the operating field unfamiliar. The position of the ureters
may be disturbed, and they should if possible be identified.

UTEROVAGINAL PROLAPSE

Herniation of the genital tract through the pelvic diaphragm.

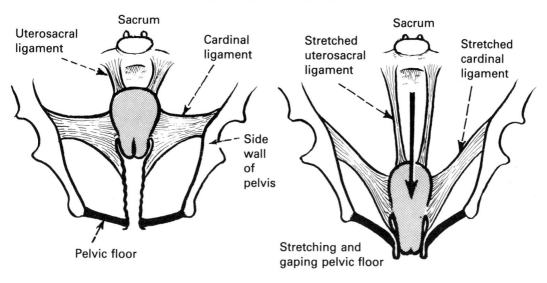

The uterus and vagina are held in the pelvis by the cardinal and utero-sacral ligaments and by the pelvic floor musculature, mainly the levatores ani.

When these ligaments and muscles become ineffective, the uterus and vagina descend (prolapse) through the gap between the muscles.

The Causes of Prolapse are:

1. The stretching of muscle and fibrous tissue which occurs with repeated childbirth and damage to the innervation of the pelvic floor.

2. Increased intra-abdominal pressure (as in fat women with chronic coughs) and in women who undertake heavy industrial work.

3. A constitutional predisposition to stretching of the ligaments as a response presumably to years in the erect position. (Thus nulliparous women can develop prolapse: cf. the constitutional factor in the development of varicose veins.)

The incidence of this condition in the United Kingdom is greatly reduced with improvement in obstetric techniques. The more liberal use of caesarean section and the elimination of long labours are probably the two most important factors.

269

UTEROVAGINAL PROLAPSE

The uterus gradually descends in the axis of the vagina taking the vaginal wall with it. It may present clinically at any level, but is usually classified as one of three degrees.

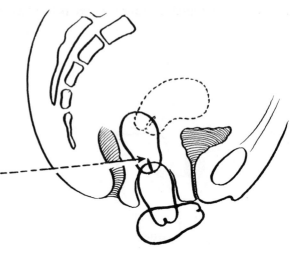

First degree: cervix still inside vagina.

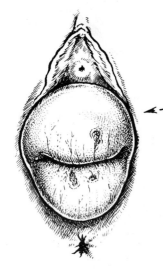

Second degree: the cervix appears outside the vulva. The cervical lips become congested and ulcerated.

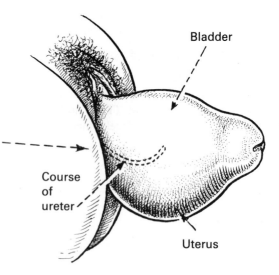

Bladder

Course of ureter

Uterus

Third degree: complete prolapse. In the picture the uterus is retroflexed, and the outline of bladder can be seen. There may be a rectal prolapse as well. This is sometimes called complete procidentia.

VAGINAL PROLAPSE

The prolapse is confined to the vaginal walls and the related viscera. The cervix may come down as well because of elongation of the supravaginal cervix (see p. 273) but the uterus stays in the pelvis.

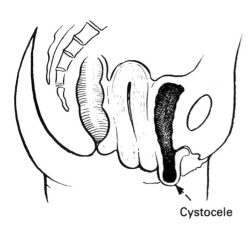

Cystocele

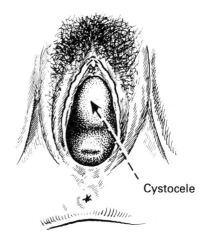

Cystocele

Anterior Prolapse

When the upper part of the anterior wall prolapses, there is an underlying failure of the investing fascia, and the bladder base also descends. This is called a cystocele.

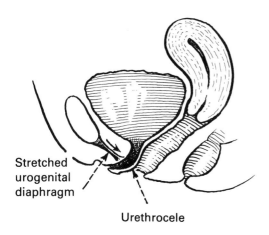

Stretched urogenital diaphragm

Urethrocele

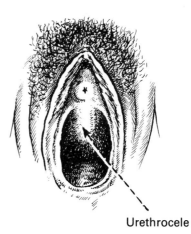

Urethrocele

Sometimes the lower part of the vaginal wall prolapses and the urethra also descends. This is called a urethrocele and indicates stretching of the urogenital diaphragm which holds the urethra to the pubic bone.

PROLAPSE OF THE POSTERIOR WALL

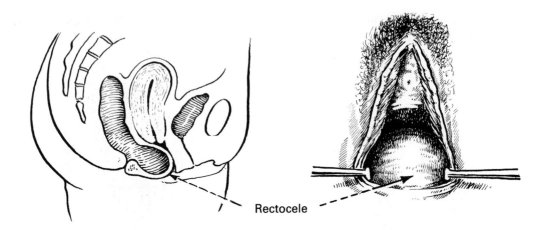

Rectocele

If the prolapse is at the level of the middle third of the vagina, the recto-vaginal septum is often involved and rectum prolapses with vaginal wall. This is called a rectocele. If the lowest part of the vagina prolapses, the perineal body is involved rather than the rectum.

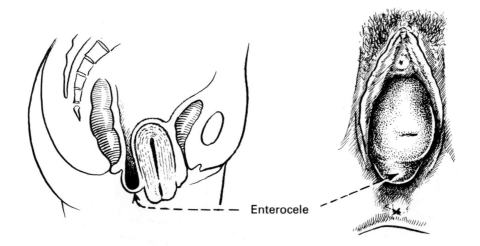

Enterocele

If the upper part of the posterior vaginal wall prolapses, the Pouch of Douglas is elongated and small bowel or omentum may descend. This is called an enterocele. Enterocele is usually associated with uterine prolapse, as in the picture, and is sometimes called 'vault prolapse' or 'hernia of the Pouch of Douglas'. The vaginal vault may prolapse after hysterectomy. This is a difficult condition to treat. One technique suspends the vault from the sacro-iliac ligaments using non-absorbable sutures.

CERVICAL PROLAPSE

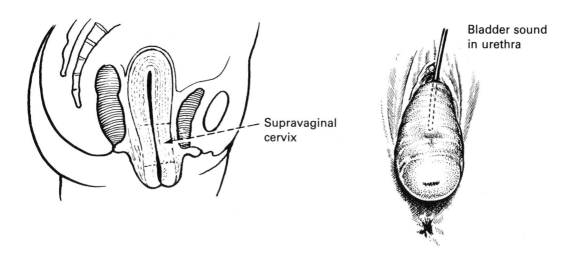

Bladder sound
in urethra

Supravaginal
cervix

Most vaginal prolapse is associated with some degree of cervical descent, even though there is no uterine prolapse. This is due to elongation of the supra-vaginal cervix and may be so marked as to suggest uterine prolapse: but the uterus stays in the pelvis.

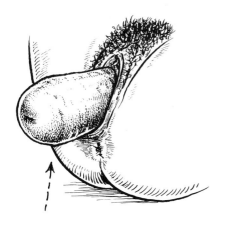

NULLIPAROUS UTERINE PROLAPSE is due to failure of the cardinal ligaments. The vaginal wall prolapses as well but there is no cystocele or rectocele. This prolapse is sometimes called 'vault' prolapse, confusing it with enterocele.

Diagnosis of Prolapse

This is most accurately made when the patient is anaesthetised. Prolapse of any kind is often not apparent until the woman has been walking about for some time, and the surgeon confirms the diagnosis only when he can apply traction with a volsellum. An enterocele sometimes cannot be identified until after the start of the operation. Rectal examination may be helpful.

CLINICAL FEATURES OF PROLAPSE

The common complaints are:

1. **'Something coming down'** when the patient is on her feet. The sensation is not there when she lies down.

2. **Backache.** This is often due simply to the patient being overweight.

3. **Increased frequency of micturition.** This is at first due to incomplete emptying, but sooner or later is aggravated by cystitis.

4. **A 'bearing down' sensation,** analogous to the parturient woman's desire to push. This is probably caused by pelvic venous congestion, and pressure from the abdominal contents on an inadequate pelvic floor.

5. **Stress Incontinence.** This is by no means always present. Sometimes it is found that reduction of the prolapse causes stress incontinence.

6. **Difficulty in voiding urine and defaecating.** The patient may find that it is impossible to initiate micturition except by pushing up the cystocele with her finger. In the same way the rectocele must be pushed back to allow emptying of the rectum.

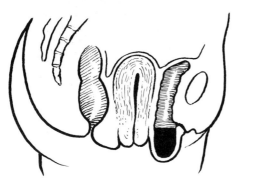 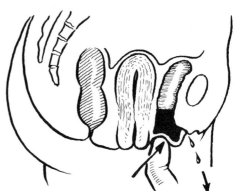

The onset may be gradual or quite sudden and is commoner after the menopause when the genital tract tissues begin to atrophy. Women tend to put off complaints of prolapse until they find their movements really inhibited, and their domestic duties have lightened sufficiently to allow them to spend some time in hospital.

DIFFERENTIAL DIAGNOSIS OF PROLAPSE

Prolapse may be complained of without being present, and not too much reliance may be placed on the history. The discomfort of atrophic vaginitis may suggest prolapse to the patient; or she is simply too fat and is feeling her weight at the most dependent part. The following conditions resemble prolapse on superficial examination.

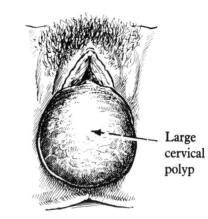

Large cervical polyp

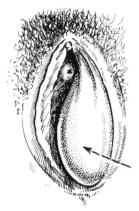

Cyst of Bartholin's gland

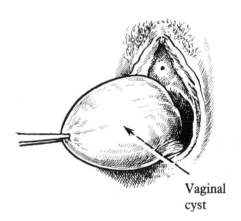

Vaginal cyst

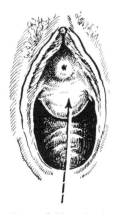

Cyst of Skene's duct

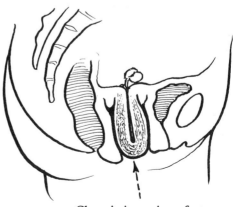

Chronic inversion of uterus

275

PESSARY TREATMENT

A ring pessary, usually of semi-rigid plastic, is inserted into the vagina and so stretches the vaginal walls that they cannot prolapse through the introitus.

The pessary is compressed into a long ovoid shape, lubricated and gently pushed into the vagina, where it resumes its circular shape and takes up a position in the coronal plane. It must not be too tight; and correct fitting is learnt by experience.

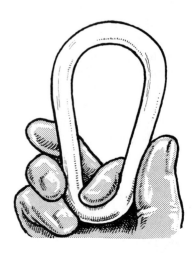

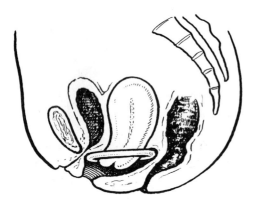

Indications for Pessary Treatment

1. The patient prefers a pessary. Pelvic surgery with its unavoidable risks should only be applied to a willing patient.

2. The prolapse is amenable to pessary support. If the perineal muscles are very deficient they will not hold a pessary. If too big a ring is required, the vaginal wall or cervix will prolapse through it.

3. The patient is not fit for surgery.

4. The patient wishes to delay operation temporarily (for example another pregnancy is anticipated).

The pessary has acquired a bad reputation as a 'dirty thing' because of the profuse purulent discharge caused by the rubber rings of the past. Plastic rings need only be changed once or twice a year, and if it has been properly fitted the patient will be unaware of its presence in her vagina even during coitus. An ill-fitting pessary is ineffective and may cause dyspareunia and discomfort. If it is too tight or left too long, ulceration of the vaginal wall will occur, and malignant change has been reported. Vaginal oestriol cream or oestradiol tablets help prevent atrophic vaginitis.

PESSARY TREATMENT

TYPES of PESSARY

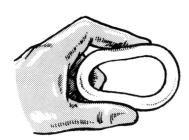

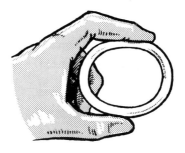

The semi-soft vinyl ring, useful when there is senile shrinkage of the introitus, making insertion of a big enough ring difficult. Vinyl rings also come out easily.

The semi-rigid polythene ring. This goes in easily but may be difficult to extract.

PROLAPSE in FRAIL OLD WOMEN

Such patients are unfit for surgery and the pelvic muscles are often too slack to contain a ring pessary. In these circumstances, the prolapse may be contained and the patient kept ambulant by a Cup and Stem pessary attached to a waist belt. These are rarely seen outside of museums now.

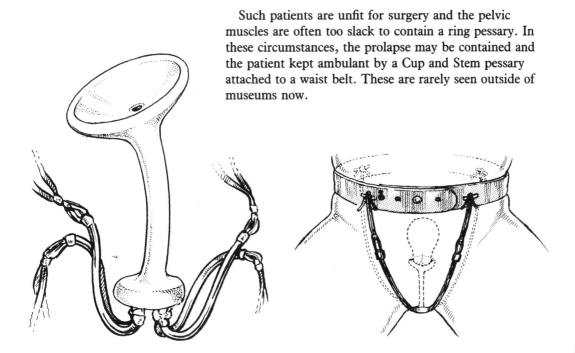

ANTERIOR COLPORRHAPHY (AND REPAIR OF CYSTOCELE)

Surgical restoration of the normal anatomy is the best treatment. Reconstitution of the fibrous 'scaffolding' of the pelvic organs allows the musculature to function efficiently, provided it is not itself too fibrotic from prolonged stretching.

Cystocele, rectocele and vaginal wall prolapse are dealt with by anterior and posterior colporrhaphy. Uterine prolapse calls for shortening of the cardinal and uterosacral ligaments. Each 'repair' must be adapted to the extent of the prolapse, and perineal repair is often required as well.

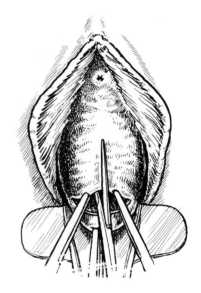

ANTERIOR REPAIR 1. Opening up the anterior vaginal wall.

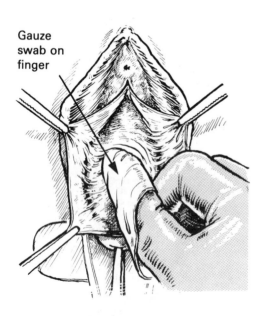

Gauze swab on finger

2. Mobilising cystocele from vaginal walls.

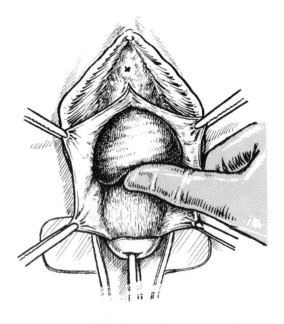

3. Mobilising cystocele from cervix.

278

ANTERIOR COLPORRHAPHY (AND REPAIR OF CYSTOCELE)

Anterior repair (*contd*)

The next step is obliteration of the
cystocele protrusion by tightening
the fascial layer between it and the
vaginal wall, a layer which is often
very difficult to identify. It has various
names – pubovesical fascia, pubocervical
ligaments (equating them with an anterior
continuation of the transverse cervical
ligaments), even fascia of Denonvillier. In
practice, the bladder has a fascial envelope
which can be used for the purpose.

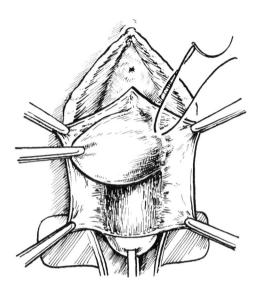

4. Placing the tightening suture as far
laterally as possible.

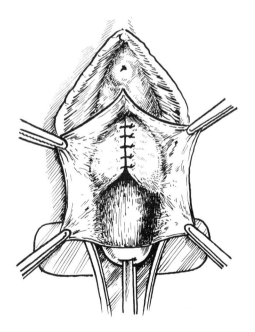

5. Obliteration of the cystocele
completed.

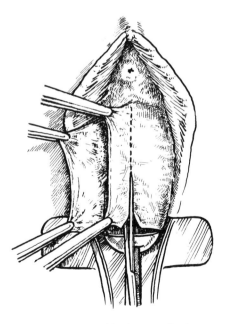

6. Removing redundant vaginal
wall. This is followed by closure with
interrupted absorbable sutures.

REPAIR OF UTERINE PROLAPSE

This involves at the least some shortening of the transverse cervical ligaments and usually amputation of the elongated supravaginal cervix. It is often done in conjunction with anterior and posterior repairs – the so-called Manchester or Donald-Fothergill operation – but only the operation for uterine prolapse would be required in, for example, nulliparous prolapse.

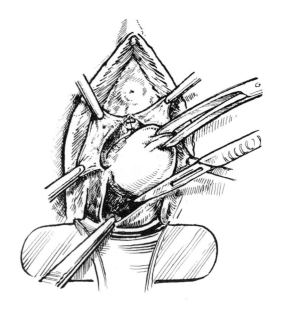

1. The cystocele has been repaired. The cervix is being stripped of vaginal wall.

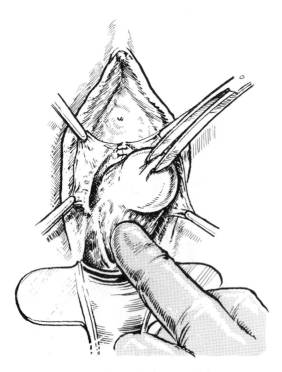

2. Posterior vaginal wall being stripped back.

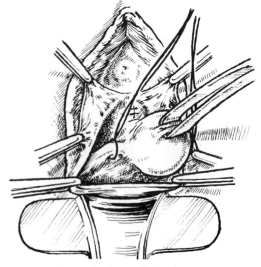

3. Elongated transverse cervical and uterosacral ligaments are sutured and divided.

REPAIR OF UTERINE PROLAPSE

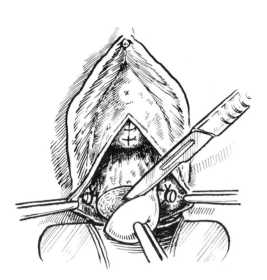

4. Amputation of cervix.

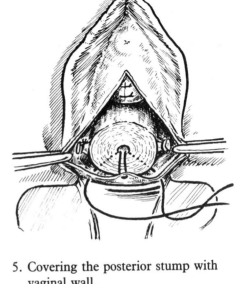

5. Covering the posterior stump with vaginal wall.

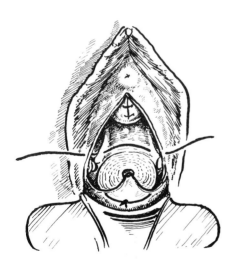

6. Tying the transverse cervical ligaments in front of the cervix and so shortening them and raising the uterus. (This is the so-called Fothergill suture: sometimes two are put in.)

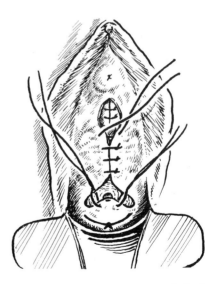

7. Covering cervical stump and closing the vaginal wall. On release of the cervical stump the uterus returns to the pelvis.

281

POSTERIOR COLPOPERINEORRHAPHY
(INCLUDING REPAIR OF RECTOCELE)

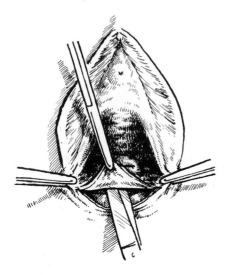

1. Mobilisation of the posterior vaginal wall.

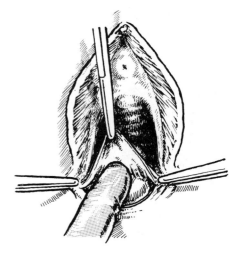

2. Separating rectocele from posterior vaginal wall.

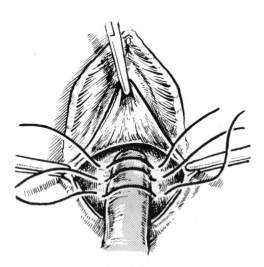

3. Obliterating the rectocele by tightening the fascial layer (cf. obliterating the cystocele.)

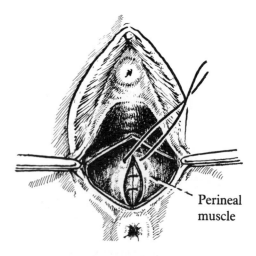

Perineal muscle

4. Excess vaginal skin is removed. The perineal muscles are sutured over the obliterated rectocele. The skin and vagina are closed as in perineorrhaphy (p.197).

REPAIR OF ENTEROCELE

An enterocele is a prolapse of the Pouch of Douglas peritoneum in between the upper vagina and rectum, and must be distinguished from a rectocele. Repair of enterocele is usually combined with repair of uterine prolapse which is not shown here.

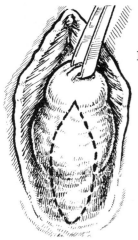

1. Dotted lines show the area of vaginal wall which will be removed.

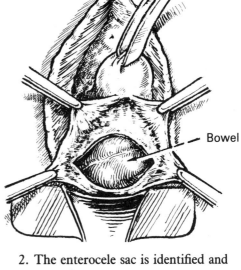

2. The enterocele sac is identified and opened.

Bowel

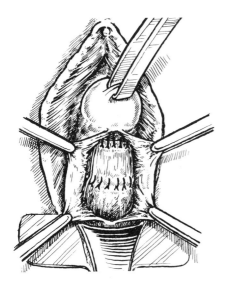

3. Once the sac is mobilised the neck is sutured up as far as possible to obliterate the enterocele. The sac is then sutured to the neck of the cervix. Alternatively a high purse-string suture may be employed.

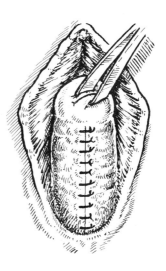

4. The vaginal wall is closed in the usual way.

283

REPAIR BY VAGINAL HYSTERECTOMY

Indications

1. When the prolapse is complete. In such cases the ligaments are very attenuated and a better result may be obtained by removal of the uterus.

2. When there is some non-malignant uterine condition – small fibroids, menorrhagia.

Some surgeons will always remove a uterus rather than leave it, when doing a repair. It may be difficult to remove the ovaries by the vaginal route.

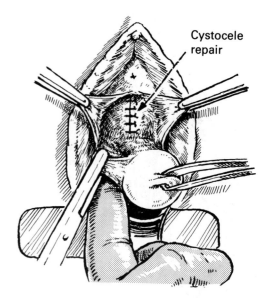

1. The bladder has been mobilised. The uterine ligaments are put on the stretch and divided.

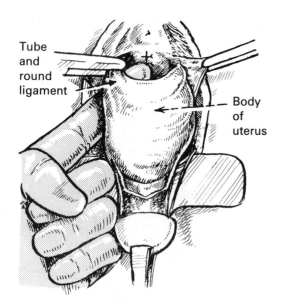

2. Utero-vesical pouch has been entered. Broad ligament structures are put on the stretch and divided.

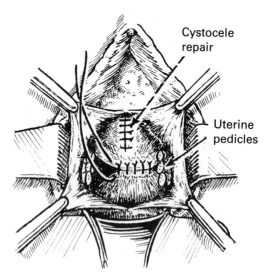

3. The uterus is removed and posterior peritoneal leaf is sutured to the peritoneum of the bladder.

REPAIR BY VAGINAL HYSTERECTOMY

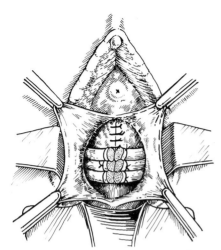

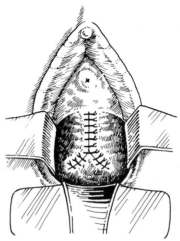

4. The lateral pedicles are sutured together to support the Pouch of Douglas.

5. The cystocele has been obliterated in the usual manner and the vaginal vault and anterior wall closed. Posterior colporrhaphy follows.

RECTOVAGINAL FISTULA

This condition is a rare complication of radiotherapy usually for carcinoma of the cervix, but will occasionally arise as a complication of repair of rectocele or colpoperineorrhaphy (page 195). Such fistulae are very unlikely to close spontaneously and should always be dealt with surgically. The technique depends on the site of the fistula.

VAGINAL REPAIR

A fistula in the lower half of the vagina or near the perineum is usually quite accessible and should be repaired by the vaginal route.

The principle is as for vesical fistula – mobilisation of the skin and rectal wall layers, and closure without tension. If the fistula is very low in the vagina it may be best to convert it into a complete tear (p. 198) and repair the tear and the fistula together.

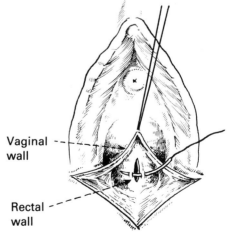

Vaginal wall

Rectal wall

ABDOMINAL REPAIR

This approach would be used by a general surgeon when repairing a rectovaginal fistula arising in the vault after hysterectomy or radiotherapy. If the fistula were large and especially if the continuing presence of malignant tissue were suspected, a temporary colostomy might be necessary.

285

ENTEROCELE – REPAIR BY VAGINAL HYSTERECTOMY

OPERATIVE AND POST-OPERATIVE COMPLICATIONS

Selection of patients
1. Neither youth nor age are contraindications but the patient must be reasonably fit, with adequate cardio-respiratory and renal function. Oestrogen vaginal cream may be used to treat atrophic vaginitis prior to surgery.
2. The patient must complain. If she does not find her prolapse inconvenient no treatment should be offered.
3. Beware of causing dyspareunia or apareunia by performing a tight repair, especially in a younger woman.

During operation
1. Bleeding pedicles are more difficult to control than during abdominal surgery. The parametric structures should be clamped, divided and ligated in small rather than large bites.
2. With the uterus gone, there is a risk of distorting the ureters if the bladder fascia is tightened too much during repair of the cystocele.

After operation
There is a tendency to vault haematoma which becomes infected and ultimately discharges per vaginam; but otherwise vaginal hysterectomy if done properly is not liable to any more complications than a repair operation.

1. **Urinary tract**

   Urinary infection is very common, and dysuria is the rule. Catheterisation is always required, and it is best to leave a catheter in the bladder until the patient is able to void urine spontaneously.

   Infection can at least be delayed by routine bladder irrigation twice daily with a urinary antiseptic. Specimens of urine should be sent regularly for culture and antibiotic sensitivity.

   Once micturition is spontaneous the amount of residual urine left in the bladder after voiding should be checked once or even twice even if it does involve further catheterisation. The amount left should not be more than 30ml.

2. **Bleeding**

   This may occur soon after operation or about the 10th day when the sutures begin to disintegrate. Rarely, it may be necessary to return the patient to theatre.

3. **Recto-anal symptoms**

   Haemorrhoids are temporarily aggravated by colpoperineorrhaphy, but respond to Anusol cream. If there is no bowel movement by the 5th day an enema should be given.

4. **Thrombosis**

   Some form of prophylaxis is now obligatory even if it is only early ambulation, and determined physiotherapy is required. Any sign of thrombosis should be treated at once with anticoagulants and antibiotics, and the possibility of embolism must be borne in mind (see page 388).

LATE COMPLICATIONS

1. Recurrence of Prolapse

(a) **Due to continuing extension of fibrous supports.** This may be a congenital weakness or a result of excessive intra-abdominal pressure as from chronic bronchitis in a fat woman. (Cf. recurrence of inguinal hernia due to imperfect healing.)

(b) **Faulty Technique**

Vaginal repair operations call for some experience. An unsuspected and unlooked for enterocele may appear.

(c) **Faulty Indications for Operation**

The patient's symptoms may have been due to vaginitis, or a neurotic response to stress, or even chronic constipation.

2. Stress Incontinence

Sometimes this appears for the first time after a repair operation, or it is not specifically complained of and ignored during operation.

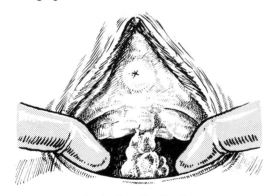

Vaginal wall adhesions.

3. Dyspareunia

The surgeon must enquire before the operation about the patient's sexual activity and must be careful to leave a functional vagina where this is required (even although this may make support of the prolapse more difficult).

Causes are:

(a) Too early resumption of intercourse before healing is complete and vaginal epithelium normal.

(b) Too small a vaginal orifice. Usually stretching will occur, but if necessary a perineoplasty can be done (page 199).

(c) Too narrow or too short a vagina. A narrow vagina can sometimes be widened at the expense of length by the equivalent of a perineoplasty. Nothing can be done if the vagina is too short beyond prescribing an oestrogen cream and counselling perseverance.

(d) Adhesions between vaginal walls. To prevent this the vagina may be packed for 24 hours post-operatively. They are caused by sepsis, and are occasionally so tough that they have to be divided under anaesthesia. Adhesions are not common and are most likely to occur in older women who are not sexually active.

CHAPTER 13

DISEASES OF THE OVARY AND FALLOPIAN TUBE

CLINICAL FEATURES OF OVARIAN TUMOURS

Symptoms due to Size

Because of the lack of any specific symptoms, ovarian tumours are often large by the time the doctor is consulted. Menstrual function is seldom upset, and any irregularity is attributed to the patient's 'time of life'. She may have noticed that her clothes are getting tight, and if the abdominal swelling has coincided with amenorrhoea, she may believe herself pregnant.

Pressure Symptoms

These are commonly an increased frequency of micturition and a dull pain in the lower abdomen. If the tumour becomes very big, there may be respiratory embarrassment and oedema or varicosities in the legs, and a characteristic 'ovarian cachexia' develops, due perhaps to interference with alimentary function.

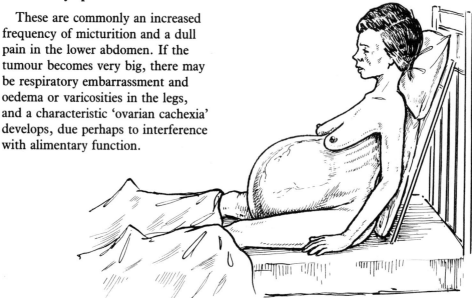

Very large tumours are in one sense reassuring, since they are less likely to be malignant. In the time taken to achieve such size, an ovarian cancer would as a rule have already declared itself by some other sign such as ascites or pain.

CLINICAL FEATURES OF OVARIAN TUMOURS

Small tumours remain in the pelvis
and will only be detected on bimanual
examination or by ultrasound.

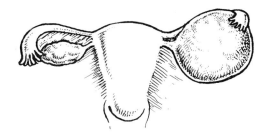

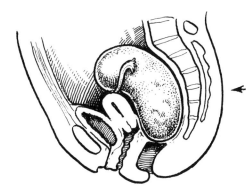

Larger tumours fill the pelvis and
usually lie between the uterus and
sacrum. If the patient is not too fat
the uterus can be distinguished on
palpation as separate from the tumour.

A tumour occupying the abdomen causes a midline swelling and is usually tense.

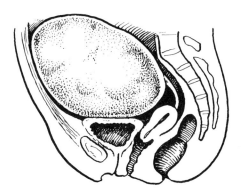

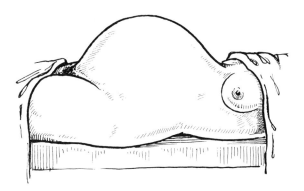

Little can be done at this stage to classify the tumour or exclude malignancy; but very large
tumours are likely to be benign; a primarily malignant tumour would have killed the patient
before reaching such a size.

CLINICAL FEATURES OF OVARIAN TUMOURS

If the patient is very thin irregularities may be palpated, and sometimes two tumours may be suspected.

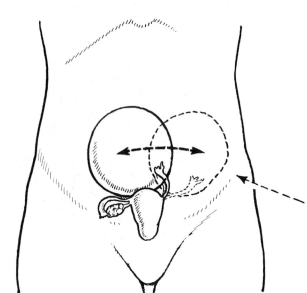

Some tumours of moderate size have a long pedicle composed of the attenuated broad ligament and fallopian tube, which allows the tumour to be displaced from side to side, or to occupy a high abdominal position.

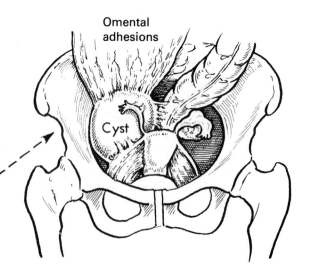

Omental adhesions

Cyst

The upper pole can usually be distinguished, and the lower pole can be palpated per vaginam.

Adhesions, inflammation and displacement of pelvic organs may all exist along with a tumour and confuse the examiner.

DIFFERENTIAL DIAGNOSIS

An experienced examiner will recognise an ovarian tumour, mainly because ovarian tumour is, in the circumstances, the most likely diagnosis. All abdominal swellings should be subjected to ultrasound and X-ray examination.

Two very obvious mistakes must be avoided.

1. The midline swelling due to a full bladder.

2. The 16-week pregnancy. The gravid uterus at this stage has a very soft isthmic region which can resemble the pedicle of a cyst.

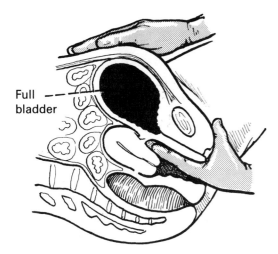

Full bladder

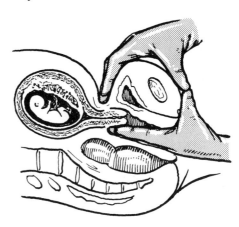

ASCITES. A fluid thrill may be elicited from an ovarian cyst, and ascites and tumour may coexist; but as a rule the distinction should be easily made.

(See 'Shifting Dullness', page 82).

Ascites
The bowel floats on the fluid. The percussion note is resonant over the top of the swelling and dull over the flanks.

Tumour
Percussion note is dull over the top of the swelling and resonant in the flanks.

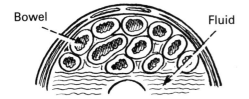

Bowel — Fluid

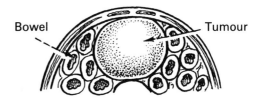

Bowel — Tumour

DIFFERENTIAL DIAGNOSIS

Uterine Fibroids

A large midline intramural fibroid (p.241) may be impossible to distinguish from a solid ovarian tumour until the abdomen is opened and an entirely different surgical problem encountered.

An ovarian tumour will displace the uterus forwards or downwards where it may sometimes be made out separately on vaginal examination.

An intramural fibroid will obscure the uterus. The cavity is often elongated.

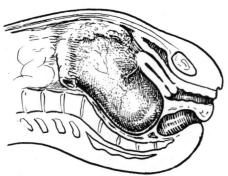

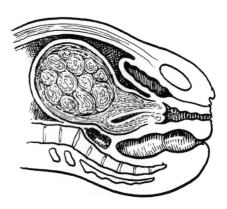

Ultrasound examination should be able to distinguish between fibroid and ovarian cyst; but many ovarian tumours are solid, and some fibroids undergo cystic degeneration. Vaginal ultrasound gives a more detailed picture of the pelvic contents and more precise diagnosis.

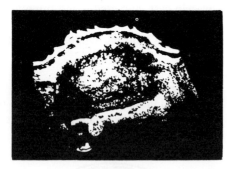

Scan of fibroid

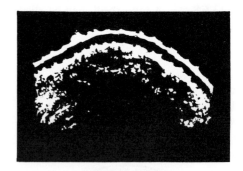

Scan of cyst

DIFFERENTIAL DIAGNOSIS

Pelvic Inflammation

The swelling palpated *per vaginam* may be due to an adherent mass of uterus, tubes, 'chocolate' ovarian cysts, and bowel.

A pyosalpinx, tuberculous or otherwise, may give the same sensation.

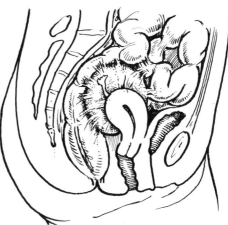

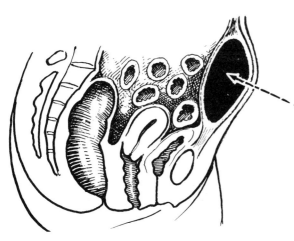

Rectus Sheath Haematoma

This rare condition presents as a fixed abdominal mass, accompanied by pain; and usually follows sudden exertion such as severe coughing. It should be thought of when the pelvis is found to be empty of any tumour.

The Atonic Abdominal Wall

This is seen in old women who display a tense and distended abdomen. There is however resonance to percussion in every area.

Fluid Retention Syndrome

This may cause considerable abdominal distension, particularly in the evening or pre-menstrually.

The Fat Abdominal Wall

The fat patient may be convinced she has a tumour although she is only putting on weight (phantom tumour). Palpation is difficult; but the percussion note in the lower half of the abdomen will be resonant.

Hydatid Cyst
Pancreatic Cyst
Large Hydronephrotic
 Kidney
⎫
⎬
⎭
These are all rarities in the U.K. but must be considered if the physical signs are equivocal and especially if the swelling is not in the midline.

DIFFERENTIAL DIAGNOSIS

Broad Ligament Cysts

The distinction is not likely to be made before laparotomy, when the intact ovary is observed on the back of the swelling.

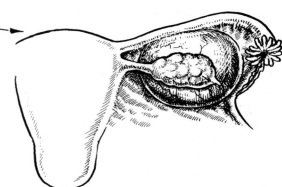

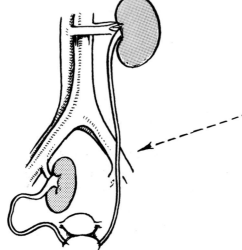

Ectopic Kidney or Spleen

These abnormalities are rare but as they are usually detected for the first time on bimanual examination they must be borne in mind. The ectopic kidney can lie anywhere in the pelvis and derives its blood supply from the iliac vessels. The ureter often runs a tortuous course.

Retroperitoneal Tumours

Retroperitoneal in the surgical sense means behind the peritoneum of the posterior abdominal wall. Such tumours are rare but may arise from any connective tissue, lipoma being the commonest. Examination reveals a fixed tumour; but the lipoma may be deceptively fluctuant. The tumour may displace the ureter and is in close relation to large vessels.

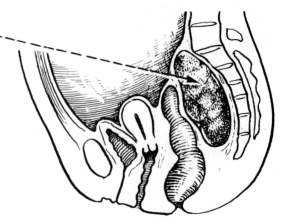

TORSION OF THE PEDICLE

Complications of Ovarian Tumours

TORSION of the PEDICLE
(Axial rotation)
This is the commonest complication
and may occur with any tumour except
those with adhesions. The thin-walled
veins of the pedicle are obstructed first
while the arterial supply continues.
As a result there is haemorrhage into
the tumour and into the peritoneum,
and if not treated gangrene will occur.
Very rarely the pedicle atrophies
and the tumour obtains a new blood
supply through its adhesions to
surrounding viscera (parasitic tumour).

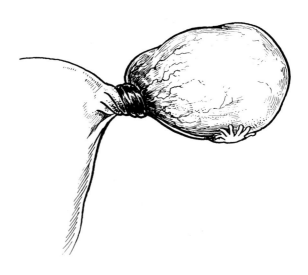

Clinical Features

Subacute

The patient complains of recurrent
abdominal pain which passes off as
the pedicle untwists. There is a rise
in pulse and temperature during the
bleeding; and over a period anaemia
develops.

Acute

The signs and symptoms are those
of an acute abdominal condition. The
problem becomes one of differential
diagnosis to exclude those conditions
in which laparotomy is not needed, and
laparoscopy may be useful.

Pain tends to be intense and
continuous.

Differential Diagnosis

1. 'Surgical Conditions' (i.e. those
conditions commonly seen and dealt
with by a general surgeon.)

Acute appendicitis
Obstruction
Diverticulitis

2. **Ruptured Cyst**

This may occur alone or in
conjunction with torsion. Rupture is
not particularly upsetting to the patient
unless the contents are irritant.

TORSION OF PEDICLE

Differential Diagnosis

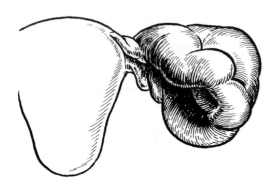

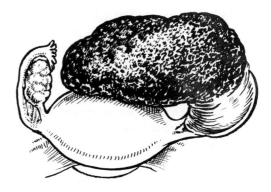

Acute Pelvic Inflammation with tubo-ovarian abscess.
Signs of infection are more marked. A cyst which has undergone rotation is usually larger than the diffuse swelling of pelvic inflammation.

Ectopic Pregnancy

The swelling is usually small although extremely tender and the history suggestive; but in a young woman this condition must always be considered.

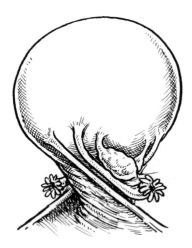

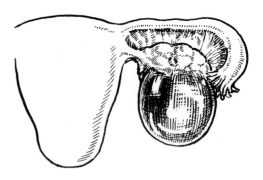

Torsion of a Fibroid

Normal organs very rarely if ever develop axial rotation, but a uterus enlarged by a fibroid may do so.

Ovulation Bleeding

If the ovulation bleeding is greater than usual the woman may show quite marked signs of peritonism. The corpus luteum may thereafter become exaggeratedly cystic and mislead the examiner.

RUPTURE OF OVARIAN CYST

Rupture may be either traumatic or spontaneous.

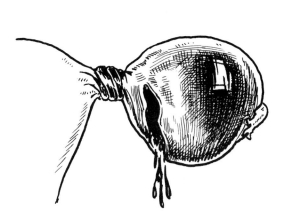

1. Following torsion of a pedicle.

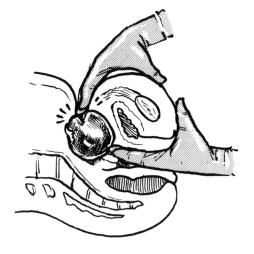

2. During bimanual examination.

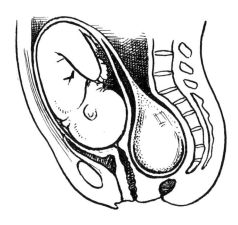

3. During labour when the cyst is impacted in the pelvis.

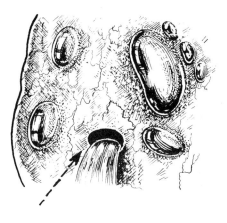

4. Spontaneous rupture. This is not uncommon, especially with malignant cysts, when the epithelial tissue outgrows the connective tissue.

RUPTURE OF OVARIAN CYST

PSEUDOMYXOMA PERITONEI

This rare condition occasionally but not inevitably follows the rupture of a mucinous cystadenoma (page 302). The epithelial cells implant on the peritoneum and continue to secrete a gelatinous pseudomucin; this material is not absorbed, or secretion is faster than absorption; and the abdominal cavity is eventually filled with the jelly, while the secreting cells spread over the parietal and visceral peritoneum. A reactive peritonitis with adhesions is a sequel, and the patient must be operated on at intervals for removal of as much of the exudate as possible. The disease develops slowly over several years, but will eventually cause the patient's death from cachexia or obstruction. A similar condition is reported chiefly in males, from a ruptured mucocele of the appendix vermiformis.

ASCITES

Ascites (Gk. askos: a wine skin) means free fluid in the peritoneal cavity, and its presence in association with an ovarian tumour is strongly suggestive of malignancy. The cause is unknown; but any large tumour may be accompanied by ascites (cf. the small quantities of free fluid sometimes seen at caesarean section).

ASCITES and HYDROTHORAX

The fluid may track via the lymphatic system from the peritoneal to the pleural cavity. Hydrothorax may accompany ascites due to any cause, or may occur as an accompaniment of a lung tumour. The so-called Meigs' syndrome describes the specific condition of ascites and hydrothorax in conjunction with a benign ovarian fibroma.

Features suggestive of malignancy

1. *Age.* If the patient is over 50 the chance of malignancy is over 50%. Tumours in childhood are usually malignant.
2. *Rapid growth.*
3. *Ascites* (almost pathognomonic).
4. *Solid tumours*, especially when bilateral.
5. *Multilocular cysts with solid areas.* (At least 10% of cysts are malignant.)
6. *Pain.* Pressure pain can occur with any tumour; but referred pain suggests malignant involvement of nerve roots.
7. In some centres tumour markers, such as CA125, may be measured in the blood.

OVARIAN TUMOURS

Ovarian tumours may arise at any age, but are commonest between 30 and 60. Their clinical significance is threefold:

1. Ovarian tumours are particularly liable to be or to become malignant.
2. In their early stages they are asymptomatic and painless.
3. They may grow to a large size and tend to undergo mechanical complications such as torsion and perforation.

Histological Classification

Most tumours arise from the ovarian stroma and germinal epithelium. The embryonic coelom from which that epithelium develops also gives rise to the Müllerian duct from which develop the structures of the genital tract, and it is this common origin which explains the great variety of epithelial patterns which are met with.

PRIMARY EPITHELIAL TUMOURS

1. Mucinous cystadenoma orcystadenocarcinoma (cf. cervical epithelium).
2. Serous cystadenoma or cystadenocarcinoma (cf. tubal epithelium).
3. Endometrioma or Endometrioid carcinoma (cf. endometrium).
4. Clear cell carcinoma.
5. Brenner tumour.

STROMATOUS TUMOURS

Fibroma or sarcoma.

GERM CELL TUMOURS

1. Dysgerminoma.
2. Teratoma.
3. Gonadoblastoma.
4. Yolk sac tumour.
5. Carcinoid
6. Thyroid tumour } Hormone-
7. Choriocarcinoma } producing

HORMONE-PRODUCING TUMOURS

Oestrogen-producing:
1. Granulosa cell tumour.
2. Thecoma.
Androgen-producing:
3. Sertoli-Leydig cell tumour (Arrhenoblastoma).
4. Hilar cell tumour.
5. Lipoid cell tumour.

There is one well-known secondary tumour of the ovary, the Krükenberg tumour, a secondary of a stomach carcinoma.

It is now recognised that all ovarian tumours may secrete hormones, especially oestrogens.

MUCINOUS CYSTADENOMA

A unilocular or multilocular cyst of ovary lined by tall columnar epithelium resembling that of the cervix or large intestine. It is usually large and may reach immense proportions, occupying the whole peritoneal cavity and compressing other organs. It may occur at any age. Together with dermoids they are the commonest cystic neoplasms of the ovary.

The surface of the cyst is completely smooth and round but may be slightly nodular due to projecting loculi.

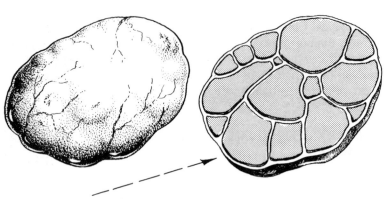

The cut surface of the cyst is multilocular and has a mosaic pattern.

Microscopically the tumour has an outer fibrous capsule from which extend septa supporting the walls of the cysts. The latter are lined by tall columnar epithelium with basal nuclei and contain a gelatinous glycoprotein or mucin.

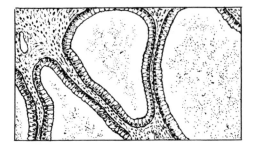

The signs and symptoms are those generally associated with any non-functioning ovarian tumour. Rupture may occur and seeding of the epithelium on the peritoneal surface will cause pseudomyxoma peritonei.

MUCINOUS CYSTADENOCARCINOMA

This is only a third as common as the serous variety. Malignancy in a mucinous cyst is characterised by the formation of areas of solid carcinoma in the wall. The cells are columnar, show mitoses and tend to form glandular structures.

SEROUS CYSTADENOMA

A unilocular or multilocular cyst lined by epithelium similar to the fallopian tube. They are common and form 20% of all ovarian neoplasms. In a third of cases they are bilateral. It is uncommon to find them larger than a fetal head. They show one of three structures:-

(1) A simple cystic form with smooth surface and smooth lining.

(2) A cystic structure with intra-cystic papillary formations. The latter may be sessile buttons or pedunculated frond-like projections.

(3) An adenomatous form where many of the loculi are small and papillary structures are solid and complex.

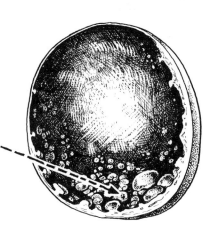

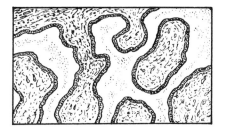

Microscopically the tumour has a fibrous capsule. Septa support the cysts which are lined by cubical epithelium and contain thin serous fluid.

They present no distinctive symptoms.

If rupture occurs papillary structures may land on the peritoneal surface where they may grow or lie dormant for years.

SEROUS CYSTADENOCARCINOMA

This is by far the commonest primary carcinoma, accounting for 60% of all cases, and in half the cases it is bilateral. The cysts are always of papillary type and the epithelium burrowing through the capsule produces papillary processes on the serous surface. Extension of the growth to the pelvis and adjacent organs fixes the tumour. Ascites is always present.

The papillomata are always more fleshy than in the simple cysts and microscopically the epithelial cells are several layers thick and show numerous mitoses. When they invade the capsule they frequently take an acinar form.

CARCINOMA OF THE OVARY

Nearly 25% of all ovarian neoplasms are malignant. Approximately 80% of them are primary growths of the ovary, the remainder being secondary, usually carcinomata.

Primary Carcinoma of the Ovary   80% of all cases of primary carcinoma of the ovary arise in serous or mucinous cysts. These cysts may however be malignant from the outset. Reference has already been made to these forms of malignancy.

Solid Carcinoma of the Ovary   This accounts for 10% of primary carcinoma. It is commonly bilateral but one tumour is usually larger than the other. The ovarian shape is retained for a time and there is a well-marked pedicle but soon the tumours become fixed, secondary deposits occur in the omentum and ascites develops.

Microscopically the growth may take the form of an adenocarcinoma but more commonly it shows solid alveoli or anaplastic epithelial cells in a fibrous stroma.

Endometrioid Carcinoma of the Ovary   It is now recognised that carcinoma of the ovary may be of endometrial type, sometimes arising in endometrioma. Attacks of pain, unusual with ovarian cancer, are common. Sometimes there is uterine bleeding in post-menopausal cases.

Usually the lesion is cystic and chocolate brown in colour. If such a cyst ruptures spontaneously malignancy should be suspected. The histology varies as in uterine carcinoma. It may be a well-differentiated adenocarcinoma, an adeno-acanthoma, mucinous adenocarcinoma or clear-celled carcinoma.

Clear Cell Carcinoma   It is doubtful if this exists as a distinct entity. Clear cells may be seen in almost any variety of ovarian carcinoma, but occasionally a carcinoma, usually solid, consists almost entirely of polygonal cells with clear cytoplasm. It behaves in the same way as any other solid carcinoma and has the same prognosis.

Secondary Carcinoma of the Ovary   The ovary may be the site of secondary deposits from growths arising in other parts of the genital tract. These are usually overshadowed by the clinical manifestation of primary growth.

Ovarian metastases from extra-genital tumours are not uncommon. The commonest sites of primary growth are breast, stomach and large intestine. They usually occur in functioning ovaries and their importance lies in the fact that the metastatic growths reach a large size while the primary growth is small and gives rise to no clinical manifestations. They usually reproduce the histological characteristics of the primary cancer. Owing to their rapid growth they tend to be friable and haemorrhagic giving rise to blood-stained peritoneal exudate.

BRENNER TUMOUR

A benign tumour mainly solid and most common in the 6th decade, composed of fibrous and epithelial elements in varying proportions. It forms 2% of all solid ovarian neoplasms.

It is usually solid and resembles a fibroma. Occasionally there may be microcysts or even an associated large mucinous cyst. Microscopically it is composed mainly of fibrous tissue with small islands of clear epithelial cells of squamous appearance. Sometimes the islands become cystic and the epithelial cells become mucinous.

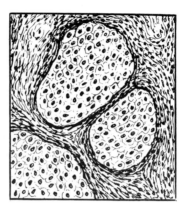

FIBROMA

This is composed of fibrous tissue and resembles fibromata found elsewhere. It is most common in the elderly and accounts for 4–5% of all ovarian neoplasms.

The fibroma is believed by many to be a thecoma which has undergone fibrous transformation. It is sometimes associated with Meig's syndrome.

GERM CELL TUMOURS

There are four main types of germ cell tumour:-

(1) Dysgerminoma; (2) Tumours of tissues found in the embryo or adult – the teratomata; (3) Tumours of dysgenetic gonads – commonly a gonadoblastoma; (4) Tumours of extra-embryonic tissues such as choriocarcinoma or yolk sac tumour.

DYSGERMINOMA

This is the only solid ovarian tumour of characteristic appearance. Usually ovoid with a smooth capsule, it is of rubbery consistency and greyish colour. It is commonest in younger age groups, under 30 years as a rule, and is often bilateral. Sometimes it is found in cases of intersex.

GERM CELL TUMOURS

Dysgerminoma (*contd*)

Microscopically it consists of masses of large clear epithelial cells with large nuclei, resembling primitive germ cells, in cords or alveoli. Fine connective tissue infiltrated by lymphocytes separates the bundles of epithelial cells. The malignancy varies but many appear to be relatively benign and do not recur. Those in children tend to be more malignant.

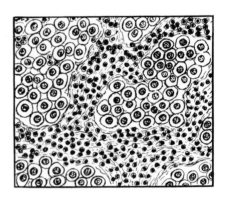

TERATOMATA

These are broadly divided into (a) cystic and (b) solid forms.

  (a) **Cystic teratoma or dermoid**

    This is one of the commonest ovarian tumours and is usually diagnosed during the child-bearing period but may be found at any age and is frequently bilateral.

    It is ovoid and unilocular with on one aspect a rounded eminence from which hairs grow and on or in which teeth may be found. The wall consists of dense fibrous tissue lined by stratified squamous epithelium. The eminence may contain sebaceous glands, teeth, hair, nervous tissues, cartilage, bone, respiratory and intestinal epithelium and thyroid gland tissue. Thick yellow sebaceous material fills the cyst.

    They are particularly liable to have a long pedicle and easily undergo torsion or interfere with the movement of the pregnant uterus.

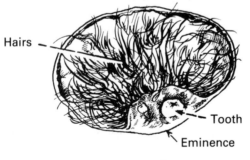

Hairs

Tooth

Eminence

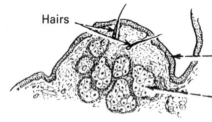

Hairs

Stratified squamous epithelium

Sebaceous glands

GERM CELL TUMOURS

(b) Solid teratoma

These occur at an earlier age than dermoids, often in childhood. They are solid and may contain any tissue from the three germinal layers, mixed in a completely disorderly fashion. They are particularly liable to undergo malignant change, the malignancy arising in any one of the tissues present.

Gonadoblastoma

This is a tumour associated with dysgenetic gonads, usually streak gonads. The patient is an apparent female and may have a diminutive uterus, tubes and vagina, but usually there is a sex chromosome anomaly such as XO/XY.

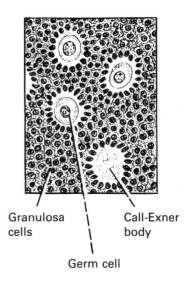

Granulosa cells

Call-Exner body

Germ cell

The tumour is composed of two types of cell: (a) a large primitive germ cell and (b) small cells of granulosa cell type. Call-Exner bodies (small rosettes) may be seen in the latter. These two types of cell form epithelial islands in a stroma which may contain Leydig-like cells. Sometimes the germ cells may undergo rapid proliferation and give rise to a dysgerminoma. Some of the dysgerminomata in children probably arise in this way. Choriocarcinoma may also take origin in a gonadoblastoma. There are frequently some signs of masculinisation and 17-ketosteroid excretion may be raised.

Yolk sac tumour

This is a rare tumour found in children and young adults. It has a variable histological structure and is highly malignant. The main interest lies in the fact that it produces alpha-fetoprotein and the blood levels can be used as a diagnostic test and as a means of monitoring response to treatment.

Choriocarcinoma is mentioned in the succeeding part dealing with hormone-producing tumours.

KRUKENBERG TUMOUR

This is a secondary carcinoma of the ovary. It is remarkable for its characteristic histological appearance and the fact that the primary growth, usually in the stomach, less commonly in the large intestine, is often clinically silent. The ovarian tumours are bilateral, of equal size, smooth and lobulated. They remain freely mobile with no adhesions. Being firm and fibrous in appearance they are frequently mistaken for fibromata, but these are usually unilateral. The patient is usually between 30 and 40 years of age, younger than the usual gastric carcinoma patient.

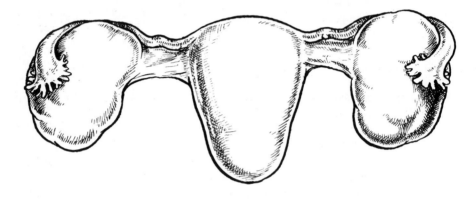

Histologically they have a well-defined appearance. There is a very cellular stroma, resembling a sarcoma, in which are large epithelial cells lying singly or in alveoli. These epithelial cells have a clear cytoplasm with a crescentic nucleus pushed to one side giving a signet-ring appearance which is typical. The cytoplasm is full of mucin.

The majority of patients with this tumour succumb within 1 year of diagnosis.

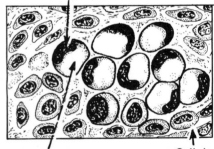

Nucleus of 'signet-ring' cell

Clear mucin-filled cytoplasm

Cellular stroma

HORMONE-PRODUCING TUMOURS

AMENORRHOEA and OVARIAN TUMOURS

Disturbance of menstruation is unusual with the commoner forms of ovarian tumour such as cystadenomas. Amenorrhoea is much more likely to occur in cases of functioning tumours producing steroids.

HORMONE-PRODUCING TUMOURS

The commonest tumours of this kind are steroid-producing, particularly sex steroids. Both androgenic and oestrogenic effects have been described with every histological variety but certain tumours of well defined histological structures are commonly associated with the production of one type of steroid.

OESTROGEN-PRODUCING TUMOURS

These belong to the granulosa-theca cell group and are found at all ages. They account for 3% of all solid tumours of the ovary.

Oestrogen excess causes:

1. Hyperplasia of myometrium ⟶ enlarged uterus.
2. Hyperplasia of endometrium ⟶ irregular bleeding. Occasionally amenorrhoea occurs if the production of oestrogen does not fluctuate.
3. Hyperplasia of mammary gland tissue ⟶ enlargement, tenderness of breasts.
4. Oestrogenic vaginal smear.

In childhood there is accelerated skeletal growth and appearance of sex hair.

5% occur in children ⟶ precocious puberty.

60% occur in child-bearing years ⟶ irregular menstruation.

30% occur in post-menopausal women ⟶ post-menopausal bleeding.

Diagnosis

Granulosa cell tumour in childhood is the usual cause of female precocity and diagnosis is obvious. In child-bearing and post-menopausal years diagnosis is difficult owing to the multiplicity of causes of irregular vaginal bleeding. Laparoscopy and ovarian biopsy may be useful.

Pathology

These tumours vary very much in function. Large tumours may be virtually functionless. In childhood and early adult life the tumours are composed mainly of granulosa cells. In later life they are usually thecomata. The granulosa cell type of growth should be considered as carcinoma. Recurrence may occur many years after removal of the primary growth. It is not possible to correlate accurately malignancy with histological appearances. In 14% of cases endometrial hyperplasia becomes atypical and carcinoma develops.

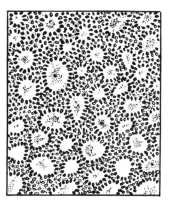

ANDROGEN-PRODUCING TUMOURS

Three distinct types of masculinising ovarian tumour are recognised: (a) Sertoli-Leydig cell tumour (Arrhenoblastoma), (b) Hilar cell tumour, (c) Lipoid cell tumour. All three cause amenorrhoea.

SERTOLI-LEYDIG CELL TUMOUR (Arrhenoblastoma)

This is a rare tumour and forms less than 1% of all ovarian tumours. It occurs in young adult females. Clinically two stages are recognised:

1. Period of defeminisation   2. Period of masculinisation

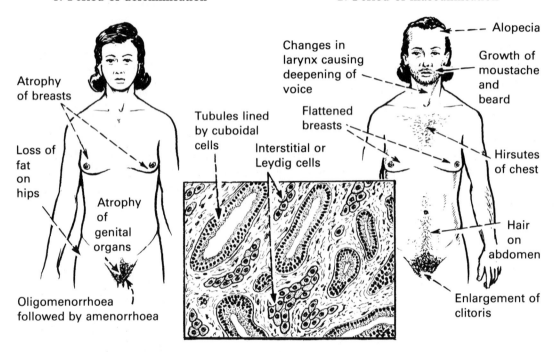

Atrophy of breasts

Loss of fat on hips

Atrophy of genital organs

Oligomenorrhoea followed by amenorrhoea

Tubules lined by cuboidal cells

Interstitial or Leydig cells

Changes in larynx causing deepening of voice

Flattened breasts

Alopecia

Growth of moustache and beard

Hirsutes of chest

Hair on abdomen

Enlargement of clitoris

Pathology

Usually appears as a small white or yellowish tumour within the ovarian substance. Cystic degeneration may occur. In 20% the tumour is malignant and behaves like a carcinoma producing widespread metastases.

Histologically it consists of primitive tubules surrounded by Leydig cells which contain crystalloids of Reinke. These are rod-shaped structures in the cytoplasm of Leydig cells and said to be diagnostic of these cells.

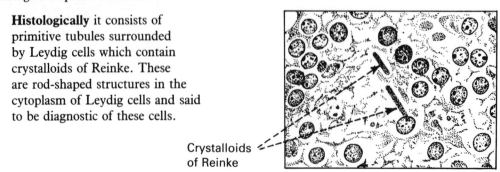

Crystalloids of Reinke

ANDROGEN-PRODUCING TUMOURS

SERTOLI-LEYDIG CELL TUMOUR (*contd*)

Biochemistry

The symptoms are due to the secretion of testosterone. The quantities are small and therefore the output of metabolites such as 17-ketosteroids is within the normal range. Direct estimations of blood testosterone can be made but this requires very sophisticated laboratory procedures.

Removal of the tumour results in regression of symptoms in the same order as their appearance. Menstruation returns within a month or two. Voice changes tend to be permanent.

HILAR CELL TUMOUR

This is a very rare tumour found in post-menopausal women. Defeminisation occurs but signs of virilism are usually mild, consisting of hirsutes, alopecia and enlargement of the clitoris.

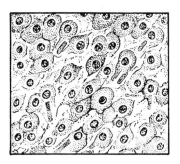

Pathology

Hilar cell tumours are small, brown, simple tumours in the ovarian hilum consisting of polyhedral Leydig cells. Crystalloids of Reinke are occasionally present. 17-ketosteroids are usually within the normal post-menopausal range. Small quantities of androgen are produced.

LIPOID CELL TUMOUR (ovoblastoma, masculinovoblastoma, adrenal-like tumour)

This is also a rare tumour causing masculinisation and producing symptoms and signs of hyper-corticoidism such as skin striae, obesity, polycythaemia, a diabetic glucose tolerance curve and hypertension.

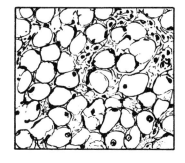

Pathology

The tumour consists of cells with a high content of lipoid and is commonly large and yellowish.

Unlike other virilising tumours the 17-ketosteroid output is greatly increased and the excretion of 17-hydroxycorticosteroids is also raised. ACTH or chorionic gonadotrophin will cause a further increase, but dexamethasone does not diminish the output, thus helping to differentiate the condition from virilism of adrenal origin.

OTHER HORMONE-PRODUCING TUMOURS

CARCINOID (Argentaffinoma: serotonin-producing tumour)

This tumour arises in association with cystic teratoma of the ovary from cells related to respiratory or intestinal epithelium sometimes found in these cysts.

It may give rise to a typical carcinoid syndrome with patchy cyanosis, flushing, diarrhoea, intestinal colic, oedema and cardiac failure due to tricuspid valve lesion. Sometimes the syndrome does not appear until the tumour has metastasised to the liver.

Thyroid Tumour (Struma Ovarii)

Small foci of thyroid tissue are common in ovarian teratomata but large amounts are rare and functioning thyroid tissue is still more rare. When the thyroid tissue actually proliferates and forms a tumour 5-10% become malignant.

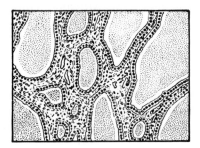

CHORIOCARCINOMA of the Ovary

This is an extremely rare tumour of the ovary. Most commonly it is associated with dysgerminoma and both in turn may be derived from germinal cells in a dysgenetic gonad. Syncytiotrophoblast is always present, but sometimes cytotrophoblast is also formed. The hormones produced are those normally associated with chorionic tissue – chorionic gonadotrophin, oestrogens, etc. Metastases may occur as in any choriocarcinoma.

HORMONE-PRODUCTION by NON-FUNCTIONING TUMOURS

Occasionally the presence of tumour growth in the ovary induces a thecal transformation of the ovarian stroma which in turn produces steroids, sometimes androgenic but more commonly oestrogenic. This has been reported in association with benign and malignant cysts, Brenner tumours, fibroma and secondary carcinoma of ovary. The secretion of steroids results in menstrual upset and in the case of androgens, virilism.

SURGICAL TREATMENT OF OVARIAN TUMOURS

Ovarian tumours must be removed; but this maxim will occasionally be modified by circumstances. Three degrees of excision are recognised:

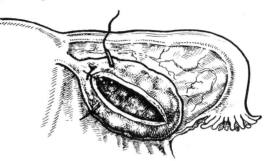

1. **Resection:**   A portion of the ovarian cortex is removed. This procedure is restricted to some cases of polycystic ovary disease.

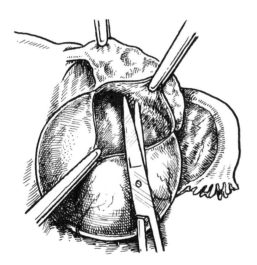

2. **Cystectomy:**   Enucleation of the tumour from its capsule of ovarian tissue, thus preserving ovarian function.

   Indications: A tumour apparently benign in a woman under 45.

   This operation would not be feasible in the case of a very large tumour, or where there had been previous inflammation.

3. **Ovariotomy:**   Removal of an ovary containing a tumour. (Removal of an ovary not containing a tumour is called oophorectomy.)

   Indications: (a) Malignancy. (The uterus and other ovary are also removed.)

   (b) The patient is over 45, or she wishes no more children and the other ovary is normal.

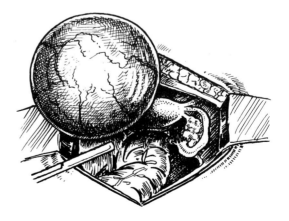

DEALING WITH THE TUMOUR PEDICLE

The pedicle is made up of the fallopian tube, broad and ovarian ligaments and the infundibulopelvic fold; and contains the anastomosing uterine and ovarian vessels which will be much distended if the tumour is large.

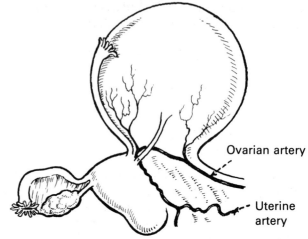

Ovarian artery

Uterine artery

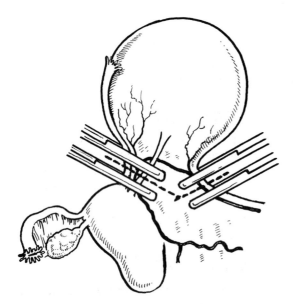

Once the pedicle is clamped and cut, care must be taken to prevent retraction of ovarian vessels with a consequent retroperitoneal haematoma.

If the pedicle is of any size it should be secured with – – – – – – –➤ three or four ligatures.

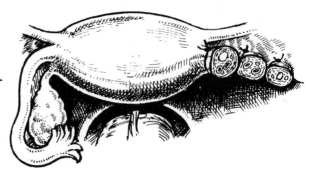

TREATMENT OF OVARIAN CANCER

Much attention is being directed towards the treatment of epithelial ovarian cancer which is now the most frequent cause of death from gynaecological malignancy. The principles of treatment are:

1. Surgical removal of as much malignant tissue as possible, even if this should call for resection of structures outside the normal field of the gynaecologist.

2. Follow-up with intensive chemotherapy, using various combinations of antineoplastic drugs.

3. A 'second look' laparotomy or laparoscopy operation (SLO), to determine the actual effectiveness of the chemotherapy and to decide whether it should be stopped. The second look also allows the removal of any remaining cancerous tissue. It is less practised now.

It will be seen that treatment of this intensity is beyond the scope of the gynaecologist working on his own. Co-operation with a general surgeon may be necessary for the first operation, and experience in the field of chemotherapy lies mainly with the oncologist or radiotherapist. Treatment by radiotherapy itself is probably of use only in palliation, or in specific circumstances such as a localised malignant deposit.

SPREAD of OVARIAN CANCER

It is essential to know the direction of spread of ovarian cancers, so that the true extent of the disease may be recognised.

1. Direct

The first spread is directly into neighbouring structures – peritoneum, uterus, bladder, bowel and omentum.

2. Transcoelomic

Cancer cells are carried across the peritoneum and along paracolonic gutters by the serous fluid, and achieve widespread seeding.

3. Lymphatics

Ovarian drainage is to the para-aortic glands, but sometimes to the pelvic and even inguinal groups. Cells seeded on to the peritoneum are drained via the lymphatic channels on the underside of the diaphragm into the subpleural glands and thence to the pleura.

4. Blood stream

Blood spread is usually late, to the liver and lungs.

SURGICAL PROCEDURES IN OVARIAN CANCER

The objectives are:
1.   To classify the growth according to its extent of spread (staging) as accurately as possible.
2.   To remove as much cancerous tissue as possible ('surgical debulking'; 'cyto-reductive treatment').

Incision   A vertical incision that can be extended is essential to allow a full inspection. Reduction of a cyst by tapping and extraction through a suprapubic incision is more cosmetic, but liable to disseminate malignant cells.

Inspection   The whole cavity must be palpated, including liver, subdiaphragm, bowel and mesenteries, omentum and aortic nodes. Suspicious areas are biopsied.

Organs removed   These must always include the uterus, tubes, ovaries, appendix and omentum. Partial resection of bladder and bowel may also be required, but epithelial cancer tends to spread over invaded tissue rather than penetrate it, and a plane of cleavage can often be found.

Cytology   Specimens of ascitic fluid or peritoneal washings (saline flooded in and withdrawn) must be taken for cytological examination. A cytology smear should be taken from the underside of the diaphragm.

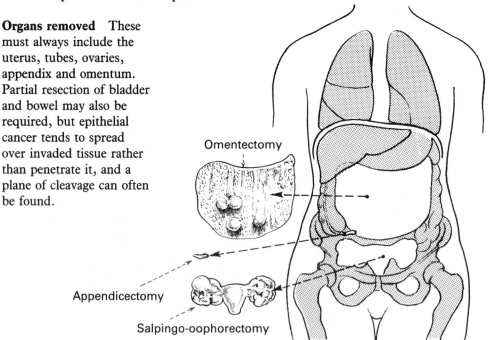

Omentectomy

Appendicectomy

Salpingo-oophorectomy

Very large cysts
    These have to be tapped before surgical removal is attempted and this must be done by drainage through the abdominal wall which reduces the risk of dissemination. Tapping also allows a gradual reduction in the size of the abdominal swelling and diminishes the risk of cardio-respiratory failure when the support of the diaphragm is removed.

STAGING OF OVARIAN CANCER

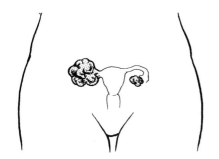

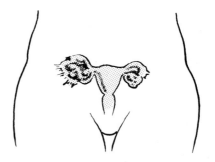

STAGE I Growth limited to ovaries.
Ia. Limited to one ovary. No ascites.
Ib. Limited to both ovaries. No ascites.
Ic. Ascites or positive peritoneal washings also present.
Treatment: Surgery alone for Ia and Ib. Add chemotherapy if Ic.

STAGE II Pelvic extension.
IIa. Spread to uterus/tubes.
IIb. Spread to other pelvic tissues.
IIc. IIb with ascites.
Treatment: Surgery and chemotherapy.

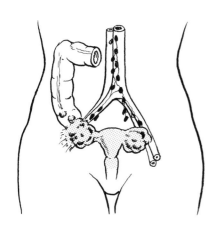

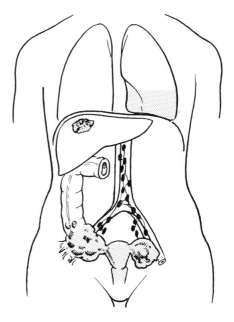

STAGE III Extrapelvic intraperitoneal spread and/or retroperitoneal positive nodes.
OR: No extrapelvic spread but involvement of intestines or omentum.
Treatment: Surgery as extensive as necessary and possible, followed by chemotherapy.

STAGE IV Distant metastases. Pleural effusion with positive cytology.
Treatment: As much surgical extirpation as possible, perhaps with colostomy, followed by chemotherapy. Palliative radiotherapy may be used here.

ANTINEOPLASTIC DRUGS

Antineoplastic drugs act by inhibiting cell division – both normal and malignant – and thus reducing the number of new cells formed.

TUMOUR GROWTH   Tumour cells multiply at the same rate or more slowly than normal cells, but are not subjected to the same physiological control of numbers of cells, so that a cancer gradually develops.

The Cell Cycle (for both normal and tumour cells)

The time taken for a cell to divide into two daughter cells is between 40 and 80 hours, and the chief variable factor is the initial resting phase (G_1).

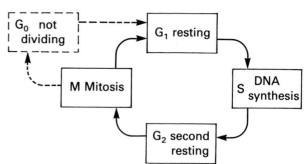

The time taken for a tumour to double its mass is theoretically the same 40–80 hours, but in practice is found to be between 4 and 500 days.

The variable factors in tumour development are the cell-cycle time, the number of cells dividing, and the number lost or incapable of dividing.

	Normal Cells	*Tumour Cells*
Cell-cycle Time	40–80 hours.	40–80 hours. (Tends to be longer than normal cells.)
Cell Loss Factor	100%. Every cell lost is replaced by one cell only and there is no increase in numbers.	Cells are lost through shedding into body cavities, necrosis, immune defences etc. and biologically inadequate cells which cannot divide or only for a few generations ('doomed cells'). Up to 99% may be lost but there is always some growth.
Growth Fraction	Even in normal bone marrow which is a very active tissue only about 20% of the cells (stem cells) are dividing, the remainder being in the G_0 phase.	The growth fraction in tumours varies between 20 and 90.

PHARMACOLOGY OF ANTINEOPLASTIC DRUGS

ALKYLATING AGENTS

These compounds have a bivalent alkyl group R-CH which combines with the guanine base in DNA and prevents replication.

    Cyclophosphamide (Endoxana)
    Chlorambucil (Leukeran)
    Melphalan (Alkeran)

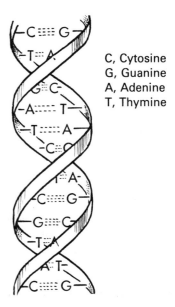

C, Cytosine
G, Guanine
A, Adenine
T, Thymine

ANTIMITOTIC ANTIBIOTICS

These compounds were discovered in the search for active antibiotics. They act against human cells by combining with single strands of DNA to prevent protein synthesis.

    Actinomycin D (Cosmegen)
    Doxorubicin (Adriamycin)

ANTIMETABOLITES

Metabolites in this context are the chemical groups required for the synthesis of nucleic acid and protein. An antimetabolite has a similar structure although functionally different, and is preferentially taken up by the enzyme system, thus preventing the synthesis of nucleoprotein.

    Methotrexate resembles folic acid.
    5-fluorouracil resembles uracil which is a metabolite of RNA.

VINCA ALKALOIDS

These drugs are derived from the periwinkle plant (vinca) and inhibit growth by interfering with mitosis.

    Vincristine (Oncovin)
    Vinblastine (Velbe)

OTHER NON-ALKYLATING AGENTS

Cis-Platin

Carboplatin is a derivative of Cis-Platin. It is better tolerated than Cis-Platin but is more myelosuppressive.

TOXICITY

All antineoplastic drugs are extremely toxic when given in effective dosage, and there is invariably some depression of the bone marrow and the gastro-intestinal tract. **Cis-Platin** is particularly neurotoxic and nephrotoxic and must be preceded by intravenous hydration and accompanied by mannitol to ensure diuresis. **Doxorubicin** is cardiotoxic and the patient must be given a wig for the alopecia. Other complications include tissue necrosis of the veins, and liver failure. Patients taking antineoplastic drugs must be kept under continual supervision, with regular checks on marrow and liver function.

ANTINEOPLASTIC DRUGS

Rationale of Antineoplastic Drug Therapy

It is at present believed that after assault by an antineoplastic drug, tumour cells replace themselves more slowly than normal cells. Treatment is therefore interrupted by rest periods (pulsed therapy) to allow the normal tissues time to recover.

Administration

The drugs are given as the primary treatment when surgery is not feasible, and as supportive therapy after adequate extirpative surgery. The alkylating agents are usually given orally, but others such as Cis-Platin and doxorubicin require intravenous infusion with many precautions. Combinations of one or more agents have the merit of increasing the likelihood of response. Cis-Platin based combinations may improve survival. There is an associated increase in toxicity and probably no true synergic effect.

PRESENT PROGNOSIS FOR OVARIAN CANCER

Stage	5-year survival
I	60–70%
II	40–50%
III	5–10%
IV	Nil

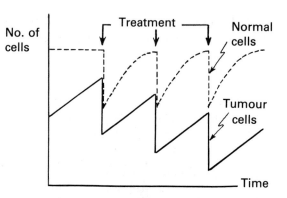

Results of Treatment

Chemotherapy has been used in ovarian cancer for about 30 years, but only relatively recently have mean survival rates beyond 18 months or speculation on cure seemed possible. Patients showing complete regression could survive 2 1/2 years, partial regression up to 18 months and non-responders perhaps 12 months, depending on the extent of surgery. 'Second look laparotomy' is now regarded as of dubious value.

Survival in advanced ovarian cancer may possibly be improved by Platinum combination therapy, which certainly produces the greatest respite rate. This is the basis of the ICON 2 trial (International Collaborative trial, Ovarian Neoplasm) using either Carboplatin or CAP (Cyclophosphamide Adriamycin and Cis-Platin). *B.M.J.* (1991) **303**, 884–893.

Cis-Platin has a dose response curve in advanced (Stages III and IV) ovarian cancer, though with increased toxicity in higher doses. Neuro-toxicity is the principal obstacle to continued use of high dose Cis-Platin.

Median survival:
114 weeks 100mg/m^2 Cis-Platin
69 weeks 50mg/m^2 Cis-Platin
+ 750mg/m^2 Cyclophosphamide

Kaye, S.B. et al. *Lancet* (1992), **340**, 329–33.

COMPUTERISED AXIAL TOMOGRAPHY (CAT SCANNING)

The CAT scanner will demonstrate the presence of lymph node metastases not detectable even by laparotomy, and it will increase the accuracy of staging of ovarian cancer, and of assessing the response to treatment.

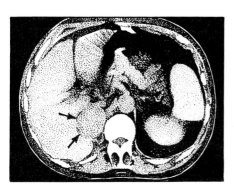

Liver metastasis from
ovarian carcinoma

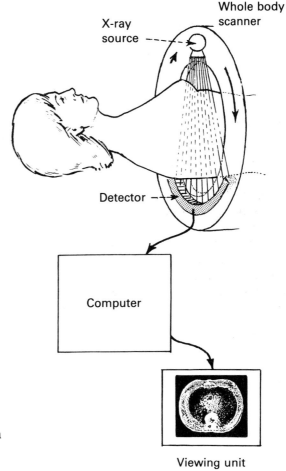

The scanner takes repeated X-ray pictures of a cross-section of the body (nearly 300 pictures within 5 seconds) as the X-ray tube is rotated round the patient.

Some absorption of X-rays takes place according to the density of the tissues through which the X-rays pass. Thus the difference between the amount of radiation entering the body and the amount measured by the detectors is equivalent to the density of the tissues.

These measurements are passed to a computer which performs millions of calculations within a few minutes, and reconstructs from the detector readings a cross-section picture of the viscera.

Magnetic Resonance Imaging (MRI) is also a useful technique, though less widely available.

IMMUNOLOGICAL SCANNING

Advantage is taken of two facts. Firstly, certain strains of mice are prone to develop malignant myeloma. The cells of these tumours can be fused with mouse antibody-producing cells to form hybrid cells which continue to form antibodies. Secondly, most human tumours produce substances, either peculiar to the tumour, or normal but in excessive quantities. These substances can be used as antigens to raise antibodies. The process can be visualised as follows:

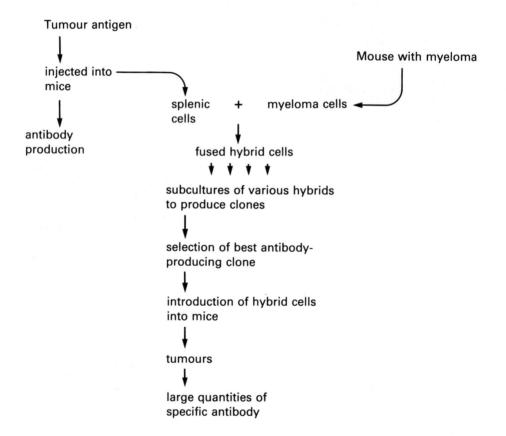

Clinical use

The antibody is tagged with a small quantity of radioactive substance e.g. I_{123}. This is injected intravenously into the patient. After a short time the tagged antibody will be concentrated in tumour cells of the main growth and secondary deposits. The radioactive tumour masses can then be visualised using a gamma-camera.

A further development may be the combination of an antibody with an anti-neoplastic drug. Such a combination would hopefully concentrate in tumour cells and kill them.

BROAD LIGAMENT CYSTS

BROAD LIGAMENT CYSTS (Parovarian cysts)

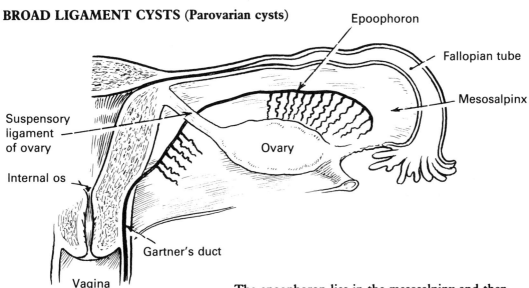

The epoophoron lies in the mesosalpinx and then parallel to the uterus. At about the level of the internal os it penetrates the muscle of the uterus and descends in cervix and vaginal wall to the hymen.

Parovarian cysts derived from the epoophoron are unilocular and contain watery fluid without mucin. The wall is thin and lined with a layer of cuboidal cells – sometimes ciliated.

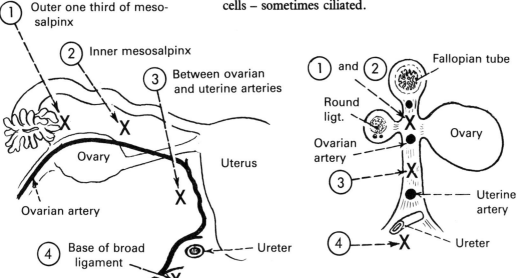

Original location of cyst.

If one imagines any of these locations (marked X) expanding like a balloon the resulting displacement of tissues is easily understood.

323

BROAD LIGAMENT CYSTS

Diagnosis

On palpation the cyst, which is not mobile, may displace the uterus and is closely related to it. An ovarian cyst with adhesions may feel very similar and it is seldom possible to distinguish between the two before laparotomy.

Operation

Great care must be taken in identifying tissues as the location of the original site of cyst determines displacement and characteristics.

In the outer third of the broad ligament the cyst tends to develop a pedicle.

In the middle of the broad ligament the tumour is sessile but relatively fixed.

The ovarian vessels are displaced and may be stretched leading to interference with ovarian blood supply.

It is possible for the ureter and uterine artery to be displaced outwards, but usually they are below and medial to the cyst.

The tumour may increase in size and strip the peritoneum off the pelvic walls and spread laterally and posteriorly obliterating the Pouch of Douglas.

The broad ligament is incised anteriorly where the blood vessels are few and the cyst is enucleated digitally. The oozing area is now exposed and should be obliterated. Care is necessary to avoid damage to blood vessels, ureter and bladder. Redundant broad ligament may require to be excised.

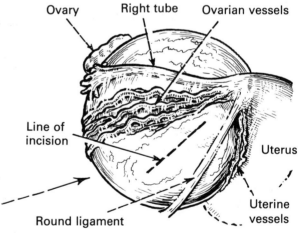

Ovary Right tube Ovarian vessels

Line of incision

Uterus

Broad ligament cyst of right side displacing uterus to left

Round ligament

Uterine vessels

CYSTS of KOBELT's TUBULES, HYDATIDS of MORGAGNI, FIMBRIAL CYSTS

These are names given to small cysts found in the mesosalpinx and around the terminal portion of the fallopian tubes. They are of indeterminate embryonic origin and are of no clinical significance.

CARCINOMA OF FALLOPIAN TUBES

The fallopian tubes, which are so prone to infection, are extremely resistant to malignant change, and the gynaecologist may, in his professional lifetime, expect to see perhaps one case of carcinoma of the tube.

Pathology

The growth is usually an adenocarcinoma of the tubal epithelium which grows inwards and secretes a copious serosanguinous fluid which characteristically discharges per vaginam if the proximal tube remains patent. This classical sign of tubal carcinoma is rare.

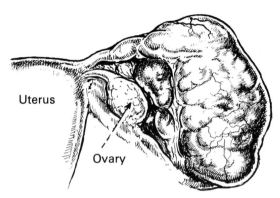

Uterus

Ovary

Clinical Features

The patient is usually in her fifties and there is an association with low parity. Her complaints are of pain and sometimes discharge, and in the absence of definite symptoms the diagnosis is often made rather late. Pelvic signs suggestive of infection in a post-menopausal woman should always be investigated. The differential diagnosis includes carcinoma of the uterus or ovary.

Aetiology is unknown, since the condition is too rare to attract much attention.

Clinical Staging

Stage I   confined to one or both tubes.
Stage II pelvic extension.
Stage III spread to other structures (omentum, bowel, etc.).
Stage IV distant metastases (including bladder).

5-year survival rate	
Stage I	40–60%
Stage II	20–40%
Stage III	10–25%

Treatment

Total hysterectomy and bilateral salpingo-oophorectomy should be done as a minimum, followed by external beam radiation. If the surgeon has the experience an extended hysterectomy and lymphadenectomy would be justified, but the disease is usually not diagnosed before laparotomy.

Prognosis depends on the stage of diagnosis and on the degree of differentiation of the tumour.

STERILISATION

Many women seek sterilisation once they decide that they want no more children, even when still in their early twenties, and the free provision of an operation of such social consequence must inevitably give rise to controversy. The doctor should make certain that his patient knows exactly what the operation involves, its consequences, and the possibilities that may exist for a later recanalisation.

The WOMAN should be as certain as a woman can be that she wants no more pregnancies, come what may. The decision should be taken with deliberation and not during pregnancy or the immediate post-natal period.

The MALE partner should have a clear understanding of the consequences of the operation, and should if possible be brought to agree. Among the more conservative sections of the community there will sometimes be found a reluctance to allow the woman the freedom that sterilisation brings, along with a refusal to consider the alternative of vasectomy.

TECHNIQUES

Occlusion of the fallopian tubes is carried out by the application of ligatures, clips or rings, and the object is to traumatise the tube and bring about a permanent blockage by fibrosis. Destruction of a portion of the tube by diathermy is also effective, but has too small an operative safety margin.

1. **Laparotomy and Tubal Ligation**   This is the most reliable method but requires several days in hospital, and carries the risk of chronic salpingitis.
2. **Occlusion of the tubes by clips or rings under laparoscopic vision**   There is virtually no morbidity and hospital stay is short, but the technique is not quite so reliable.

POST-STERILISATION SYNDROME

This uncertain entity consists of pelvic adhesions and salpingitis, and irregular patterns of menstruation. Women who have been sterilised seem more likely to undergo hysterectomy in later years, especially after tubal ligation, and reductions in plasma progesterone have been shown in such patients. This may be due to interference with the utero-ovarian circulation and would explain the irregular bleeding.

STERILISATION FAILURE

The only certain method of sterilisation is removal of the ovaries, and as more tubal occlusions are done, more failures will appear. Laparoscopic techniques have a failure rate about the same as oral contraceptives, probably 1%, and tubal ligation rather less.

Failure is more likely when the operation is done at the time of abortion or term delivery, and there is a higher than normal risk of ectopic pregnancy. Points of technique are important in sterilisation operations and experience is required.

STERILISATION

TUBAL LIGATION

The easiest way to interrupt the continuity of the fallopian tubes is to tie them with a ligature. The tubes have some powers of resistance (cf. recanalisation of veins) and it is necessary to crush the muscle coat, although the endosalpinx is probably not divided. Failure is very rare and can be due to recanalisation, or to the development of a fistulous opening.

The incision can be small and so placed as to be covered by the pubic hair. If there is any laxity of the vagina and uterine ligaments, it is often possible to reach the tubes through an incision in the posterior fornix. With either route there are small risks of sepsis and embolism.

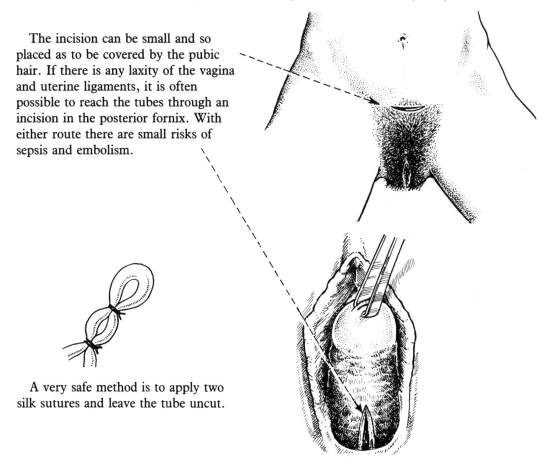

A very safe method is to apply two silk sutures and leave the tube uncut.

Type of Ligature

The material used probably does not matter.

In the Pomeroy method, catgut is used and the tube is then cut so that the ends fall apart. In the Madlener method silk is used after crushing the tube. Burial of the proximal end of the ligated tube is also practised, but this technique is no more immune from fistula formation than any other.

LAPAROSCOPIC STERILISATION

The tubes can be occluded by the application of clips or rings under laparoscopic vision. (Two clips are applied to each tube by some operators.)

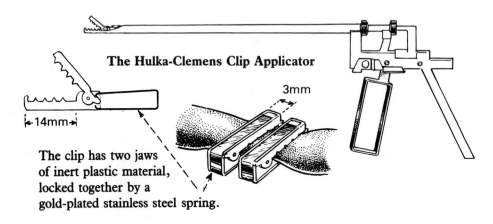

The Hulka-Clemens Clip Applicator

The clip has two jaws of inert plastic material, locked together by a gold-plated stainless steel spring.

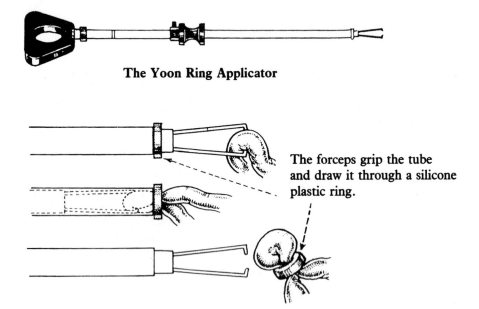

The Yoon Ring Applicator

The forceps grip the tube and draw it through a silicone plastic ring.

These applicators, whether for clips or rings, are passed into the abdominal cavity through a trocar after passage of a laparoscope. The clips should be placed about 1cm from the cornu, and the rings as near that point as possible. Thick and vascular tubes are more difficult to occlude by these methods.

RESTORING TUBAL PATENCY

Once the tube is blocked by infection and adhesions, the chances of restoring patency are poor. There is a tendency for the blockage to recur, and tubal function is never as good as in the pristine state. Nevertheless several techniques have been developed.

SALPINGOSTOMY

This is done when the fimbriae have been destroyed, and the artificial opening will not be as effective as the fimbriae. The polyethylene splint should be removed after a week and since splints tend themselves to stimulate fibrosis some surgeons will not use them, but rely on large doses of intraperitoneal hydrocortisone acetate (up to 1.5g) to inhibit adhesion formation.

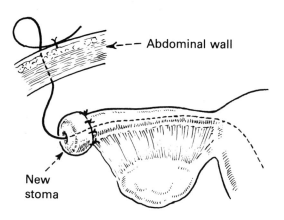

UTEROTUBAL IMPLANTATION

If the interstitial portion of the tube is blocked, the isthmus can be resutured to the cornu after a fresh passage has been made. It is hoped that the passage will become lined with tubal mucosa.

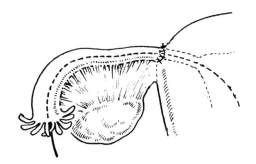

The tube is guided into the uterus and sutured in place.

RESTORING TUBAL PATENCY

This is done by cutting out the occluded and fibrotic portions of tube and anastomosing the ends. The less amount of destruction done to the tube during the sterilisation operation the better, and in this respect the Hulka-Clemens clip, which crushes only 3mm of tube, has a distinct advantage over other methods. Anastomosis in the isthmic portion gives the best results as the opposing ends of tube are the same diameter.

TUBAL ANASTOMOSIS

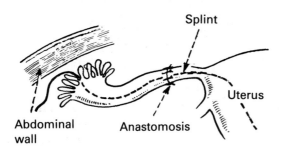

Fibrotic tissue is cut out, and the ends of tube are sutured together over a thin plastic splint, usually an epidural catheter.

This splint should be removed per vaginam a week later.

MICROSURGICAL TECHNIQUES

The use of the operating microscope and suitable instruments for performing tubal anastomosis is becoming more popular but this technique has not yet been shown to be invariably superior to 'macro-anastomosis'. It is particularly recommended when the isthmus has been destroyed and the tubal lumen has to be anastomosed to the cornu.

Under about x20 magnification all fibrotic tissue is removed, bleeding points stopped with fine diathermy, and the lumina anastomosed with very fine multiple sutures.

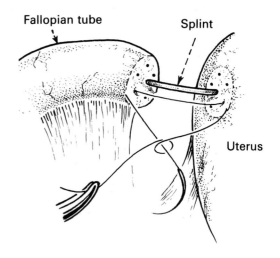

ECTOPIC PREGNANCY

Implantation of the fertilised ovum outside the uterus, nearly always in the fallopian tube.

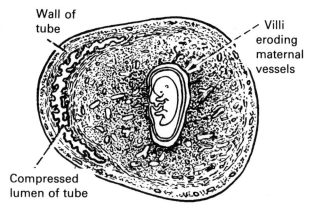

Wall of tube

Villi eroding maternal vessels

Compressed lumen of tube

Incidence

It is impossible to compute the number of ectopic implantations per conception, but in practice the incidence seems to be about one case for every 300 deliveries.

Site The trophoblast can successfully implant on any tissue with an adequate blood supply, but ectopics anywhere other than the tube are a great rarity. The commonest site for an 'ectopic ectopic' is the pelvic peritoneum, but the literature contains accounts of implantation in the liver, the spleen, the lower sac, the stomach and the intestine.

Aetiology

Often unknown, but there are a number of associated factors:

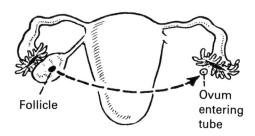

Follicle

Ovum entering tube

1. Pelvic Inflammatory Disease

About half the patients will have signs of salpingitis or a history of infection, including gonorrhoea or tuberculosis.

2. Intra-Uterine Devices

The IUD may introduce infection or have some unknown effect. Since the probable action of the IUD is to cause an abortion every cycle, a relative increase in ectopic pregnancy is to be expected.

3. Migration of the Ovum

The corpus luteum is occasionally seen on the side opposite the ectopic, and it has been assumed for many years that the ovum, growing as it crosses the pelvis, reaches the stage of implantation while still in the other tube.

4. Endocrine Causes

There is no definite evidence of hormonal causation but the tube, like the uterus, is under hormonal control and it is known for example that the rate at which the cilia make their waving motions is increased after ovulation (the 'ciliary beat' is about 7 per second). Prolactin is said to reduce motility, and a higher incidence of tubal pregnancy has been observed after HPG/HCG treatment for infertility.

331

SITES OF IMPLANTATION

Sites of Implantation

The ampulla is the commonest followed by the isthmus, but the developing ovum can implant anywhere in or out of the uterus.

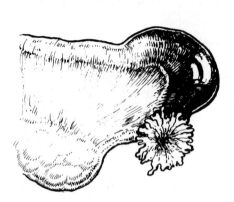

Ampullary implantation. Note the thinning of the tube wall.

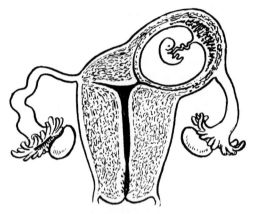

Interstitial implantation is very rare but very dangerous because rupture is accompanied by bleeding from uterine arteries.

Effect on the Uterus

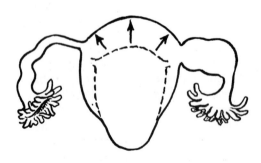

In the first 3 months the uterus enlarges almost as if the implantation were normal. This is a source of confusion in diagnosis.

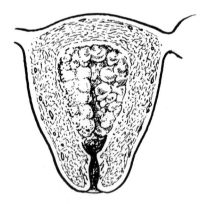

Decidua grows abundantly, and degenerates and bleeds when the ovum dies. Rarely is it expelled entire as a decidual cast.

RUPTURE OF THE TUBE

The muscle wall of the tube has not the capacity of uterine muscle for hypertrophy and distension, and tubal pregnancy nearly always ends in rupture and the death of the ovum.

RUPTURE into LUMEN of TUBE
Tubal Abortion

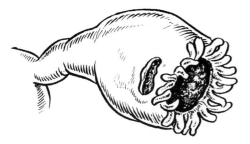

This is usual in ampullary pregnancy at about 8 weeks. The conceptus is extruded, complete or incomplete, towards the fimbriated end of the tube, probably by the pressure of accumulated blood. There is a trickle of bleeding into the peritoneal cavity, and this may collect as a clot in the Pouch of Douglas. It is then called a pelvic haematocele.

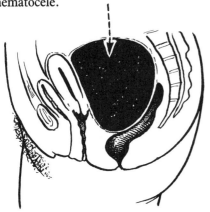

RUPTURE into the PERITONEAL CAVITY

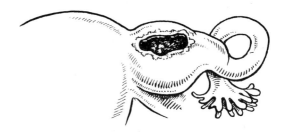

This may occur spontaneously, or from pressure (such as straining at stool, coitus or pelvic examination) and occurs mainly from the narrow isthmus before 8 weeks, or from the interstitial portion at 12 weeks. Haemorrhage is likely to be severe.

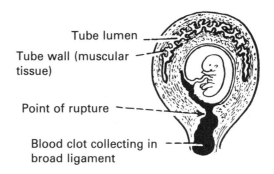

Tube lumen

Tube wall (muscular tissue)

Point of rupture

Blood clot collecting in broad ligament

Sometimes rupture is retroperitoneal between the leaves of the broad ligament – broad ligament haematoma. Haemorrhage in this site is more likely to be controlled.

DIAGNOSIS OF TUBAL PREGNANCY

Tubal pregnancy can present in many ways and misdiagnosis is common.

PAIN in the lower abdomen is always present and may be either stabbing or cramp-like – 'uterine colic'. It may be referred to the shoulder if blood tracks to the diaphragm and stimulates the phrenic nerve, and it may be so severe as to cause fainting. The pain is caused by distension of the gravid tube, by its efforts to contract and expel the ovum, and by irritation of the peritoneum by leakage of blood. More than 50% of ectopics present as chronic rather than acute episodes.

VAGINAL BLEEDING occurs usually after the death of the ovum and is an effect of oestrogen withdrawal. It is dark brown and scanty ('vaginal spotting') and its irregularity may lead the patient to confuse it with the menstrual flow. In about 25% of cases tubal pregnancy presents without any vaginal bleeding.

INTERNAL BLOOD LOSS will, if gradual, lead to anaemia. If haemorrhage is severe and rapid (as when a large vessel is eroded) the usual signs of collapse and shock will appear. Acute internal bleeding is the most dramatic and dangerous consequence of tubal pregnancy but it is less common than the condition presented by a slow trickle of blood into the pelvic cavity.

PELVIC EXAMINATION in the conscious patient will demonstrate extreme tenderness over the gravid tube or in the Pouch of Douglas if a haematocele has collected. If the pregnancy is sufficiently advanced and rupture has not occurred, a cystic (and very tender) mass may be felt in the fornix; but often tenderness is the only sign elicited.

PERITONEAL IRRITATION may produce muscle guarding, frequency of micturition, and later a degree of fever, all leading towards a misdiagnosis of appendicitis.

ßCHG PREGNANCY TESTS are positive early in pregnancy. A negative result almost completely excludes a diagnosis of ectopic pregnancy.

SIGNS and SYMPTOMS of EARLY PREGNANCY must be expected, all of which can confuse the clinical picture. When implantation occurs in the isthmus, tubal rupture may occur before the patient has missed a period, and pregnancy tests may be negative until the 40th day.

ABDOMINAL EXAMINATION will demonstrate tenderness in one or other fossa. If there has been much intra-peritoneal bleeding there will be general tenderness and resistance to palpation over the whole abdomen.

DIAGNOSIS OF TUBAL PREGNANCY

Differential Diagnosis

This includes salpingitis, abortion, torsion of the pedicle of a cyst or rupture of a cyst and perhaps appendicitis.

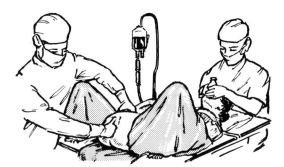

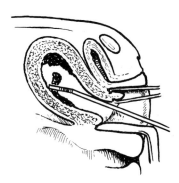

1. **Examination under Anaesthesia**
   This is not likely to yield more information than in the conscious patient. It should always be done in theatre because of the risk of starting haemorrhage.

2. **Curettage**
   If products of conception are obtained, a co-existing tubal pregnancy is very unlikely. Decidua alone means an ectopic but the histological report must be awaited. Marked decidual reaction with absence of chorionic villi suggests ectopic pregnancy.

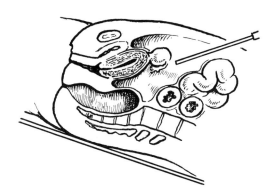

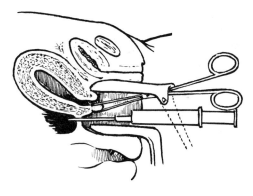

3. **Laparoscopy**
   This is the most useful method of diagnosis in doubtful cases, and is especially useful in excluding tubal pregnancy.

4. **Culdocentesis**
   The passing of a wide-bore needle through the posterior fornix. Old blood is very suggestive, but the absence of blood does not exclude an ectopic pregnancy.

335

TREATMENT OF TUBAL PREGNANCY

1. Haemorrhage and shock must be treated but if there is delay in obtaining blood the operation should be proceeded with. The patient's condition will improve as soon as internal bleeding is controlled.

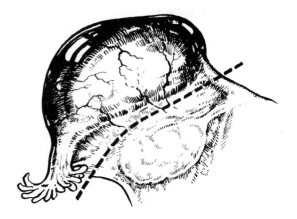

2. Salpingectomy or even salpingo-oophorectomy may be necessary to control the bleeding. The risk of conservation is of course the theoretically increased chance of another ectopic; but if there are no obvious signs of infection in the intact tube, and if the affected tube is not too damaged by haemorrhage and oedema, then conservation should be attempted.

3. Conservative laparoscopic surgery has been employed using RU 486 (Mifepristone) and prostaglandins to abort the ectopic through the fimbriated end of the tube.

Natural History of Ectopic Pregnancies

Rupture or abortion is almost inevitable in tubal pregnancy but absorption must very occasionally occur, and 40 years ago it was common practice to encourage natural resolution by vaginal drainage of a pelvic haematocele.

Abdominal pregnancies usually present as obstetrical problems, but in such cases the fetus may also be absorbed or passed per rectum or present as a bizarre gynaecological problem with lithopaedion formation.

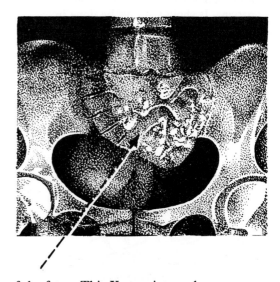

Lithopaedion is the name given to calcification of the fetus. This X-ray picture shows a lithopaedion which took 4^{1}/2 years to develop.

CERVICAL PREGNANCY

This is a rare variant of ectopic pregnancy, which carries a considerable risk of severe bleeding.

Clinical Features

The patient is likely to be misdiagnosed as a case of inevitable abortion.

1. The cervix is dilated and thin-walled and contains products of conception.

2. A small firm uterine corpus can be palpated, resting on the swollen cervix.

3. Attempts at evacuating the 'abortion' cause increased bleeding.

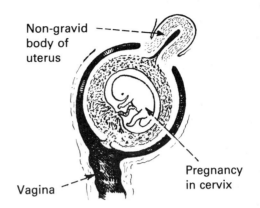

Management   This is a dangerous condition. The choice is between hysterectomy and local excision, and the former is strongly indicated if the bleeding is heavy and not controllable, especially if the maturity is beyond 8 weeks.

If local excision is attempted, the cervix must be clamped laterally to occlude the lateral vessels. After the pregnancy is dissected out, any cervical tears must be repaired, and the vagina should be packed.

OVARIAN PREGNANCY

Implantation of the fertilised ovum in the ovary makes up 1% of all ectopics. The symptoms and course of the condition are much the same as for other ectopics, but the ovarian tissue is perhaps less likely to rupture than is the muscular wall of the tube. An enlarged ovary is found at operation and if an ectopic is suspected, the tumour should be excised. It should be possible to preserve the ovary.

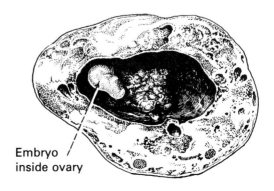

337

CHAPTER 14

THE URINARY TRACT IN GYNAECOLOGICAL PRACTICE

THE URETERS

The ureter enters the pelvis retroperitoneally by crossing over or near the bifurcation of the common iliac artery.

It is itself crossed by the ovarian vessels and is near the fold of peritoneum which forms the infundibulopelvic ligament.

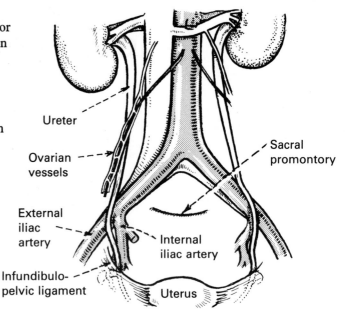

It passes down and medially behind the ovarian fossa and is in close relation to the internal iliac artery. In the healthy subject its shape can be made out beneath the peritoneum and its movements observed (vermiculation).

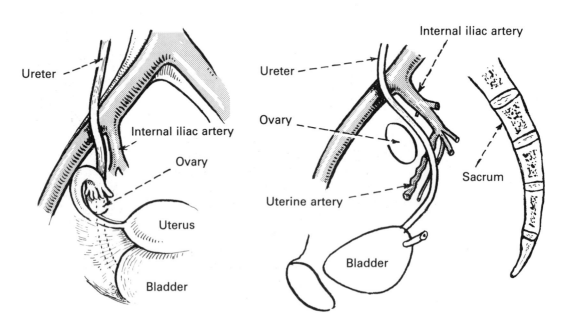

THE URETERS

The ureter then passes beneath the base of the broad ligament, through the transverse uterine ligament and into the bladder. In this parametrial part of its course it lies alongside the vaginal fornix and passes under the uterine artery.

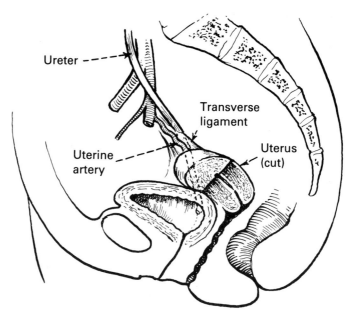

This picture shows the parametrial part of the ureter with the connective tissue removed. Note that the assymmetry of the uterus and vagina makes the left ureter have a much closer relationship with the vaginal fornix than the right.

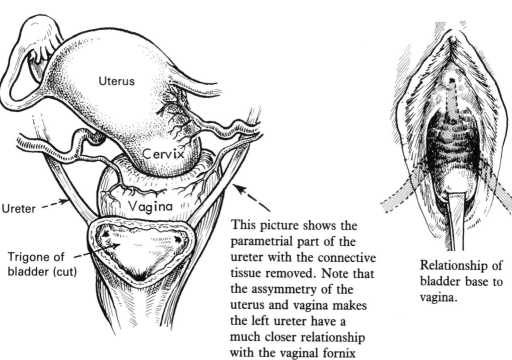

Relationship of bladder base to vagina.

341

BLOOD SUPPLY

The ureter is supplied by branches from the main arteries with which it is in relation, principally the renal and ovarian arteries. The pelvic vessels are variable; and because the blood enters mostly at the upper and lower ends the peri-ureteric anastomoses are important.

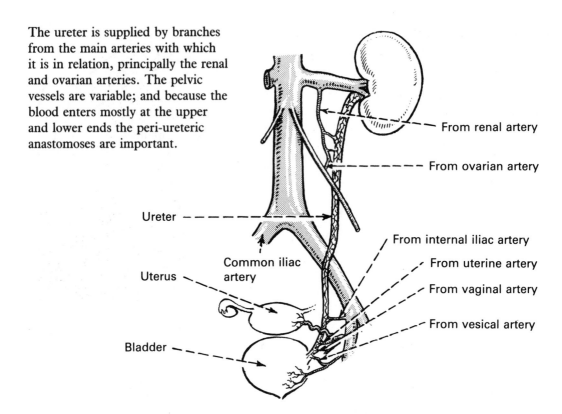

From renal artery

From ovarian artery

Ureter

Common iliac artery

Uterus

Bladder

From internal iliac artery

From uterine artery

From vaginal artery

From vesical artery

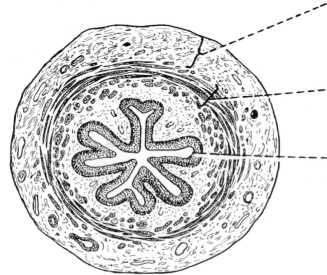

The Adventitia is a fibrous sheath containing the peri-ureteral arterial network, the autonomic nerves and the lymphatics.

The Muscularis consists of two or three layers of smooth muscle irregularly arranged.

The lumen is lined by plicated transitional epithelium on a loose areolar stroma. This arrangement allows for distension of the ureter as required (cf. the fallopian tube).

INJURY TO THE URETER

The ureter will occasionally be damaged no matter how much skill and care are exercised.

1. The ureter is not easily demonstrated or dissected where it is in closest relationship to the genital tract; and not always easily palpated.

2. The ureter's course is to some extent variable, and under pressure it will gradually change its position in the pelvis. A large tumour filling the pelvis will displace it laterally; a tumour in the broad ligament may displace the ureter outwards and upwards; and double ureters are occasionally met with.

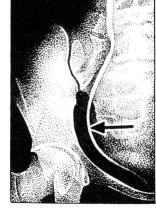

IVP
showing lateral displacement

Ureter displaced by a fibroid which has occupied the broad ligament

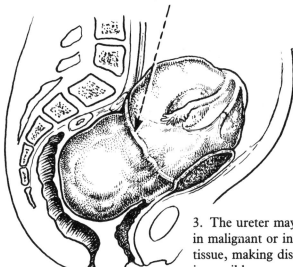

3. The ureter may be embedded in malignant or inflammatory tissue, making dissection almost impossible.

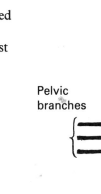

Pelvic branches

4. Radical surgery may destroy so much of the pelvic blood supply that the pelvic ureter becomes ischaemic, leading to fibrotic narrowing or fistula. Damage to the blood vessels may also be produced by pelvic irradiation.

INJURY TO THE URETER

The ureter is most commonly injured:

1. Entering the Pelvis.
The ureter descends medial to the
infundibulopelvic ligament, and if
displaced by inflammation or tumour,
may be so close as to be caught in a
clamp applied to the ligament.

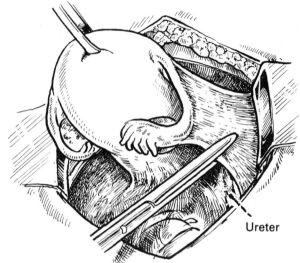

Ureter

Ureter

**2. Passing through the Transverse
   Ligament.**
If the clamp is applied too far out from
the uterus the ureter will be included.
The uterosacral ligament also must be
clamped close to the cervix.

Vesico-uterine
ligament

3. In the vesico-uterine ligament
as the ureter turns round the vagina
into the bladder. This ligament must
be displaced laterally before excision
of the uterus if the ureter is to be
safe. Unfortunately the more the
lateral displacement the greater the
disturbance of the venous plexus and
the greater the bleeding.

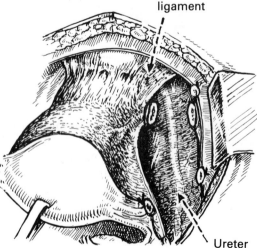

Ureter

PREVENTION OF INJURY TO THE URETER

In simple hysterectomy where the ureter is not exposed, it should be palpated if possible where it lies alongside the vaginal fornix. It conveys a rubbery incompressible sensation to the fingers; but some engorged veins feel similar, and much fat or inflamed tissue make the palpation difficult. Great care is taken to free the bladder from the front of the cervix, to which it may be adherent after Caesarean section. It is then pushed downwards, before applying clamps to the uterine arteries.

In radical hysterectomy the ureter must be dissected clear of the uterine artery before the artery is divided.

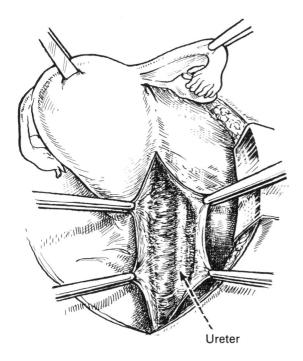

Ureter

The course of the ureter should be examined before starting the dissection. Vermiculation can usually be observed through the peritoneum, but if there is any doubt the peritoneum should be incised and reflected medially so that the ureter may be traced down to where it enters the transverse ligament.

Never pass pedicle ligatures deeper than necessary.

Do not apply haemostatic forceps blindly when there is sudden haemorrhage. Apply swab pressure and try to identify the bleeding point.

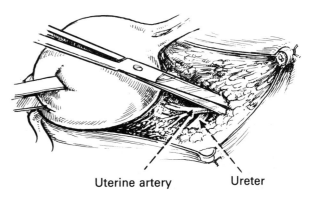

Uterine artery   Ureter

URETER IN VAGINAL OPERATIONS

When there is prolapse and when the cervix is drawn down, the position of the adjacent ureters is also altered. The prolapsed uterus pulls down its arteries which in turn displace the ureters, and the bladder base is also involved in the prolapse.

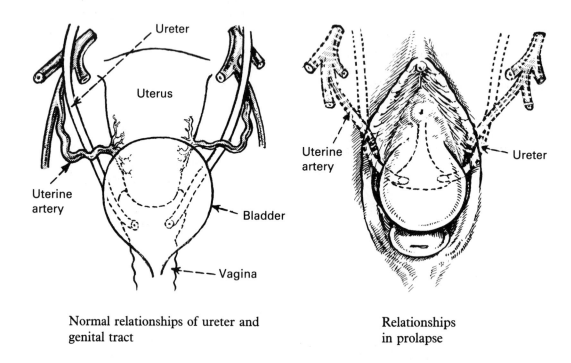

Normal relationships of ureter and genital tract

Relationships in prolapse

During vaginal hysterectomy or in 'complete procidentia' (page 270) the ureter can sometimes be palpated laterally, and when the cystocele is being obliterated, sutures placed too deeply or too far laterally will catch the ureter. The removal of the uterus removes the 'splint' and support of the trigone; and too much infolding of the bladder may distort and obstruct the ureters in their passage through the bladder wall.

REPAIR OF DAMAGED URETER

DAMAGE OBSERVED AT OPERATION

Bruising by Clamp or Ligature

A fistula is likely to follow such damage, and the correct treatment is to excise the bruised portion and re-anastomose over a T-tube catheter. If urological help is not immediately available, the gynaecologist might find it easiest to open the bladder and pass a catheter up to the renal pelvis. Silastic 'pigtail' catheters can be left for up to 3 months, to allow for spontaneous healing.

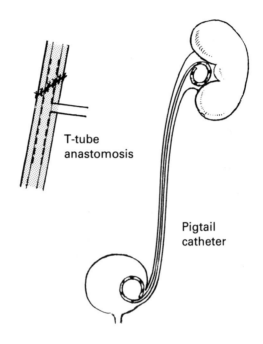

T-tube
anastomosis

Pigtail
catheter

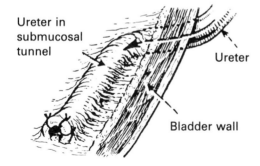

Ureter in
submucosal
tunnel

Ureter

Bladder wall

Division of Ureter

If possible, a primary anastomosis should be done over a T-tube, but if more than 2–3cm of ureter have been removed, and no urological help is available, the gynaecologist should be able to re-implant the ureter in the bladder, which has more mobility.

If he is unable to restore continuity he must provide external drainage of the proximal ureter by means of a T-tube (ligating the end of the ureter) and get the patient to a urologist as soon as possible.

All operations on the ureter must be supported by external peritoneal drainage when the abdomen is closed.

REPAIR OF DAMAGED URETER

DAMAGE NOT OBSERVED AT OPERATION

Clinical Features

a. If only one ureter is occluded there may be no disturbance and the kidney silently atrophies.

b. Occlusion of both ureters will result in anuria or the development of fistula, vaginal or through the abdominal wound.

c. Often the patient is acutely ill for no obvious reason, and at this stage ureteric damage should be considered. Signs include pyrexia, high pulse, loin pain if hydronephrosis is developing, and abdominal pain and ileus if urine is leaking internally through fistula.

Management

Anuria without fistula   Both kidneys are involved, and the first step must be decompression of the kidneys and the establishment of renal drainage.

Fistula without obstruction   This usually results in early recognition of damage. The fistula should be repaired as soon as possible, but there is unlikely to be advancing upper urinary tract damage.

Fistula associated with progressive renal damage   This is often the case when there is late recognition of ureteric damage. Renal drainage must be established immediately, the site and extent of the ureteric damage assessed and a definitive repair carried out when the patient's condition has improved.

Investigation

The first step is an intravenous pyelogram whether or not fistula is present. This will confirm the presence of ureteric obstruction and demonstrate the degree of renal back-pressure.

If facilities are available, a percutaneous nephrostomy can be carried out under X-ray or ultrasound control. A catheter is passed through the skin using local anaesthesia and into the renal pelvis and ureter. Besides draining the kidney this approach allows the injection of contrast medium (antegrade pyelography) which gives further information about ureteric damage.

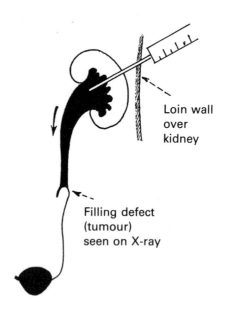

Loin wall over kidney

Filling defect (tumour) seen on X-ray

URETERIC OBSTRUCTION – RENAL DRAINAGE

1. The first step should be an attempt to pass a retrograde catheter past the obstruction. A pigtail catheter can be left in situ for several months to allow spontaneous healing, but this method of drainage is not feasible in a case of complete obstruction.

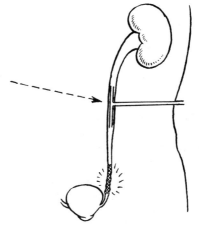

2. In gynaecological work, where the ureteric damage is low down in the pelvis, it is usually possible to insert a T-tube into healthy ureter in the flank or loin (through an extraperitoneal incision) and provide external drainage.

3. **Percutaneous nephrostomy** is described on the previous page and is most useful because the drainage so established can be used as a safety mechanism when the definitive ureteric repair is attempted.

4. **Tube nephrostomy.** This operation is being superseded by percutaneous nephrostomy, but may be required as a last resort. The kidney is exposed through a flank incision and a Malecot or Foley catheter drawn into the kidney as shown. This kind of nephrostomy does not always drain as it should and it is uncomfortable for the patient.

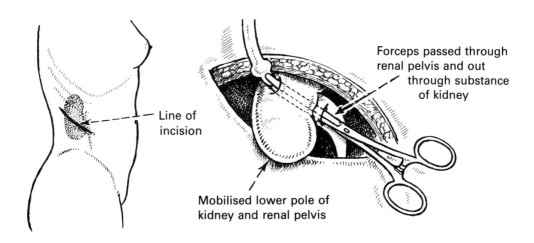

Line of incision

Forceps passed through renal pelvis and out through substance of kidney

Mobilised lower pole of kidney and renal pelvis

REPAIR OF URETERIC FISTULA

If the damaged area cannot be traversed by a pigtail catheter which can then be left in situ for several months, the urologist will preferably carry out an end-to-end anastomosis. If too much ureter has been destroyed, the choices are bladder implantation (the bladder is more mobile), use of a segment of ileum, or transverse implantation into the other ureter.

BLADDER IMPLANTATION
(Boari operation)

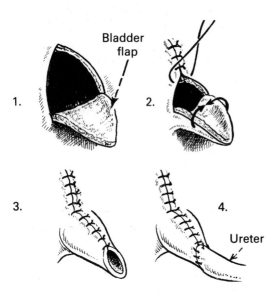

If the anastomosis is still under tension, the bladder can be mobilised and sutured to the iliopsoas muscle ('psoas hitch').

USE OF A SEGMENT OF ILEUM

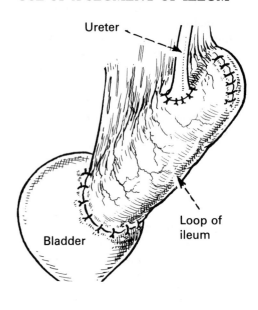

This procedure carries obvious risks of infection.

TRANSVERSE URETERIC IMPLANTATION

This requires one intact ureter and there may be complications if the anastomosis is under tension or if the blood supply is poor. It has the advantage of avoiding the infection risk associated with the use of segments of bowel.

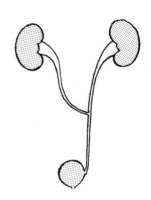

PERMANENT URINARY DIVERSION

If the ureteric damage is irreparable the urinary stream must be permanently diverted. The procedure most frequently used is the ileal conduit or ileal bladder.

The ureters are anastomosed to an isolated loop of ileum which is implanted in the skin as an ileostomy.

This not inconsiderable surgical procedure helps to avoid the pyelonephritis and chloride absorption which follow bowel implantation, and the many complications of permanent cutaneous ureterostomy which include stenosis, pyelonephritis, abscess formation and difficulties in collecting urine.

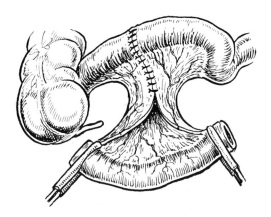

Isolating loop of ileum

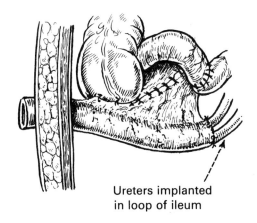

Ureters implanted
in loop of ileum

The ileal conduit is fashioned with wide stomata (both skin and ureteric) and in theory merely acts as a pipe carrying a free flow of urine, so that there is no stenosis and no stasis, no absorption and no acidaemia, no reflux and no ascending infection.

The collecting apparatus consists of a rubber or plastic flange held to the skin by a watertight adhesive, and supported by a belt. The urine passes into a bag which can be drained without being taken off.

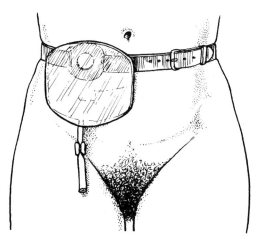

PHYSIOLOGY OF MICTURITION

The involuntary voiding of small amounts of urine is very common in women. It is known perhaps wrongly as 'stress incontinence' and its treatment calls for an understanding of bladder and urethral physiology.

Intravesical Pressure

The bladder displays the phenomenon of adaptation to increased urinary volume. Pressure remains below 10cm H_2O until over 500ml of urine are contained.

Intra-urethral Pressure

Urethral pressure is maintained by the 'internal sphincter' made up of longitudinal and circular plain muscle and elastic tissue; and an 'external sphincter' which contributes striated muscle.

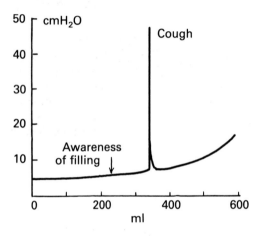

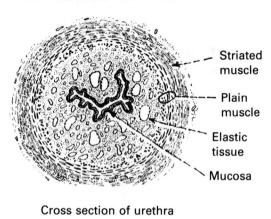

Cross section of urethra

A 'urethral pressure profile' shows the changes in pressure along the length of the urethra. This is normally much greater than the intravesical pressure, thus ensuring continence.

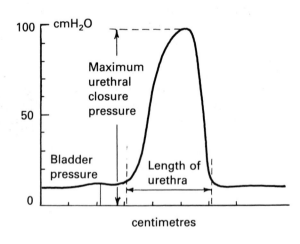

PHYSIOLOGY OF MICTURITION

Innervation of Bladder and Urethra

There is an intercommunicating sympathetic, parasympathetic and somatic supply. The parasympathetic stimulates detrusor contraction, and the sympathetic fibres (chiefly through the alpha receptors) stimulate contraction of the bladder neck and urethra. There is thus some degree of reciprocal activity, but the precise function of each type of nerve and the exact control of the mechanism of bladder neck opening are not yet known.

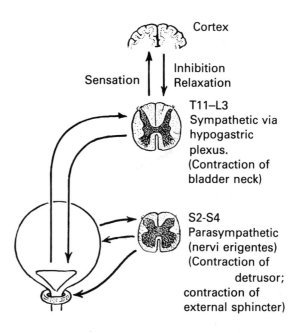

Cortex

Sensation

Inhibition
Relaxation

T11–L3
Sympathetic via hypogastric plexus.
(Contraction of bladder neck)

S2-S4
Parasympathetic (nervi erigentes)
(Contraction of detrusor;
contraction of external sphincter)

The striated muscle has been shown to have a dual autonomic/somatic supply via the pelvic plexus, and the long-held concept of pudendal innervation is being questioned. In normal urethral closure all the components of the sphincter mechanism must function together and the striated muscle has more to do than merely contract voluntarily when the desire to micturate must be resisted.

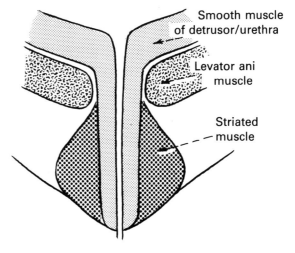

Smooth muscle of detrusor/urethra

Levator ani muscle

Striated muscle

Diagram of urethral closure mechanism

MECHANISM OF VOIDING

Cystometry recording demonstrates the timing of events.

1. Intra-abdominal pressure increase.
   (Measured per rectum.)

2. Detrusor contracts.
   (Intravesical pressure increase.)

3. Sphincter relaxes.
   (Electromyogram of anal sphincter.)

4. Urine flow begins.

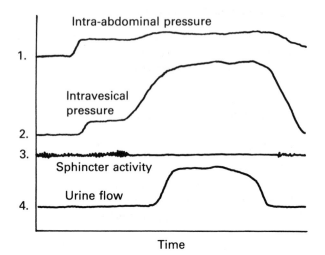

The urethra and bladder neck are maintained in the closed state by the trigonal condensation of muscle (the base plate) and the urethral sphincter (plain and striated muscle).

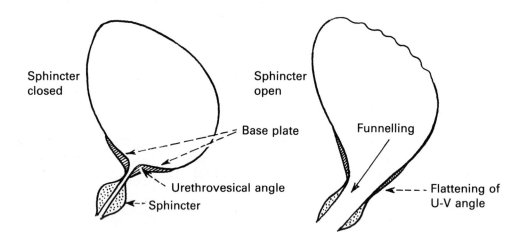

When cortical inhibition is withdrawn the detrusor contracts, and the bladder neck relaxes (funnelling). The sphincter also relaxes and urine is voided. As the flow continues, the bladder neck moves downwards and backwards and the urethrovesical (UV) angle is obliterated.

INCONTINENCE OF URINE

Urgency Incontinence

The patient experiences an irresistible desire to micturate. Detrusor instability is the commonest cause, but it may also be due to inflammatory disease of the bladder without detrusor contraction. All forms of bladder pathology must be considered including calculus and carcinoma. There is usually an associated complaint of frequency.

Fistula Incontinence is described on page 370 et seq.

Overflow Incontinence

Sudden retention is rare in women except after pelvic floor operations. Spasmodic detrusor contractions force a little urine into the urethra, and the stretched muscle takes several days to regain its tone.

When obstruction to outflow occurs gradually, as from pressure by a pelvic tumour or an incarcerated retroverted gravid uterus, the detrusor has time to hypertrophy and for a time forces urine out; but eventually the bladder become atonic and painless and urine dribbles out only when the intra-abdominal pressure is raised.

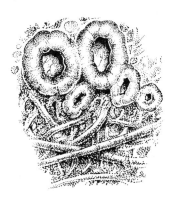

Atonic, distended, trabeculated bladder due to tumour.

Neurological Disease

Failure of detrusor inhibition is the commonest symptom and is the cause of senile incontinence. It is also a symptom, although not usually the presenting one, of multiple sclerosis. Full sensation is present, but the incontinence is of the urgency type and cannot be resisted.

Failure of bladder sensation is a result of diseases which interrupt the posterior columns of the cord, e.g. tabes, syringomyelia, occasionally multiple sclerosis. Chronic overdistension leads to an atonic bladder and overflow incontinence, and infection is a common complication.

INCONTINENCE OF URINE

When a sudden increase in intravesicular pressure is caused by a contraction of the detrusor muscle or by an increase in intra-abdominal pressure as by coughing or straining, the stimulus is usually applied to the intra-abdominal urethra as well, and there is no leakage of urine. If urine does escape, the condition is called *stress incontinence*.

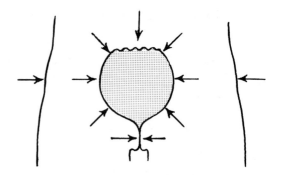

Genuine Stress Incontinence

Involuntary leakage occurring in the absence of a detrusor contraction. This leakage is attributed to some displacement of the bladder neck so that it cannot respond normally to a sudden increase in intra-abdominal pressure. The cause is likely to be a pelvic floor weakness as a result of parturition, prolapse, ageing or a combination of all three.

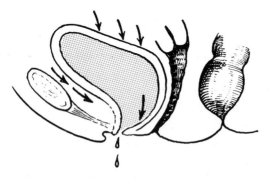

Detrusor Instability

Defined as a contraction exceeding 15cm of water in pressure, occurring during filling of the bladder, or standing erect or coughing and straining. This may also cause involuntary incontinence, but the mechanism is altogether different from that of genuine stress incontinence.

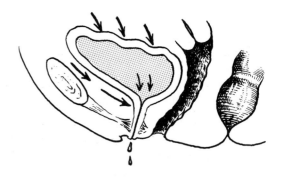

Both these causes of involuntary or stress incontinence can exist together, making for difficulty in diagnosis.

INCONTINENCE

SYMPTOMS AND SIGNS ASSOCIATED WITH INCONTINENCE

Frequency
Increased frequency of micturition is defined as the passage of urine seven or more times during the day, and twice or more during the night. It may arise from any source of irritation including infection, detrusor instability, tumour or incomplete emptying. It is usually diurnal – during waking hours only – but in severe cases will awaken the patient from her sleep. It is one of the earliest symptoms of pregnancy.

Urgency
This is defined as a desire to void urine before the bladder contains 50ml of urine. True urgency occurs in the absence of a detrusor contraction, and is often associated with infection. Severe urgency leads to 'urge incontinence'.

Dysuria
This means pain associated with micturition, and indicates either an infection of the bladder and urethra, or of the vulval and perineal epithelium which is irritated by the dribbling of urine.

Incidence of Stress Incontinence
One survey found an incidence of 10% of inappropriate leakage of urine in women between the ages of 35 and 64. It is more common after child-bearing, but occurs also in nulliparous women who are more prone to detrusor instability than to genuine stress incontinence. The shortness of the female urethra may be a factor.

THE URETHRAL SYNDROME

The urethral syndrome includes complaints of frequency, dysuria, urgency and a sensation of incomplete emptying in a patient in whose urine no evidence of infection can be demonstrated. The cause is not known and there are several views.

Urinary infection is strictly defined as being present only when 10^4 or more typical urinary pathogens are grown per ml of freshly voided mid-stream urine, and it may be that the urethral syndrome is simply a condition caused by fewer than the usual number of organisms, or by organisms which cannot be cultured in the media used for conventional organisms. Clinically these patients must be regarded as suffering from a urinary tract infection and investigation must be persevered with. Even if no evidence of infection is obtained some empirical treatment will have to be given.

INVESTIGATION OF INCONTINENCE

It is necessary to distinguish between urethral and bladder dysfunction since their treatment is different, and this cannot be done with certainty on the history and clinical examination alone.

Stress Incontinence due to:

1. BLADDER NECK INCOMPETENCE
('Genuine Stress Incontinence')

Gradual onset after one or more pregnancies.

Urine appears only after effort (stress) such as coughing, laughing, running for a bus.

Only small quantities of urine are passed, whether the bladder is full or not.

2. DETRUSOR INSTABILITY

History of a weak bladder even before pregnancies if any.

History of enuresis especially in childhood.

Complaints of urge incontinence and frequency, especially at night (nocturia).

Stress incontinence combined with urgency incontinence due to bladder infection or cystocele is quite common. Continuous incontinence suggests fistula (page 370).

The degree of severity is indicated by the extent to which the patient feels socially restricted.

Examination Signs of infection (urethritis) and scarring from previous surgery are looked for, and the usual bimanual and speculum examinations are made (pages 84–86).

Demonstration of Stress Incontinence

The patient is asked to strain and cough and, if stress incontinence is present, small drops of urine will be observed escaping from the urethral meatus. Unfortunately this test is really valid only in the erect position when observation of the meatus becomes almost impossible.

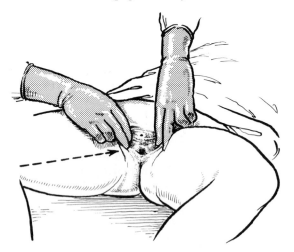

URODYNAMIC INVESTIGATION OF BLADDER FUNCTION

This means an investigation of bladder movements and tensions during different levels of filling, and involves measurement of bladder activity (cystometry) and urethral flow (uroflowmetry). Modern apparatus is sophisticated and expensive.

Cystometry
The intravenous pressures are continuously recorded as the bladder is filled. The diagram illustrates single-channel cystometry which does not record intra-abdominal pressures.

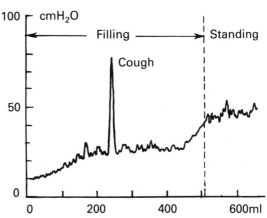

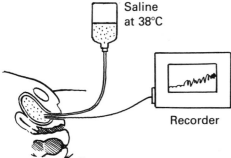

Twin-Channel Cystometry
The rectal pressure which represents intra-abdominal pressure is simultaneously recorded by a transducer in the rectum. Electronic circuitry subtracts one channel from the other, thus recording the true intravesical pressure.

Modern urodynamic apparatus will also measure detrusor pressure and urethral activity.

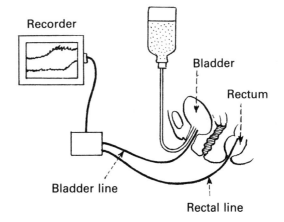

VIDEOCYSTOURETHROGRAPHY (VCU)

This elaborate technique demonstrates bladder neck activity by means of cine-radiography and at the same time measures changes in intravesical pressure. It gives the most reliable evidence of the pressure or absence of detrusor instability but its cost is against its use for routine screening.

1. The bladder is filled with contrast medium and is seen on the left half of the screen.

Bladder neck incompetence is diagnosed by the presence of an open bladder neck at rest or on coughing.

2. Electrodes in bladder and rectum record the required pressures.

3. The flowmeter records the rate at which urine is voided.

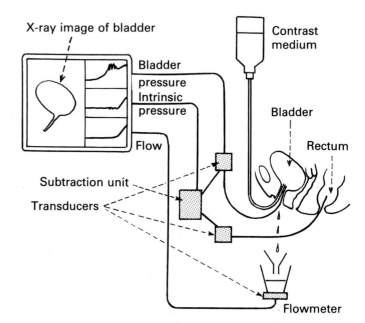

Indications for Urodynamic Assessment

These investigations are invasive (carrying a 2% risk of infection) and also costly, but their application would be justified in the presence of the following indications:

1. Continuing difficulty in distinguishing genuine stress incontinence from detrusor instability.

2. After failure of surgery to relieve a complaint of incontinence.

3. Where there are other complicating factors such as neurological disease.

4. Where difficulty in voiding urine is complained of or is suspected. Such a condition may be met with after pelvic surgery and leads to incomplete emptying and perhaps retention overflow.

OTHER INVESTIGATIONS FOR INCONTINENCE

Bacteriological Culture of Urine

This must be carried out in every case.

Neurological Disease

This possibility must always be borne in mind, and the gynaecologist should test for reflexes in the usual manner. The integrity of the sacral reflexes is demonstrated by contraction of the anal sphincter in response to a perineal skin prick. Where there is doubt, the patient must be referred to a neurologist.

Endocrine Diseases

Diseases such as diabetes mellitus and insipidus may present with frequency and hormonal assays may be required.

X-Ray Investigation

X-ray urethrocystography may be undertaken independently of urodynamic investigations.

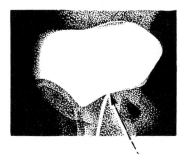

Normal resting X-ray.
Note the well-formed UV angle.

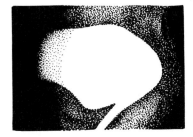

Normal micturating X-ray.
Note the funnelling, downward displacement and flattening of the UV angle.

The bladder is filled with contrast medium and radiographs are taken at rest, straining and micturating.

This investigation can be carried out with normal X-ray facilities, but it does not distinguish between sphincter weakness and detrusor instability. The relationship between incontinence and urethrovesical angles as shown by this technique is unpredictable.

TREATMENT OF STRESS INCONTINENCE

Complete cure is probably impossible and the aim of treatment should be to leave the patient better than she was.

General measures

There are three well-known conditions contributing to stress incontinence which do not readily yield to treatment.

1. **Chronic Urinary Tract Infection**

   This must be dealt with before any other treatment can be worthwhile. Urinary infection by itself is often complicated by urgency incontinence.

2. **Obesity**

   If an obese woman can shed about 25% of her weight she will experience a definite improvement in bladder control.

3. **Chronic Cough and Dyspnoea**

   There is some evidence that leakage during dyspnoea is due to partial loss of sphincter control or to the initiation of detrusor contraction rather than simple stress. Such patients should be advised to stop smoking.

Principles of Treatment

The physiology of the bladder is not yet fully understood nor is the difference between bladder and urethral dysfunction invariably distinguishable. It is even impossible sometimes to be absolutely sure that the patient is in fact incontinent. It is best therefore to investigate as thoroughly as possible, preferably in association with a urologist or employing urological techniques, and to start with simple treatment such as physiotherapy and drugs. Surgery should be restricted to those patients with prolapse or with evidence of bladder neck descent.

Physiotherapy – Exercises

Pelvic floor exercises may be of value, especially in the puerperium. These include repeated pressing together of the buttocks and thighs, and the stopping of the urine stream during micturition. The patient might also practise contracting the vaginal sphincter over her two fingers. Lead cones are available which may be placed temporarily in the vagina and retained by contracting the perineal muscles.

Bladder Training

Bladder training ('Bladder Drill') is advocated as the first treatment for detrusor instability. It is a psychological approach to a condition the cause of which is often in doubt, and although it involves about 10 days in hospital and much supervision, it is well worth a trial in resistant cases.

After a full explanation, the patient is instructed to pass urine only at hourly intervals which are gradually increased to 3 hours if possible. Fluid balance and times of micturition are recorded, and obviously the patient must be motivated to persist with the treatment. This drill is followed only during the day-time, but is continued in modified form after returning home.

DRUG TREATMENT FOR STRESS INCONTINENCE

Surgical treatment (colposuspension) may cure or improve stress incontinence but does not cure urge incontinence due to detrusor instability. Urodynamic studies are important when a mixture of urinary symptoms exists.

Oxybutinin Hydrochloride (CYSTRIN, DITROPAN) 5mg 2–4 times daily may help urinary frequency and urge incontinence, neurogenic bladder instability and nocturnal enuresis. It is contraindicated in glaucoma, intestinal atony and significant bladder outflow obstruction, having atropine-like side effects.

Propantheline Bromide (PROBANTHINE) 15mg 3 times daily may reduce urgency.

Flavoxate Hydrochloride (URISPAS) 200mg 3 times daily is another urinary antispasmodic, with less marked antimuscarinic side effects.

Amitryptiline, which is used for nocturnal enuresis in children, may help urinary urgency.

Oestriol (OVESTIN) or **Oestradiol** (VAGIFEM) local preparations may improve urgency and frequency due to atrophic vaginitis. Systemic HRT may also help.

Bethanechol Chloride 10–25 mg or Carbachol 2mg given 3 times daily may be employed where there is retention of urine due to bladder atony.

Treatment of urgency and frequency often gives poor results.

SURGICAL TREATMENT OF STRESS INCONTINENCE

All operations attempt to elevate the bladder neck above the pelvic floor and behind the symphysis so that increases in intra-abdominal pressure will compress the urethra and not force it downwards. There are 3 methods, each with several variations.

1. Vaginal urethroplasty

The urethra is plicated and secured as much as possible behind the symphysis through a vaginal incision. This is the simplest method, but the least likely to achieve adequate elevation.

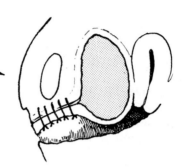

2. Urethropexy

The bladder neck is approached through a suprapubic incision and elevated by suturing the paraurethral tissues to adjacent structure such as the rectus sheath or the ilio-pectineal ligament.

These operations are more difficult than vaginal urethroplasty, especially in obese women.

3. Urethral Sling Operations

A sling of synthetic material, sutures or tendon is passed under the urethra and attached to the rectus muscles or adjacent ligaments. This requires a combined vaginal-suprapubic approach and is the most difficult of the 3 methods.

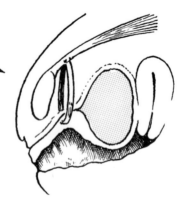

The urethropexy operations are probably most likely to be successful provided the incontinence is due to urethral inadequacy and not detrusor instability.

VAGINAL URETHROPLASTY

This simple operation, sometimes called 'buttressing of the urethrovesical junction', is usually the first choice, although the propriety of this is now being questioned. It is an attempt to elevate the urethrovesical area by suturing fascia beneath it.

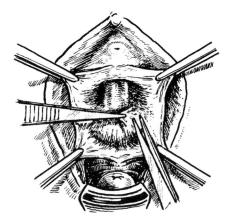

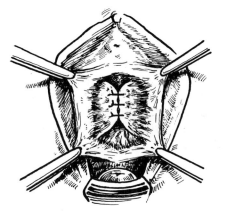

1. Anterior vaginal wall is carefully dissected from the urethrovesical area.

2. The bladder fascia on either side is sutured together in the mid-line. The vaginal wall is now closed.

MARSHALL-MARCHETTI-KRANTZ URETHROPEXY

The urethrovesical junction is made to adhere firmly to the anterior vaginal wall by suturing the vaginal tissue to the back of the symphysis pubis.

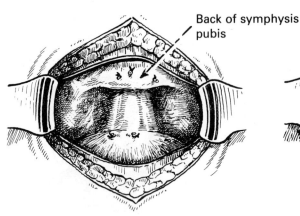

Back of symphysis pubis

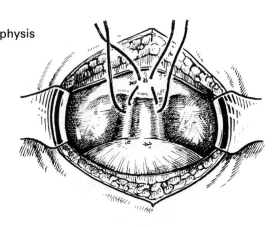

1. The urethrovesical junction is exposed in the space of Retzius. Adhesions are divided and all bleeding points picked up. The urethra must be dissected to within 1cm of the external meatus.

2. A Foley's catheter in the bladder helps to identify the urethrovesical junction. Silk sutures pick up vaginal tissue on either side and suture it to the pubic periosteum.

   Closure is with a Redi-Vac drain for 48 hours in case of urinary leakage or haematoma formation. Haematuria is common and continuous catheterisation is required for 7 days.

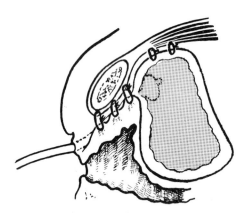

3. Additional sutures are added between bladder muscle and rectus muscles. (This step is sometimes unnecessary.)

Periosteitis is sometimes a late complication and the operation is difficult in the presence of excessive obesity. If too acute an angle is produced, the patient may have difficulty in emptying her bladder.

BURCH'S COLPOSUSPENSION OPERATION

This operation elevates the anterior vaginal wall, bringing the urethra up with it. A vaginal urethropexy can be done at the same time but is probably not necessary.

1. Through a suprapubic incision the bladder neck area is mobilised from the paravaginal fascia. This procedure is accompanied by a good deal of bleeding which must be controlled.

2. The paravaginal fascia (and some vaginal tissue as well) is sutured on each side to the inguino-pectineal ligaments, using four or five Dexon sutures.

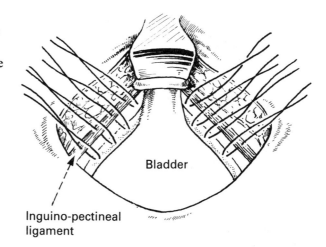

Bladder

Inguino-pectineal ligament

The wound is closed with Redi-Vac suction drainage as for the Marshall operation, and the possible complications are similar. Suprapubic operations can be difficult when the patient is very obese.

STAMEY COLPOSUSPENSION OPERATION

This is a less invasive procedure, where a long Stamey needle is passed through a small incision above the pubis on each side, *behind the pubic bones*, into the vaginal lumen. A nylon suture is attached to the vaginal wall and tied to the rectus sheath, to elevate the vagina and bladder base.

A cystoscope is passed to ensure that the needle has not entered the bladder after each pass of the Stamey needle.

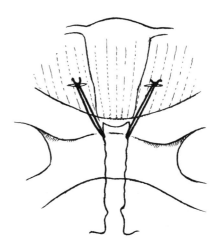

MOIR'S OPERATION

This operation makes use of a strip of mersilene gauze instead of fascial strips which may be difficult to obtain and require a wide incision in the abdominal wall.

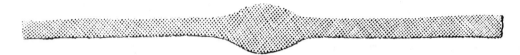

Two small suprapubic incisions are first made and the aponeurosis incised. A finger makes a passage as far down as the obturator foramen.

The vagina is then opened in the usual way and the passage completed upwards with forceps. This passage is extraperitoneal and care is necessary to avoid damage to the bladder.

The gauze hammock is sutured over the bladder neck and the ends threaded up to be sutured to the abdominal muscle aponeurosis. The sling should be slack enough to allow a finger tip to be inserted between it and the urethra.

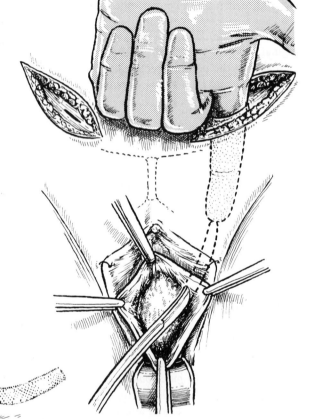

The principle and also the possible complications of this operation are the same as for Aldridge's operation, in which strips of rectus sheath were used instead of synthetic material.

OTHER TREATMENTS FOR STRESS INCONTINENCE

PROLONGED BLADDER DISTENSION

This treatment has been applied to severe cases of detrusor instability not responding to drug treatment.

Under epidural anaesthesia the bladder is filled to a pressure equal to the systolic blood pressure for interrupted periods totalling 2 hours.

The ischaemia and stretching of the muscle fibres reduces irritability and there is often a return to a normal cystogram; but the treatment resembles ECT in psychiatry in being completely empirical.

Complications include rupture of the bladder.

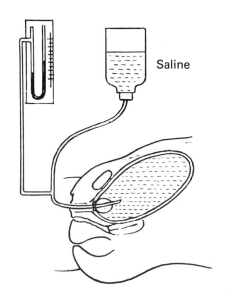

A condom is tied to the end of a Foley's catheter and gradually distended with saline at 38°C. The bladder fundus may reach above the umbilicus.

INCONTINENCE PANTS

'Kanga' marsupial pants are used in geriatric work and are acceptable to patients with severe stress incontinence.

The pants are close fitting and made of 100% polyester which is hydrophobic, and allows urine to flow through it very quickly.

There is a pouch in front over the genital area, extending backwards to the coccyx, which contains a pad of bleached wood pulp capable of absorbing 400ml of urine.

The pad can be changed easily without removing the pants.

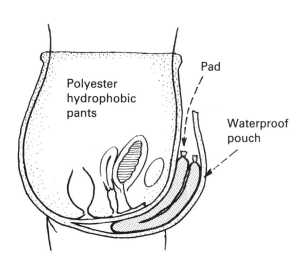

URINARY FISTULA

(L. *fistula*: a pipe) A pathological connection between the urinary tract and an adjacent structure through which urine escapes. A fistula between the bladder base and the vagina is the condition most often seen.

Aetiology

1. The exposed bladder wall is torn or penetrated during a vaginal operation, or during total abdominal hysterectomy. This is the commonest cause in this country.

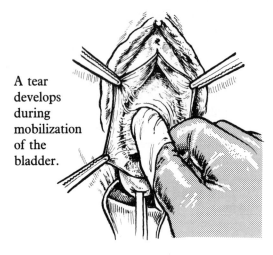

A tear develops during mobilization of the bladder.

Prolonged pressure of vertex on the vagina during obstructed labour. In a few days slough forms. (This should not occur with modern obstetrics in developed countries.)

2. The vaginal wall and bladder are torn during an obstetric operation, or pressure necrosis develops during a prolonged and difficult labour.

3. The ureter is damaged or made ischaemic during a pelvic operation, especially radical hysterectomy. This produces a ureterovaginal fistula.

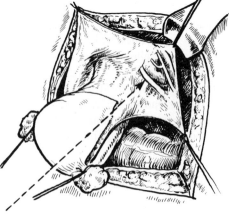

Exposing ureter in radical hysterectomy.

CAUSES OF FISTULA

Aetiology (*contd*)

4. Radiation burns following treatment for carcinoma of the cervix. This fistula may appear several years after treatment.

5. Untreated or recurrent cancer of bladder or genital tract. (This may also be complicated by radiation effects.)

6. Chronic tuberculosis or syphilis. Fistula may complicate surgical treatment of pelvic tuberculosis.

7. Congenital fistula. An accessory ectopic ureter may open into the vagina. This condition should be recognised in childhood.

SITES of urinary fistula

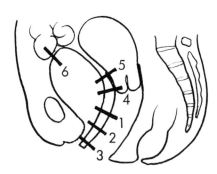

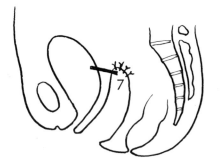

1. *Vesico-vaginal*: the commonest.

2. *Urethro-vesico-vaginal*: closure usually followed by stress incontinence.

3. *Urethro-vaginal*: the only fistula not causing incontinence.

4. *Vesico-cervico-vaginal*: due to a cervical tear during delivery.

5. *Utero-vesico-vaginal*: due to a tear of the lower segment and bladder.

6. *Vesico-intestinal*: may arise from sepsis following major surgery, or from tuberculosis.

7. *Vault* fistula following hysterectomy.

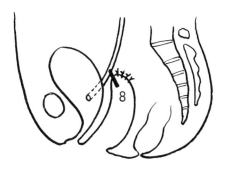

8. *Uretero-vaginal*: follows ureteric damage at hysterectomy.

PATHOLOGY OF URINARY FISTULA

If the cause is a tear, urine escapes at once but the wound may not immediately become infected, and primary union can occur in a week or two provided the urinary stream is diverted.

If the cause is pressure necrosis, the affected area will form a slough which eventually drops out leaving a fistula.

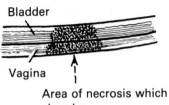

Area of necrosis which sloughs.

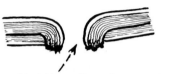

Bladder wall tends to prolapse through fistula.

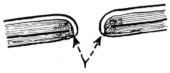

Scar tissue forms and the fistula becomes lined with transitional epithelium.

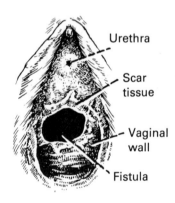

If the fistula is large (over 2cm diameter) spontaneous healing is unlikely and scar tissue gradually forms a dense white ring round the edge of the fistula, even fixing it to a pubic ramus.

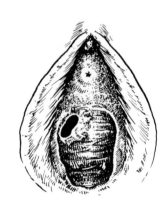

Large fistula of bladder base with much scarring.

Fistula fixed to the pubic ramus by scar tissue.

Urinary fistulae have a natural tendency to close by granulation, fibrosis and contraction. Factors interfering with this are:

1. The continual flow of urine.   2. Sepsis.

3. Persistence of a causative factor such as malignancy or radiation necrosis.

If the urinary stream is diverted by a catheter and good bladder drainage maintained, and if the sepsis is dealt with, the natural decrease in size will occur, and many fistulae of 1cm diameter or less may be expected to close in 2 or 3 months.

SYMPTOMS AND DIAGNOSIS OF FISTULA

Incontinence may immediately follow the injury, but usually the patient has several days of dysuria and haematuria with symptoms of urinary infection. A discharge appears followed by sloughing, and the patient finds her vulva and perineum are constantly wet. This is soon followed by excoriation of the skin accompanied by a strong ammoniacal smell and incrustation of vulva and vagina with urinary salts. The area becomes extremely tender.

Diagnosis

This is usually easy, but if the patient says she also passes urine normally, two conditions must be considered.

1. **A very small fistula.** Most of the urine is retained in the bladder and passed per urethram. Sometimes quite large quantities of urine may be held temporarily in the vagina while the patient is resting, and she will say that she seems to be dry at night. Small 'pinhole' fistulae may persist for years and be mistaken for stress incontinence.

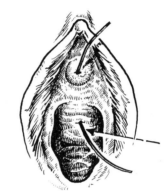

A nylon thread passed through a pinhole fistula.

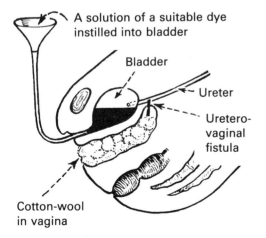

A solution of a suitable dye instilled into bladder

Bladder

Ureter

Uretero-vaginal fistula

Cotton-wool in vagina

2. **A ureterovaginal fistula** produces a constant trickle of urine, but the bladder is still intact and will continue to function. The usual test is to instil a solution of a suitable dye into the bladder. Cotton-wool in the vagina will not be stained if the fistula is ureteric. During cystoscopy the dye is injected intravenously to identify the ureteric openings, and cotton-wool in the vaginal vault will then be stained. An intravenous pyelogram will show contrast medium leaking into the vagina.

TREATMENT OF VESICOVAGINAL FISTULA

A period of bladder drainage is usual. Fistulae do have a tendency to 'grow smaller' and local infection should be dealt with. The object is to obtain as small as possible a fistula surrounded by reasonably healthy vaginal wall which will allow suturing without tension. If the fistula is small it may even heal spontaneously.

Technique of Closure

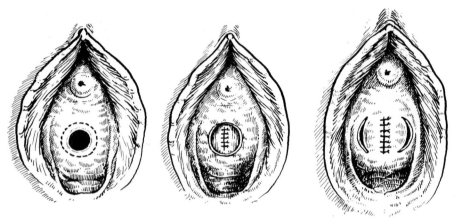

Vaginal skin is dissected as shown. This may leave a rather large wound but it is necessary to obtain healthy vascular skin edges and to avoid tension. Absorbable suture material should be used. Note the relaxation incisions which are sometimes required to allow the wound to close easily without tension.

After-Treatment

Antibiotic cover is given and catheter drainage is continued for 10–14 days depending on the size of the repair. If there is any doubt about healing, as for example if cystitis has developed, catheter drainage must be continued.

(J. Marion Sims, after whom the Sims' speculum is named, performed the first successful repair of a vesicovaginal fistula.)

URETHRAL FISTULA

FISTULA INVOLVING THE URETHRA

This type of fistula is most likely to be met with as
a complication of a buttressing operation for stress
incontinence. The same principles of treatment
are followed – prolonged catheterisation followed
if necessary by repair, but the operator may have
difficulty in obtaining a vaginal skin suture line which
is not under tension.

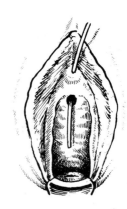

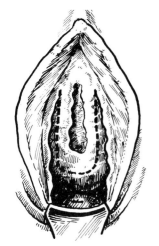

DESTRUCTION OF THE URETHRA

The reconstruction operation shown here would be
carried out by a urologist.

1. A U-shaped
   incision is
   made, and
   vaginal flaps
   mobilised.

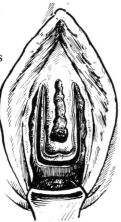

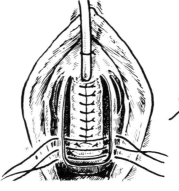

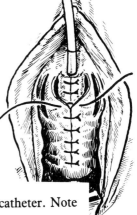

2. The flaps are sutured over a catheter. Note
   the relaxation incisions.

The new urethra will gradually become lined with epithelium, and after healing has
occurred further treatment may be needed to improve sphincter control.

INTERPOSITION OPERATIONS

Interposition operations are used when a repaired fistula requires the support of a tissue with a fresh blood supply. Such techniques would only be applied by an expert surgeon faced with extensive tissue damage.

Interposition of Bulbospongiosus Muscle (Martius' Operation). A pedicle of this muscle and attached fatty tissue is interposed.

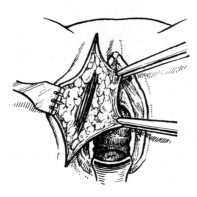

1. An incision is made lateral to the labium majus.

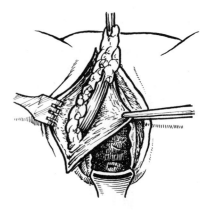

2. A pedicle of musculo-fatty tissue is prepared. Haemorrhage is troublesome.

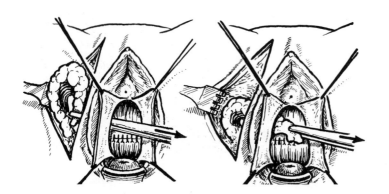

3. The pedicle is pulled medially under the labium minus and sutured over the closed fistula and bladder neck.

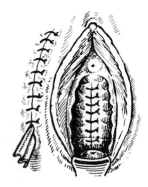

4. The incisions are closed. Note the drain in the labial wound.

TRANSVESICAL REPAIR

The transvesical approach is favoured by the urologist and often offers better access than the more old-fashioned vaginal approach. It is now the practice to ask the urologist to deal by this method with any vesicovaginal fistula (especially post-hysterectomy vault fistula) to which vaginal access is difficult.

The suprapubic space is opened and the bladder incised by a transverse incision.

Polythene catheters are inserted into the ureters. The vagina should be packed beforehand to push the bladder base upwards.

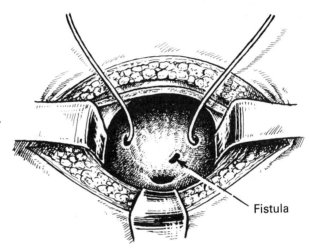

Fistula

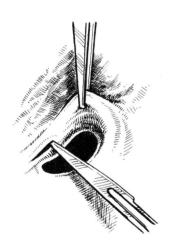

Bladder wall is mobilised from vagina.

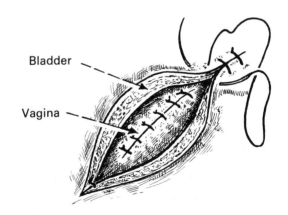

Bladder

Vagina

The vagina is closed with catgut and then the bladder wall.

CHAPTER 15

VENOUS THROMBOSIS

DEEP VEIN THROMBOSIS (DVT)

Aetiology

It is not known why or precisely how pathological thrombi develop but there are well recognised predisposing factors:

1. Any abdominal or pelvic floor operation. When contemplating hysterectomy, especially if other aetiological factors are present, it should be remembered that the risks of thrombo-embolism are greater with the abdominal than with the vaginal operation.
2. Chronic venous insufficiency (varicose veins, phlebitis).
3. Obesity.
4. Immobility leading to circulatory stasis.
5. Oral contraceptives.

Curiously, cigarette smoking which increases the risk of myocardial infarction does not seem to predispose to DVT, possibly because heavy smokers tend to eat less and so avoid obesity.

Pathology

The theory embodied in 'Virchow's Triad' is still clinically useful:

1. Changes in the vessel wall.   2. Changes in the rate of flow.   3. Changes in the blood.

1. Changes in the vessel wall

Damage to the endothelium allows platelets to adhere to the exposed collagen tissue, and then to release substances which will cause further platelet aggregation. Fibrin and leucocytes then adhere to the platelets. Research now suggests that a balance is maintained between different groups of prostaglandins.

Prostaglandin (PG1) is an *anti-aggregatory* substance secreted by intact endothelium. It also causes vasodilatation.

Thromboxane (TXA) is a *pro-aggregatory* substance released by platelets. It also causes vasoconstriction.

2. Changes in the rate of flow

Venous flow in the legs is much reduced in the post-operative period as a result of inactivity and poor muscle tone.

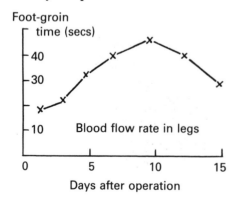

Days after operation

3. Changes in the blood

Platelet count and platelet 'stickiness' and fibrinogen levels are all increased. Fortunately there is a compensating increase in fibrinolytic activity so that nearly all thrombi are naturally broken down.

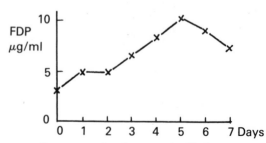

Post-operative increase in fibrin degradation products (FDP) as a result of thrombus destruction.

VENOUS THROMBOSIS

SITES OF THROMBUS FORMATION

1. Calf veins, extending to popliteal.

2. Long and short saphenous veins, especially lateral to the knee.

3. Ilio-femoral segment, extending to vena cava.

4. Superficial thrombosis in veins.

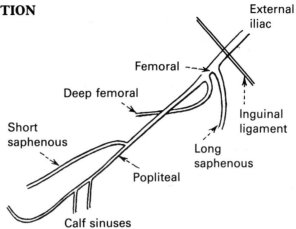

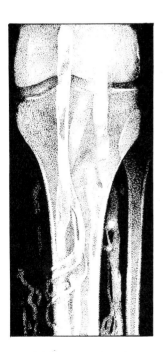

Phlebogram showing thrombi in calf veins and extending up the popliteal.

FORMATION OF THROMBUS

Some endothelial lesion allows the platelets to come in contact with the subendothelial structures to which they adhere. In the process of aggregation various substances are released, including adenosine diphosphate (ADP), which increase adherence. Liberated thromboplastins initiate the formation of fibrin clot. The vessel wall also liberates a substance, prostacyclin, which inhibits platelet adherence, and activator, which initiates fibrinolysis. If the local concentration of these substances is inadequate, thrombus formation continues, and an embolus may break off into the blood stream.

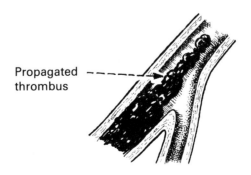

CLINICAL FEATURES OF DVT

There is very often no complaint, but silent thrombosis is now known to be a common post-operative complication, and clinical signs should be looked for. Predisposing factors are previous thrombosis, age, obesity, a history of oral contraception, sepsis and immobility.

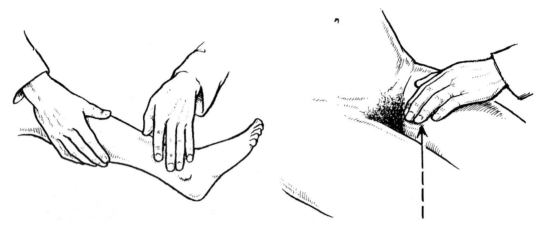

Palpation of the calf demonstrates tenderness and oedema.

The femoral vein must also be palpated in the groin.

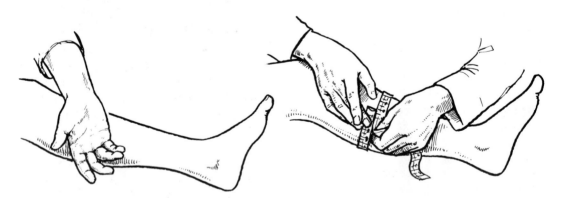

The affected leg may feel warmer to the back of the hand.

Careful measurement may reveal some swelling compared with the other leg.

SCREENING TESTS FOR DVT

DVT can be symptomless until pulmonary embolism declares itself, and various screening tests have been developed – none of them completely satisfactory.

Fibrin Degradation Products (FDP)

FDP are an indication of fibrin production, and normal levels rule out significant degrees of DVT. Raised levels are not specific and although fractions of fibrin can be measured by radioassay and give more accurate indications of thrombus formation, such tests are not universally available and at present there is no clinically available chemical test for hypercoagulability or for symptomless DVT.

^{125}I-Fibrinogen Scanning

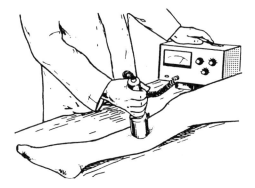

The thyroid gland is blocked with sodium iodide to prevent uptake of the iodine isotope, and 100μc of ^{125}I-fibrinogen are injected before operation. The legs are scanned at different levels for the next 6 days with a portable scintillation counter. Aggregations of fibrin in thrombus show as a raised count. Readings are more reliable at calf level than at thigh level where there are more vessels and more fat. The use of radioactive substances is controlled by regulations which have to be complied with.

Thermography

The technique of thermography demonstrates heat patterns of the skin surface by means of infra-red rays, and irregular venous patterns of heat production can be demonstrated after exercise.

 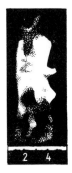

Thermogram of a normal left leg showing a cool area over the subcutaneous tibia.

Abnormal after-exercise thermogram showing irregular distribution of 'hot spots' over the tibia.

Irregular after-exercise thermograms are associated with chronic venous insufficiency and such patients are at greater risk. The technique, however, is predictive rather than diagnostic or screening.

SCREENING TESTS FOR DVT

PHLEBOGRAPHY

This is the most reliable method of demonstrating thrombi in veins, but it is time consuming and requires experience. The contrast medium may aggravate the phlebitis.

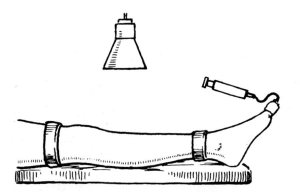

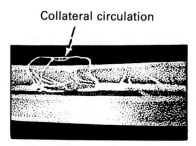

Collateral circulation

Contrast medium is injected into a vein near the big toe. Two inflated cuffs force it into the deep veins where its progress can be watched on image intensification apparatus.

A filling defect indicates the site of thrombosis. Note the opening of the collateral circulation.

ULTRASONIC DIAGNOSIS

The flowing movement of blood produces characteristic sounds when picked up by an ultrasonic transducer held over the vessel. The frequency and amplitude of the sounds are increased when the flow is accelerated by squeezing the calf.

The transducer is placed over the femoral vein in the groin, and the thigh or calf compressed with an inflatable cuff. Absence of any increased sound suggests that flow is impeded by a thrombus.

This method is less reliable than isotope scanning and will not detect small thrombi.

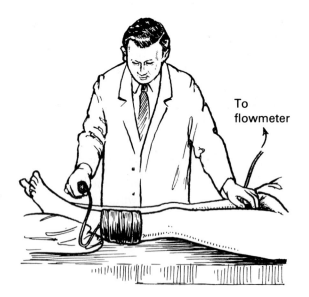

To flowmeter

PREVENTION OF DVT

When DVT occurs the immediate risk is pulmonary embolism, but there is also a likelihood of permanent damage to the veins, producing what is called the 'post-phlebitic syndrome' swelling, bursting pain, varicose veins, ulceration. In modern surgical practice there now exists an obligation to take some form of prophylactic measure.

PHYSICAL MEASURES TO PREVENT STASIS

1. Early Ambulation

All patients however frail should be 'walked round the bed' on the day following the operation, and they should be encouraged as they gain strength to walk about the wards.

2. Post-operative Physiotherapy

This is particularly valuable but is time consuming and expensive. The physiotherapist encourages the patient in deep breathing and in exercises to restore muscle tone.

3. Compression bandaging

This reduces the pooling of blood in the leg veins. A crepe bandage can be used or, more effectively, an elastic stocking.

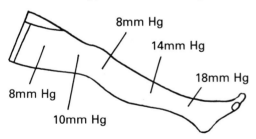

8mm Hg
14mm Hg
18mm Hg
8mm Hg
10mm Hg

Graduated static compression stockings exert a greater pressure at the ankle than at the thigh.

4. 'Pneumatic Stockings'

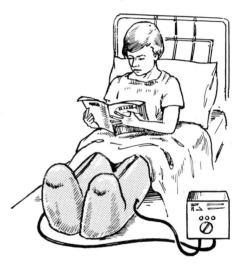

Inflatable gaiters exercise an intermittent pneumatic pressure to the legs during operation and afterwards. They are rather cumbersome and get in the way of nursing, and have to be taken off for ambulation and then reapplied.

PREVENTION OF DVT

LOW DOSE HEPARIN

Dosage: 0.2ml (5000 IU) is injected subcutaneously into the fat of the abdominal wall 3 times daily starting before operation and continuing for a week. There is a slight increase in wound haematoma but no laboratory control is required. This system of treatment is rather uncomfortable for the patient.

Rationale: Low dose heparin increases the activity of antithrombin III, the most important inhibitor of blood clotting. In high doses it directly inhibits thrombin.

ULTRA LOW DOSE HEPARIN

Dosage: 1.0 IU heparin/kgbw/hour, which is equal to 1680 IU in 24 hours for a 70kg woman. It has to be given intravenously by an infusion pump or gravity drip, and maintained for 5 days.

Rationale: This amount of heparin is almost homeopathic and must achieve its effect indirectly. It is thought that it acts by reducing the post-operative increase in platelet adhesiveness and by stimulating endogenous anticoagulant substances.

DEXTRAN 70

Dextran reduces platelet adhesiveness and blood viscosity, and it is simple to give half a litre during operation and again 48 hours later. This treatment is acceptable to the patient but carries a risk of pulmonary oedema if the heart is embarrasssed.

INTRAPULMONARY HEPARIN

This is an experimental method at present. Vascular endothelial surfaces have a high affinity for heparin, and it may some day be possible to give a single prophylactic dose of heparin via the endotracheal tube.

OTHER DRUGS MODIFYING PLATELET BEHAVIOUR

Dipyridamole ('Persantin') is a coronary vasodilator which also inhibits platelet aggregation.
Sulphinpyrazone ('Anturan') was introduced for the treatment of gout and has been found to impair platelet aggregation.
Aspirin has been found to inhibit the release of thromboxane from the platelets. However, it also inhibits prostacyclin synthesis.

None of these drugs has yet found a place in the routine prophylaxis of DVT.

TREATMENT OF DVT

ANTICOAGULANT DRUGS

These are indicated in all but the most minor and superficial degrees of thrombosis, which may be treated by elevation of the leg and tight bandaging. The patient must be encouraged to walk about as soon as she is free of pain.

HEPARIN is a mucopolysaccharide extracted from the lungs and intestines of cattle. It combines with antithrombin and in large doses interrupts the coagulation process at almost every step. The object is to prevent the further growth of a thrombus by preventing the manufacture of fibrin.

Administration of Heparin

Continuous infusion is the most effective at the rate of 30,000 IU in 24 hours. If the necessary supervision is not possible 10,000 IU may be given intravenously every 8 hours.

Side-effects   The only serious side-effect is bleeding from the operation site. This can be severe and may occur even when coagulation tests are normal. The anticoagulant action is reversed by 5ml protamine sulphate and this may take up to an hour to be effective. Prolonged heparin therapy can cause osteoporosis.

Control of Dosage   The simplest method is the *in vitro* clotting time which should not go beyond 20 minutes. A more precise monitoring is achieved by the activated partial thromboplastin time (APTT) which should be not more than twice the normal.

Duration of Treatment   Usually Warfarin treatment is begun at the same time, and heparin can then be discontinued after about 4 days.

WARFARIN, a derivative of the coumarin series, is given orally. This drug acts as a vitamin K antagonist and reduces the plasma concentrations of Factors II (prothrombin) VII, IX and XI.

Administration of Warfarin   A loading dose of 25mg is given orally and maintenance is about 5mg every second day. The drug is started at the same time as heparin infusion, and the therapeutic level is reached in about 48 hours.

Side-effects   The danger is bleeding and microhaematuria is the rule. Gastric haemorrhage, skin bruising and rectus sheath haematoma may occur with varying severity. The antidote is vitamin K, 5–30mg, which will take 24 hours to be effective. If anticoagulation is to be maintained it is better to give fresh frozen plasma to replace deficient factors.

PHENINDIONE (DINDEVAN) is a derivative of indanedione, and an alternative oral anticoagulant. It has the same action as Warfarin and the loading dose is 200mg daily. It turns the urine pink or orange.

Control of oral anticoagulants   The prothrombin time is estimated against the standard British Comparative Thromboplastin (BCT) or by the 'Thrombotest' reagent. The therapeutic test time is 10% of normal which is near the bleeding level.

Duration of Treatment depends on the severity of DVT but should extend for at least a week after complete disappearance of symptoms.

EXAMPLE OF ANTICOAGULANT TREATMENT OF DVT

Day 1. Begin heparin 10,000 units 6-hourly.
   Control by clotting time or thrombin time.
   Alternatively infuse by pump at 40,000 units in 24 hours, monitoring every 4 hours. If the thrombin time exceeds 60 seconds, give 2mg of protamine sulphate.
   Give a loading dose of 30mg of Warfarin.

Day 2. Stop heparin in the evening.

Day 3 et seq. Adjust Warfarin dosage by thrombotest.

   By the 10th day, Warfarin dosage should be stabilised with thrombotest at about 10% of normal. Urine should be tested daily for haematuria.

DRUGS INTERACTING WITH ORAL ANTICOAGULANTS

ENHANCEMENT	Mechanism
Butazolidine, Indomethacin, Alcohol.	Interfere with liver catabolism.
Salicylates, Sulphonamides.	Compete with drug at binding sites.
Broad spectrum antibiotics.	Decrease bowel synthesis of Vit.K.
INHIBITION	
Barbiturates, Oral contraceptives.	Induce liver enzyme activity.

CONTRAINDICATIONS TO ORAL ANTICOAGULANT THERAPY

Cardiovascular

   Malignant hypertension,
   Retinopathy,
   Endocarditis,
   Non-embolic cerebral haemorrhage.

Haematological

   Pre-existing haemostatic defect.

Renal

   Renal impairment of severe degree.

   Long term oral anticoagulant therapy requires good patient co-operation, and is contraindicated in mental defectives and alcoholics.

PULMONARY EMBOLISM

An embolism arises from a thrombus which is non-occlusive in the vessel in which it was formed, and is therefore symptomless. It has long been recognised that clinically florid venous thrombosis is unlikely to give rise to embolism; the danger is from the clinically silent thrombus that may be floating in the vein of the other leg.

PERIPHERAL PULMONARY EMBOLISM

Small emboli are lysed rapidly and are symptomless unless infarction occurs. They often precede a major embolism unless treatment is given.

Symptoms	Signs
1. Fever	1. Pyrexia
2. Tachypnoea	2. Pleural rub
3. Pleural pain	3. Crepitations
4. Haemoptysis (40%)	4. Perhaps opacity on lung X-ray

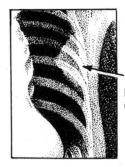

Peripheral pulmonary emboli

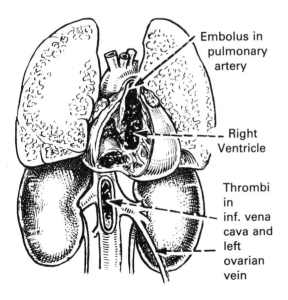

Embolus in pulmonary artery

Right Ventricle

Thrombi in inf. vena cava and left ovarian vein

CENTRAL PULMONARY EMBOLISM

A large embolus impacting in the main pulmonary artery will be immediately fatal, but if a little more peripheral, circulatory obstruction will be incomplete and there is a chance of survival.

Symptoms	Signs
1. Collapse	1. Shock
2. Faintness	– vasoconstriction
3. Respiratory distress	– hypotension
4. Pain.	2. RV failure
	– distended neck veins
	– Gallop rhythm
	3. Cyanosis.

The cardiac output drops at once and there is intense reflex vasoconstriction, leading to tachycardia, hypotension, and syncope if the patient is sat up. The respiratory distress is very severe, and the pulmonary cyanosis may be aggravated by a right-to-left shunt through the patent foramen ovale which exists in 25% of individuals.

PULMONARY EMBOLISM

INVESTIGATIONS

ECG changes consistent with right heart change will occur but last only a few hours.

SQT waves all show inversion.

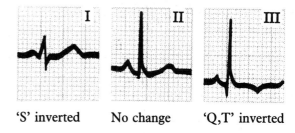

'S' inverted   No change   'Q,T' inverted

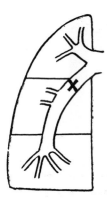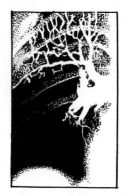

Only the upper lobe arteries are seen. The embolism has lodged at **X**.

PULMONARY ANGIOGRAPHY

Contrast medium is injected through a catheter in an arm vein. This investigation is only necessary in cases of suspected massive embolism in a very ill patient.

PERFUSION SCANS

These require special facilities. Technetium-labelled albumin is injected and the lungs scanned with a gamma camera or scintillation scanner. Different postures are required and this is not for the seriously ill patient.

It takes 1–2 hours to perform and, of course, other causes of reduced perfusion such as bronchitis will show a similar picture.

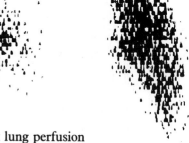

Right lung perfusion much reduced.

PULMONARY EMBOLISM

IMMEDIATE RESUSCITATION

The patient should be transferred to an intensive care unit as soon as possible, but some resuscitative measures are called for. The longer the period of survival, the better the prognosis.

Reducing the Degree of Obstruction

External massage may move the embolus onwards so that it is less obstructive.

Heparin, 15,000 units intravenously, is given as a serotonin antagonist as well as an anticoagulant, and may reduce pulmonary vasoconstriction and bronchospasm.

Improving Venous Return to the Heart

Keep the patient flat and expand blood volume with Dextran.

Oxygenation

Give oxygen by mask, and inject bicarbonate 50m.eq. to combat the inevitable acidosis.

DIFFERENTIAL DIAGNOSIS

Minor (Peripheral) Embolism

Pneumonia
Acute and chronic bronchitis
Other causes of haemoptysis
  and pleural effusion.

Recent surgery and sudden onset are highly indicative. The legs will show a positive scan.

Major (Central) Embolism

1. Other causes of collapse:
   Myocardial infarction,
   Cardiopulmonary oedema,
   Septic shock.

2. Other causes of acute dyspnoea:
   Pneumothorax,
   Asthma.

3. Minor embolism with existing
   cardiopulmonary disease.

With the exception of angiography in massive embolism, there is no specific confirmatory test for pulmonary embolism and any or all of the expected signs and symptoms may be absent.

TREATMENT OF PULMONARY EMBOLISM

USE OF THROMBOLYTIC AGENTS

This is an effective but dangerous treatment which would be resorted to only if thrombi or emboli continued to be produced.

Streptokinase is an exotoxin derived from haemolytic streptococci. The drug must first overcome the antibodies which everyone possesses against streptococcal infection.

Urokinase is a natural lytic activator manufactured in the kidneys and excreted in the urine. It is very expensive but virtually non-antigenic.

Both these drugs stimulate the conversion of plasminogen to plasmin which then lyses the fibrin in the thrombus. The dosage of streptokinase is 100,000 IU per hour, with a loading dose of 250,000 IU.

PRECAUTIONS WITH THROMBOLYTIC AGENTS

1. Treatment should not last more than 3 days.
2. Severe bleeding can be controlled by anti-fibrinolytic agents such as tranexamic acid 500mg (Cyclokapron) given 4-hourly.
3. No injections or withdrawals of blood can be carried out during treatment, so there can be no laboratory control.
4. Once treatment has stopped, anti-coagulants should be given.

CONTRAINDICATIONS TO THROMBOLYTIC AGENTS

1. Any operation within 10 days (*All* fibrin is broken down).
2. Open wound or ulcer.
3. Pregnancy or abortion.
4. Menstruation.
5. Hypertension.
6. Any tendency to be a 'bleeder'.

INTERRUPTION OF THE INFERIOR VENA CAVA

This is a cardiovascular surgeon's technique, and might be indicated in the presence of extensive iliac vein thrombosis, especially if a small non-fatal embolism has already been observed.

Many devices have been described, and the most recent is the Kim-Ray Greenfield filter which is introduced under X-ray screening through the internal jugular vein. It consists of an arrangement of steel struts fitted into an apical hub and having small hooded ends which grasp the wall of the IVC and prevent displacement.

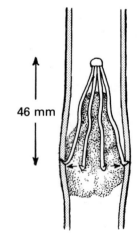

46 mm

TREATMENT OF PULMONARY EMBOLISM

SUMMARY OF MANAGEMENT

1. Massive embolism.
   Death appears imminent.

   Only embolectomy may be of use here, preferably under cardiopulmonary by-pass. Otherwise only resuscitative and supportive measures can be applied.

2. Major embolism
   with or without shock.

   Treatment of shock should be started along with heparinisation. If the patient continued to produce emboli or if the thrombosis appeared to be enlarging locally, streptokinase treatment would be considered.

3. Minor (peripheral) emboli.

   Heparinisation.

Pulmonary embolism is a catastrophe better avoided, but the patients who are going to die will do so almost at once, and complete resolution can be looked for in those who survive the first 2 hours.

CHAPTER 16

ABORTION AND ABNORMALITIES
OF EARLY PREGNANCY

ABORTION

The termination of a pregnancy before the 24th week.

The causes and prevention of abortion are matters of obstetrical concern, but gynaecological units often admit abortion patients for treatment.

THREATENED ABORTION

Technically this refers only to bleeding from the placental site which is not yet severe enough to terminate the pregnancy. In practice any case of bleeding before the 24th week may be classed as a threatened abortion in the absence of other explanation. The patient is confined to bed and the presence of a continuing pregnancy confirmed by ultrasound or positive pregnancy tests. After the bleeding has diminished, the cervix should be examined.

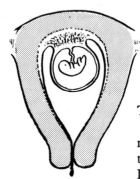

Threatened abortion
Bleeding is slight, not retro-placental and the cervix is closed. Pregnancy is likely to continue.

INEVITABLE ABORTION

Here bleeding is also slight, and the cervix is usually open. There is usually pain. Clinically the patient presents as a threatened abortion, but bleeding is retro-placental and the ovum is already dead.

Ultrasound shows no fetal vascular pulsation. The pregnancy test may still be positive as HCG is produced by the chorion, not the fetus.

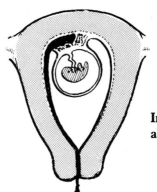

Inevitable abortion

INCOMPLETE ABORTION

The fetus and membranes are expelled but the chorionic tissue remains attached and bleeding continues. This abortion must be completed by curettage.

Ultrasound shows debris in the uterine cavity – 'mid-line echoes'.

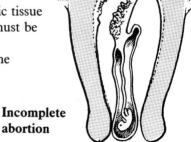

Incomplete abortion

ABORTION

MISSED ABORTION

The retention of a dead ovum for several weeks. The normal reaction of the uterus to the death of the ovum is to expel it, but for some unexplained reason this may not occur.

Up to about 12 weeks, the whole pregnancy is gradually absorbed and often presents gynaecologically as an unexplained amenorrhoea. After about 12 weeks, the formation of a carneous mole is likely, and after 18 weeks a macerated fetus is usually expelled.

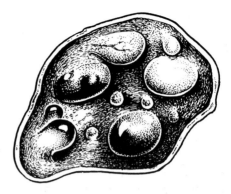

A carneous mole is a lobulated mass of laminated blood clot. The projections into the shrunken amniotic cavity are caused by repeated haemorrhages in the choriodecidual space.

Treatment

If left alone spontaneous expulsion is likely, but such management carries a risk of coagulation defect, and the patient will usually press for active treatment. Curettage is safe if the uterus is about 10 to 12 weeks' size, but otherwise the condition is better managed by induction with extra-uterine prostaglandin (p. 402).

THERAPEUTIC ABORTION

A termination of pregnancy carried out under the provision of the Abortion Act of 1967. This Act allows consideration of various social and emotional factors as well as the physical and mental state of the mother and fetus.

Menstrual regulation – curettage of the uterus before there is any evidence to suggest that a pregnancy may exist – is not with certainty covered by the Abortion Act. The *intent* to terminate a pregnancy requires to be notified.

CRIMINAL ABORTION

A termination of pregnancy not carried out under the provisions of the Abortion Act. Such abortions concern gynaecologists because of the likelihood of their being done by unskilled hands which introduce trauma and sepsis.

SEPTIC ABORTION

Any abortion which becomes infected. Such infection carries a risk of septic shock.

ANTI-D SERUM

In Rhesus-negative subjects it is necessary to administer anti-D serum to prevent Rhesus iso-immunisation. $100\mu g$ anti-D IgG immunoglobulin is given to unsensitised Rh-negative women.

CLASSIFICATION OF ABORTION

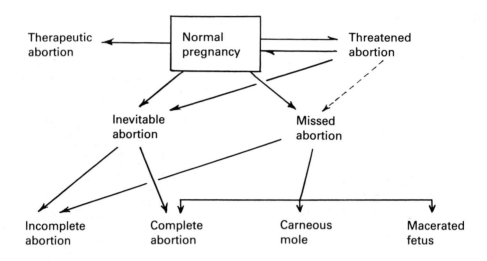

Type of abortion	Vaginal bleeding	Pain	Dilatⁿ. Cervix	Preg. Test	U/S	Treatment
Threatened	+	±	−	+ve	Fetal vascular pulsation	Conservative
Inevitable — Complete	−	−	+	±	Empty	Nil
Inevitable — Incomplete	++	+	+	±	Products of debris in uterus	Evacuation of retained products
Missed	− or dark staining	−	−	−ve	No pulsation. Products in uterus	Evacuation or Prostaglandin
Ectopic pregnancy	±	±	−	ßHCG +ve	Empty uterus. Decidua possibly adnexal mass.	Laparotomy or Laparoscopy

INCOMPLETE ABORTION

INCOMPLETE ABORTION – Dilatation and Evacuation

Once dilatation is sufficient the bulk of placental tissue may be removed with ovum forceps.

The remnants of tissue are removed with the curette. A blunt curette is ineffective and a large sharp one should be used, always with care.

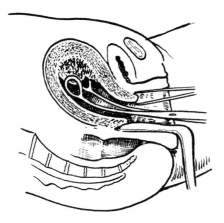

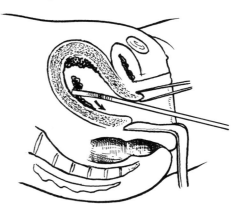

Before using any instrument inside the uterus, oxytocin 5 units should be given to contract the uterine muscle, reducing the risk of perforation.

The concave side of the curette loop is pressed against the uterine wall and pulled down. A 'clean' uterine wall gives a characteristic sensation to the operating hand.

Packing the Uterus

This is necessary if bleeding continues from an empty uterus and oxytocics are ineffective. Dry sterile gauze is used and the cervix should be dilated up to about 20mm to make it easier to get packing into the whole cavity. This is rarely necessary.

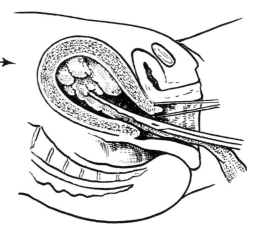

THERAPEUTIC ABORTION

Indications for Therapeutic Abortion under the Abortion Act (1967), amended 1992.

1....the continuance of the pregnancy would involve risk to the life of the pregnant woman greater than if the pregnancy were terminated.

2....the termination is necessary to prevent grave permanent injury to the physical or mental health of the pregnant woman.

3....the pregnancy has NOT exceeded its 24th week and the continuance of the pregnancy would involve risk, greater than if the pregnancy were terminated, of injury to the physical or mental health of the pregnant woman.

4....the pregnancy has NOT exceeded its 24th week and the continuance of the pregnancy would involve risk, greater than if the pregnancy were terminated, of injury to the physical or mental health of the existing child(ren) of the family of the pregnant woman.

5....there is substantial risk that if the child were born it would suffer from such physical or mental abnormalities as to be seriously handicapped.

A certificate of opinion is given by 2 medical practitioners before the commencement of treatment for the termination of pregnancy to which it refers.

A single practitioner may give an emergency certificate before termination or, where not reasonably practical, within 24 hours of termination and terminate a pregnancy if it is necessary to save the life of the pregnant woman or to prevent grave permanent injury to her physical or mental health.

THERAPEUTIC ABORTION

SUCTION TERMINATION OF PREGNANCY (STOP)

This is the best method up to 12 weeks' maturity.

The Karman plastic suction curette is commonly used and is less likely to damage the uterus than metal instruments. Plastic curettes are flexible and allow some scraping as well as suction, and they are supplied in diameters from 4 to 12mm so that dilatation of the cervix varies according to the weeks of gestation.

Softening of the cervix, making the procedure easier, may be obtained by the insertion of two prostaglandin pessaries a few hours prior to the operation.

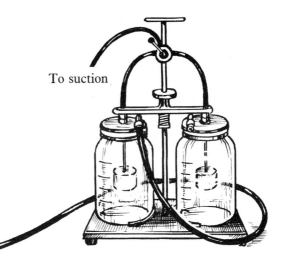

To suction

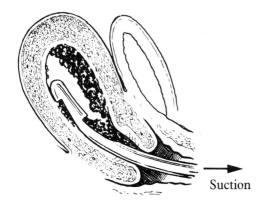

Suction

Complications

1. The main disadvantage is the likelihood of incomplete evacuation if the pregnancy is more advanced than was expected. Forceps or sponge holders may be needed to remove fetal parts which resist suction.
2. Perforation is possible although unlikely, but if it happens, a laparotomy must be carried out.
3. Sepsis. If incomplete evacuation is suspected, antibiotic cover should be provided and a repeat curettage done after 48 hours.
4. The more advanced the pregnancy, the greater the blood loss. At 12 weeks, 250–500ml loss may be expected. The use of prostaglandin pessaries reduces blood loss.

MEDICAL INDUCTION OF ABORTION

Abortion after 14 weeks can be induced by a combination of prostaglandin-2 (PGE2) applied to the cervix and oxytocin given intravenously.

EXTRA-AMNIOTIC ABORTION

PGE2 is very slowly instilled into the cervix through a Foley catheter at a rate not exceeding 2.5 ml/hour.

INTRAVENOUS OXYTOCIN

After 6–8 hours of PGE2 the cervix will be soft enough to allow the action of oxytocin given intravenously in gradually increased dosage up to 150mU/minute.

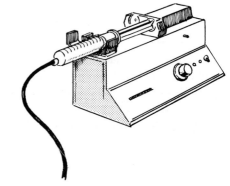

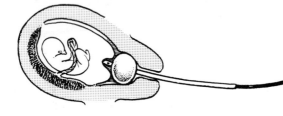

Abortion may be expected within 24 hours, and the uterus should then be curetted under general anaesthesia.

RISKS OF MEDICAL INDUCTION

1. Infection.
2. Cervical damage. Tears have been reported and the cervix should always be inspected. Oxytocic agents must always be given slowly.

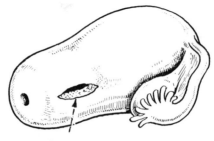

Cervical tear

THERAPEUTIC ABORTION

"MEDICAL TERMINATION"

Mifepristone (RU 486) is an anti-progestogen which offers a medical alternative to vacuum aspiration of early pregnancy, up to 63 days from the first day of LMP or dated by ultrasound.

Its use is strictly controlled to approved NHS hospitals and premises approved under the Abortion Act.

600mg oral dose is taken in the presence of the prescribing doctor and the patient observed closely for 2 hours. Unless abortion has already occurred, a 1mg Gemeprost pessary is administered vaginally 36 to 48 hours later, with 6 hours' observation because of the risk of severe hypotension. The great majority of pregnancies are aborted completely but curettage may be required for incomplete abortion. If abortion does not occur, dilatation and evacuation are mandatory.

Mifepristone is contraindicated after 64 days' gestation, in suspected ectopic pregnancy, in smokers over 35 years of age, in chronic adrenal failure, porphyria, corticosteroid therapy, coagulation disorders and in women on anticoagulant therapy.

ABDOMINAL HYSTEROTOMY

An abdominal operation, Caesarian section in miniature, this procedure was employed when the pregnancy was too far advanced for termination by dilatation and evacuation, perhaps beyond 15 weeks. Decidua is sometimes implanted in the abdominal wound, giving abdominal endometriosis. Hysterotomy has largely been replaced by extra-amniotic prostaglandin termination.

THERAPEUTIC ABORTION

LATE EFFECTS of ABORTION   These appear to be few.

1. **Chronic infection** resulting in tubal occlusion and infertility. This was common enough in the days of the backstreet abortionist, and signs of infection will still appear in about 5% of patients. The usual cause is incomplete evacuation, and antibiotics and recurettage are nearly always curative. Promiscuous women, who are the group likely to become infected venereally, are also likely to have a history of abortion.

2. **Spontaneous abortion** following cervical damage. If there are no complications this should not happen, but if the cervix is torn or excessively stretched subsequent incompetence is a possibility. Good technique is essential, and it should not be necessary to dilate the cervix beyond 12mm.

3. **Rh iso-immunisation**. Anti-D serum must be given where indicated. Even an early abortion may immunise the mother.

4. **Rupture of a hysterotomy scar** in a subsequent pregnancy. Such scars are nearly always sound if the technique is correct.

5. **Guilt and Depression**. A disturbed patient can become depressed after an abortion just as in the puerperium, but normal women will experience relief as much as remorse. Patients who have had an abortion are usually pleased to have advice about contraception, and this should be given.

6. **The Maternal Mortality Rate** for all abortions in this country is about 18 per 100,000 and this could be very much reduced if the patient would approach her doctor early in the pregnancy and there was less delay in admitting her for operation.

HABITUAL ABORTION

This condition is said to exist in a woman who has had 3 consecutive abortions.

Causes

Early abortion before 14 weeks suggests an endocrine or genetic cause. Late abortion is more likely to be due to some local uterine condition, and more likely to be susceptible to cure. In practice a definite cause is seldom found but some investigations should be done if the patient intends to start a 4th pregnancy.

1. Curettage and Laparoscopy

This will reveal any mechanical cause such as congenital uterine anomaly, fibroids, acute retroflexion, cervical laceration.

2. X-ray hysterography or Hysteroscopy

These will reveal any abnormality of the uterine cavity and may help to confirm the suspected presence of a torn and overstretched cervix ('incompetent cervix').

3. General examination should include an X-ray of lung fields, a blood count, a check of the blood pressure and blood urea level, inspection of the urine, and tests of thyroid, adrenal and ovarian function. Blood grouping, tests for syphilis and a chromosomal analysis are carried out on both partners, and chromosomal analysis on fresh aborted material if it is available. The husband should be asked to provide a specimen of seminal fluid for analysis.

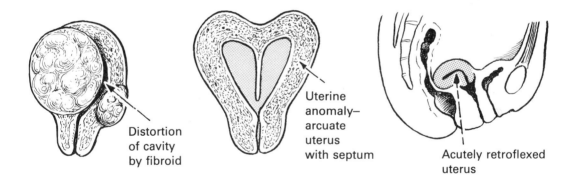

Distortion of cavity by fibroid

Uterine anomaly— arcuate uterus with septum

Acutely retroflexed uterus

These three conditions are shown as possible causes of habitual abortion; but in each case adaptation to the state of pregnancy is possible and abortion is not inevitable. It must be remembered that there is no specific investigation for habitual abortion, and a pragmatic approach is required, involving a search for any departure from the normal.

In some cases of recurrent abortion, lupus anticoagulant may be detected in the maternal serum. In others, the tissue type of the couple may be very similar. Immunisation of the woman with white blood cells from her partner has been employed but is not free of hazard immunologically.

HABITUAL ABORTION

Treatment

It is rare for a hitherto undetected systemic cause to be uncovered, but uterine abnormalities should if possible be dealt with. Fibroids should be removed and congenital defects such as a uterus septus may be corrected by plastic operations. A cervix made incompetent by previous trauma may be repaired by insertion of a suture as near as possible to the level of the internal os (McDonald's suture).

Diagnosis of this condition is made on a history of late abortions and by palpation or occasionally by hysterography.

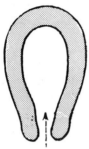

Incompetent internal os.

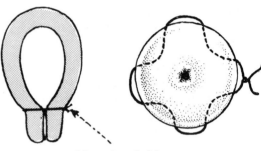

Non-absorbable suture inserted at level of the internal os.

If the cervix is much torn, a formal plastic repair can be carried out (Shirodkar's operation).

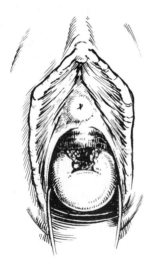

Incompetent cervix. The anterior wall has been torn right through.

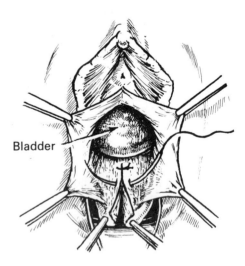

Shirodkar's repair. The vagina is opened, the bladder pushed up and the cervical edges trimmed and re-apposed.

ECTOPIC PREGNANCY – See page 331.

SEPTIC ABORTION

Uterine infection at any stage of an abortion.

Causes

1. Delay in evacuation of the uterus. Either the patient delays seeking advice, or the surgical evacuation has been incomplete. Infection occurs from vaginal organisms after 48 hours.

2. Trauma, either perforation or cervical tear. Healing is delayed and infection is more likely to be a peritonitis or cellulitis. Criminal abortions are of course particularly liable to sepsis.

Infecting Organisms

These are usually the vaginal or bowel commensals.
1. Anaerobic streptococcus
2. Coliform bacillus
3. Clostridium Welchii
4. Bacteroides fragilis.
Any of these organisms but particularly the last two may be the cause of septic shock (q.v.).

Clinical Features

Slight bleeding continues with pyrexia and a raised pulse rate. Examination reveals pelvic tenderness and the patient displays anxiety.

Treatment

This should be active to minimise the risk of septic shock. Cervical and high vaginal smears, and several blood cultures are taken and a broad spectrum antibiotic such as cephaloridine and metronidazole exhibited forthwith. Curettage should be carried out as soon as possible; there is nothing to be gained by leaving infected material *in utero*. Perforation of a septic uterus is easily done, and in a few cases hysterectomy must be resorted to. In the past, septic abortion was a relatively common cause of renal failure following septic shock. Therapeutic termination of pregnancy has virtually eliminated this.

SEPTIC SHOCK

(ENDOTOXIC or BACTERAEMIC SHOCK: GRAM-NEGATIVE SEPTICAEMIA)

Severe circulatory failure due to the toxins of bacteria. These cause vascular damage leading to increased capillary permeability; or widespread arteriolar and capillary thrombosis (Disseminated Intravascular Coagulation; DIC). The condition has a mortality of over 60% and may be a sequel of any operative procedure as well as septic abortion. A rare gynaecological form is associated with the use of vaginal tampons (see page 161).

INFECTING BACTERIA

Gram-positive
  Staphylococcus
  Streptococcus
  Clostridium

Gram-negative
  Escherichia coli
  Bacteroides fragilis
  Pseudomonas pyocyanea

Any organism including viruses and fungi can cause shock. They release foreign polysaccharides or proteins in the blood stream either as specific exotoxins or by release of endotoxins after breakdown (as in the case of gram-negative bacteria), which activate the immune system. This leads to the release of vaso-active agents such as serotonin, prostaglandins and histamine and kinins (polypeptides).

Pathology

Ischaemia of organs	Caused at first by a protective spasm as a means of preserving circulatory volume, and then by DIC.
Low cardiac output	First there is an acute fall in circulating blood volume due to peripheral vasodilatation and then myocardial failure as a result of endotoxins.
Cerebral damage	There is hypoxia which increases vasospasm, and leads to anxiety, confusion and coma.
Lungs	Low tissue perfusion follows the fall in circulatory volume, but even after this is corrected, the capillary damage may lead to pulmonary failure ('Shock lung').
Liver and Spleen	Endotoxins inhibit the phagocytic (Kupffer) cells of the liver and the reticulo-endothelial system generally, which is important in disposing of microthrombi.
Kidney	Low perfusion leads to renal failure, metabolic acidosis and further hypoxia.

SEPTIC SHOCK

SIGNS and SYMPTOMS

Early Hyperdynamic Phase

The body's first reactions to sepsis are pyrexia and local vasodilatation to improve perfusion of the affected area. The fall in peripheral resistance is countered by an increased heart rate and there may even be polyuria. At this stage the patient, although mildly hypotensive, is usually warm, alert and anxious.

Circulatory Failure Phase

The onset of this phase may be very sudden, simulating amniotic fluid embolism or myocardial infarction. The patient becomes comatose, and extreme vasoconstriction produces cold cyanosed hands and feet. Blood pressure and pulse become almost unrecordable, blood tests for DIC become positive, and signs of failure of the different organs gradually make their appearance.

TREATMENT

Infection Until bacteriological guidance is available, the antibiotic cover must be empirical. E.g. ampicillin 2g 6-hourly i.v.
gentamycin 80mg 6-hourly i.v.
metronidazole 500mg 8-hourly i.v.

Any septic focus must, if possible, be dealt with surgically. Thus if the shock is a consequence of septic abortion, the uterus must be emptied without delay.

The body's normal defence against bacteria is phagocytosis, which is inhibited in shock, and the use of antibiotics to kill bacteria in the blood stream carries a risk of increasing the amount of circulating endotoxin. Transfer to intensive care may be necessary.

Circulation

The principles are to obtain an increase in cardiac output and circulating blood volume so that tissue perfusion is restored.

Blood, plasma proteins, Dextran or polygeline (Haemacel) are given in sufficient quantity to maintain the haematocrit at about 30%.

Myocardial contractility is improved by the use of catecholamines such as isoprenaline or dobutamine, which increase cardiac output and reduce the peripheral vasospasm by dilating arterioles.

Coagulation

Tests for DIC include:-
Prothrombin Time (PT)
12–14 secs.
Partial Thromboplastin Time (PTT)
30–40 secs.
Thrombin Clotting Time (TCT)
8–11 secs.
Fibrin Degradation Products (FDP)
less than $10\mu g/ml$.
Platelet Count.

Some degree of DIC is inevitable, and if there is an inadequate response to whole blood, fresh frozen plasma must be given.

SEPTIC SHOCK

Treatment (*contd*)

LUNG

After the initial resuscitation there is a latent period of hyperventilation which may be followed by gradual pulmonary insufficiency leading to the adult respiratory distress syndrome (ARDS), which is the lung's response to prolonged vascular damage and DIC. The only treatment is ventilation through an endotracheal tube.

KIDNEY

Oliguria is the rule, and if the serum osmolarity approaches 1 (normal is over 2) a mannitol infusion should be given.

VASOCONSTRICTION

Vasodilators may be required to overcome this. E.g: thymoxamine (Opilon) 30mg, given with extreme care because of the effect of sudden vasodilatation on the central venous pressure.

CORTICOSTEROID THERAPY

Two doses of dexamethasone 30mg are given at 8-hourly intervals. Corticosteroids combat vasoconstriction and acidosis, but they also depress inflammatory responses including phagocytosis. Their use in shock conditions is debated.

NALOXONE

Naloxone hydrochloride (Narcan), an opiate antagonist, has been used with good effect in cases of shock with persistent hypotension. It counteracts the effect of the endogenous opiate beta-endorphin which is released in quantity in conditions of stress and is a hypotensive agent as well as an opiate. Such treatment is likely to uncover pain which will require exogenous analgesia.

HYDATIDIFORM MOLE

This is a peculiar condition of the placenta showing apparent degenerative changes in the stroma of the villi combined with varying degrees of neoplastic activity of the chorionic epithelium. The incidence varies in different countries, being relatively common in some equatorial regions and rather rare in the northern hemisphere. It is frequently associated with abortion and usually there is no fetus.

The true incidence is unknown in all countries since the degree of change is not constant and the aborted conceptus may be discarded as a simple abortion. The following are reported figures:

UK	1 in 1200 to 1 in 2000 pregnancies.
USA	1 in 1000 to 1 in 2500.
Russia	1 in 330.
Mexico	1 in 200.
Philippines	1 in 173.
Formosa	1 in 120.

Pathology

Five forms of the disease have been described.

1. Complete Hydatidiform Mole

Normal villus

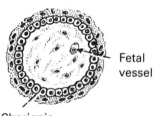

Chorionic epithelium

Fetal vessel

The normal chorionic villus in cross-section is rounded, covered by a layer of syncytial cells superimposed upon another single layer of cuboidal cells (Langhans' cells). The interior is composed of a loose connective tissue of primitive appearance in which small capillaries containing fetal red cells, many of them nucleated, are suspended.

In complete hydatid mole the villi are grossly swollen and are likened to 'bunches of grapes'.

Sometimes there are remnants which suggest that a fetus has been present but it is thought that the fetus dies before a proper utero-placental circulation develops.

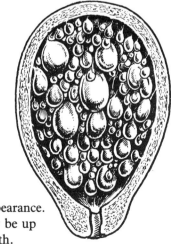

Naked eye appearance. Some villi may be up to 3cm in length.

411

HYATIDIFORM MOLE

Complete Hydatidiform Mole (*contd*)

Microscopically the enormously distended villi are mostly covered by a thin epithelial layer consisting of a single layer of syncytial cells, but in some areas of the surface both types of chorionic epithelium are present and in foci small masses of hyperplastic chorion can be seen. Special staining with antibodies shows that the syncytial cells produce ßHCG (ß Human chorionic gonadotrophin). The large surface area covered by syncytium explains the high serum concentration of the hormone in this condition.

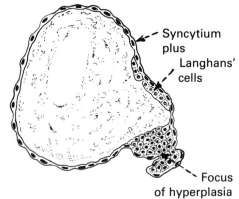

Syncytium plus Langhans' cells

Focus of hyperplasia

Fetal vessels are absent and the interior of the villi is occupied by relatively acellular myxoid stroma. Occasionally so-called 'cisterns' are present in the interior. These may be mistaken for vascular channels but they contain no cells.

The ovaries in all types of hydatid change tend to be enlarged and often contain theca lutein cysts. This is due to the activity of the high serum HCG.

2. Partial Mole

In this case there are two populations of villi. Some are of normal size and configuration, containing fetal vessels, others show the typical grape-like appearance of hydatid change, and fetal vessels are absent. Frequently an embryo is present indicating that some degree of utero-placental circulation has been established. Trophoblast hyperplasia is very focal and the serum gonadotrophin level tends to be lower than in complete hydatid condition. The fetus generally dies around 10 weeks and the uterine contents are aborted.

3. Placental site trophoblast tumour

This is a rare lesion in which few villi are formed. The bulk of the tissue consists of chorionic epithelium, much of which has not properly differentiated into the usual 2 types. Although generally benign, occasionally it can undergo malignant change and prove fatal.

4. Chorio-adenoma destruens (or Invasive Mole)

This is a molar condition with villous structure. The chorionic epithelium shows marked hyperplasia even around the villi. Langhans' cells form a multi-layered band. The syncytial cells are in irregular masses and the individual cells are greatly enlarged and are often grossly vacuolated. Fetal vessels are of course absent.

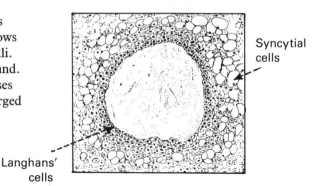

Syncytial cells

Langhans' cells

HYDATIDIFORM MOLE

Chorio-adenoma destruens *(contd)*

The molar tissue continues burrowing through the decidua and into the myometrium and associated blood vessels.

Perforation of the uterus may occur, resulting in invasion of the parametrium.

Sometimes parts of villi may form emboli and reach the lungs but only in some cases does true malignant transformation occur.

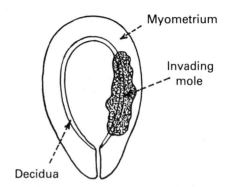

5. **Chorio-carcinoma**

This is a rare condition especially in Caucasian peoples (1 in 14000 pregnancies). It is said to be commoner in Asiatic countries but exact figures are not available.

The growth may be malignant from the very beginning but at least 50% arise from a molar condition. One of the disturbing features is that the carcinoma may arise many months after the mole has been evacuated, hence the reason for extended follow-up in all types of mole. Only about 2% of moles give rise to chorio-carcinoma but the risk is 1000 times greater than after normal delivery.

The gross appearance of the uterus containing chorio-carcinoma is of a large haemorrhagic mass showing a ragged invasion of most of the uterine wall. Section of the mass reveals that the haemorrhage is mainly central and that the uterine wall is being invaded by a layer of paler tissue.

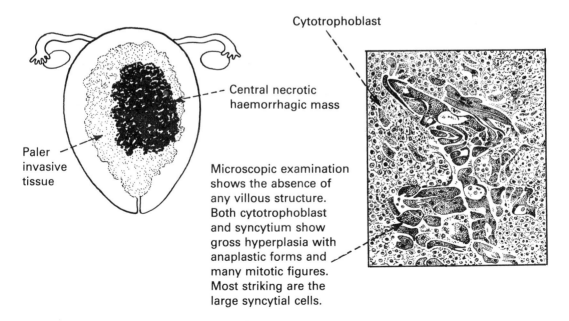

Microscopic examination shows the absence of any villous structure. Both cytotrophoblast and syncytium show gross hyperplasia with anaplastic forms and many mitotic figures. Most striking are the large syncytial cells.

413

HYDATIDIFORM MOLE

Pathogenesis of molar conditions

There are many aspects of molar change which remain wholly or only partially explained, such as:

1. The peaks of incidence are known, related to age. These occur in women under 20 and over 45.

2. The rarity of the condition in Caucasian women and its common occurrence in Asians. This difference in frequency may be part related to No 1 above. Asian women have a high pregnancy rate, start their families early and continue childbearing late in their reproductive period, thus encompassing both peaks of molar incidence.

3. Malnutrition and moles. No specific dietary factor has been identified which is related to the incidence of molar pregnancy, but congenital abnormalities are associated with malnutrition in all societies.

The formation of the molar tissue has a genetic origin although the mechanism of the genetic abnormality is not fully understood. The karyotype of complete mole is 46XX but all of the chromosomes are of paternal origin. The pronucleus of the ovum fails to develop properly and disappears. However the empty egg is fertilised by the haploid 23X sperm. This sperm duplicates its chromosomes without cell division. Why the ovum should fail to contribute to the process is not known. Since complete moles are more likely to become malignant, the karyotypes of every mole should be determined.

In partial mole, fetal tissue of some type is present and the karyotype is entirely different. Usually it is triploid – 69XXX or 69XXY. This is due to fertilisation of the empty egg by more than one sperm. Partial moles are less likely to undergo malignant change.

Mechanism of formation of the molar villi

The mechanism of the gross hydropic condition of the villi is said to be due to continued absorption of nutrients by the chorion. Since there are no fetal vessels to remove them, they accumulate in the stroma, the osmotic pressure rises and fluid is retained.

HYDATIDIFORM MOLE

Clinical course

Usually the first sign is bleeding. 50% of cases are admitted with pain and bleeding and the condition is assumed to be an ordinary abortion. The blood loss, however, is frequently high and this should raise suspicions, since a coagulation abnormality may arise.

Simple abortion usually occurs around the 10th to 12th week of pregnancy but examination will show that the uterus in a molar condition is larger than expected for the dates in 60 to 80% of patients and has a 'doughy' feel.

In addition, the expulsion of the conceptus is frequently delayed beyond the 12th week in molar conditions.

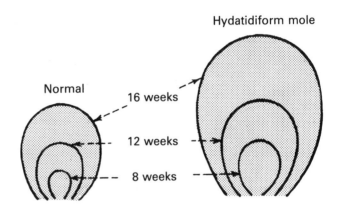

Questioning of the patient is likely to reveal that nausea and vomiting have been excessive.

The ovaries are enlarged and may equal the uterus in size. Fetal parts cannot be palpated. There may be signs of pre-eclampsia – high blood pressure and proteinuria.

A few hydatid vesicles may be passed per vaginam and confirm the diagnosis.

If not, the following examinations should be made:

1. Ultrasound

   This will reveal the absence of fetal parts. The shadow of the mole shows an irregular mass with speckled surrounding areas.

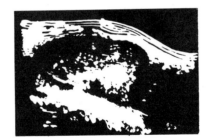

2. If ultrasound is not readily available an ordinary X-ray will show the absence of fetal parts.

3. Ordinary auscultation will reveal absence of fetal heart sounds but this often proves difficult and examination with the Doppler flowmeter will confirm the absence of a fetal heart.

4. A confirmatory but less immediately urgent test is the estimation of HCG in a urine specimen.

Differential diagnosis

A mole can mimic two common complications of early pregnancy – hyperemesis and threatened abortion – and the enlarged uterus may give rise to suspicions of twins or tumour.

415

HYDATIDIFORM MOLE

Laboratory Investigations

1. Human Chorionic Gonadotrophin

In the case of normal pregnancy the concentration of HCG in the serum and urine peaks around 60–90 days. In hydatidiform mole the curve is always steeper and continues to rise for a number of days beyond the usual time.

So long as chorionic tissue remains attached to the uterine wall HCG will continue to be produced.

It can therefore be used as a test in 2 clinical situations:

(1) To determine when molar tissue has been completely cleared from the uterus.

(2) To monitor cases where chorionic tissue persists and may be malignant. It will in these cases indicate the effects of treatment.

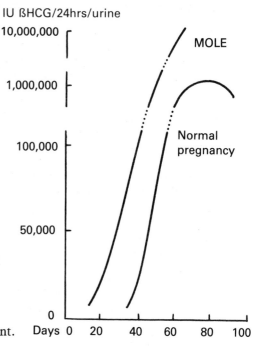

2. Thyroid Stimulating Hormone

Occasionally patients may show signs of thyrotoxicosis. It is said that thyroid stimulating hormone (TSH) is produced by the placenta but in addition HCG in large quantities possesses weak thyroid stimulating properties. Plasma TSH, T3 and T4 levels are all raised.

3. Human Prolactin (HPL)

This hormone is produced in large quantities during pregnancy but does not enter the fetal circulation. Its function is to transform maternal lipoids into glucose which is then utilised by the fetus. Although large quantities are secreted it cannot be used as a clinical test in hydatid conditions since the blood concentration does not begin to rise until ßHCG is declining, i.e. when diagnosis has already been made.

4. Oestrogens

In normal pregnancy the blood oestrogen level is high due to placental activity but its production requires a fetal enzyme input. The absence of the latter reduces the level in hydatid disease. Progesterone production is independent of fetal metabolism and the level is high.

5. Blood conditions

Due to haemorrhage severe anaemia may arise. Fibrin degradation products may be found in the blood and a fall in platelets may occur, indicating possible intra-vascular clotting.

HYDATIDIFORM MOLE

Treatment of molar conditions

If the expulsion of the mole is rapid in the 50% of cases admitted aborting, generally no further treatment is required. A gentle digital exploration may be made to make sure that all molar tissue has been expelled, but the myometrium tends to be thin and rupture may be caused. If some molar tissue has been retained, remove by digital curettage.

In some cases expulsion is delayed and suction curettage is employed. The alternatives are prostaglandins or other oxytocics. There is however a risk of intravascular dissemination of the molar tissue. Mechanical curettage must be avoided at this stage. Five days later, if there is still doubt, the following steps should be taken:

1. Repeat ultrasound examination.
2. Estimate the level of ßHCG.

If either of these indicates the persistence of molar tissue, curette the uterus.

Sometimes the diagnosis of mole is made before signs of labour appear. In such a case a decision must be made as to treatment.

If the patient has completed her family, the safest treatment is complete hysterectomy with conservation of the ovaries. The reason for such an apparently drastic measure is that 5–10% of cases undergo malignant transformation and can prove fatal.

On the other hand, the patient may be young and desire further pregnancies. This should be discussed at length with her before action is taken. After a patient has had a molar pregnancy, there is an increased risk of a repeat in a subsequent pregnancy.

Treatment in such a patient should consist of stimulation of the uterus with a dilute oxytocic solution and application of the suction curette.

Follow-up

With all types of mole and in all associated clinical situations in the UK the patient should be registered with the Tumour Registry of the Royal College of Obstetricians and Gynaecologists and followed for 2 years. The following regime should be adopted:

The follow-up of patients who have had a hydatidiform mole is based on successive estimations of ßHCG.

After delivery of the mole, bleeding should cease within 21 days and ßHCG disappear in 12–14 weeks.

HYDATIDIFORM MOLE

Follow-up (*contd*)

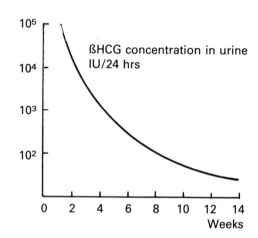

The patient should be seen at 2-weekly intervals. Evidence of persisting disease should be sought viz. clinical evidence – enlargement of uterus and ovaries. A specimen of urine must be obtained for estimation of ßHCG. If the findings fall outside the parameters indicated on the graph then more active measures must be adopted.

These may take the following pattern:

1. X-ray examination of lungs and abdominal organs to eliminate the possibility of metastatic disease.

2. Curettage of the uterus.

3. Possibly hysterectomy if there is no evidence of malignancy.

4. If curettings show any sign of malignant change, chemotherapy should be commenced.

Even if the findings indicate that the condition is simple and all clinical and laboratory results are returning to normal, the 2-weekly examinations should be continued. After 2 to 3 months, if the tests for ßHCG are negative on 3 successive visits, the examinations may be reduced to once monthly for 6 months. If the test for ßHCG remains negative for 6 months, the test may be stopped, but the patient must be seen on a regular basis for the whole period of 2 years, since malignant change may arise many months and even years after the mole has been evacuated.

Persistent Chorionic Disease

Signs of persistent chorionic disease usually indicate one of 2 conditions:

1. Chorio-adenoma destruens.

2. Chorio-carcinoma.

Both are invasive growths and it is frequently clinically impossible to differentiate one from the other.

CHORIO-ADENOMA DESTRUENS

The trophoblast retains its villous structure, but it invades the myometrium. Villi may metastasise to the vagina, or even lungs and brain.

Clinical features

1. The symptoms of mole may not clear up and the patient continues to bleed and to have ßHCG in the urine.
2. There may be no symptoms for weeks or months after evacuation of a mole: then bleeding recurs and ßHCG appears in the urine.
3. The presenting symptoms may be due to metastases, dysuria, haemoptysis, headache, visual disturbance.

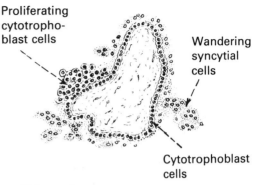

Proliferating cytotropho-blast cells

Wandering syncytial cells

Cytotrophoblast cells

Diagnosis

This is always in doubt since differentiation from carcinoma may be impossible.

1. Curettage produces friable haemorrhagic material. Histologically this usually has a benign villous structure, even when metastatic, but malignancy is a constant threat.
2. ßHCG excretion is generally high.

An X-ray of the lung fields should always be carried out if invasive mole is suspected. There may be one large shadow (Cannon-ball metastasis) or numerous emboli ('Snowstorm'). These metastases are abolished by chemotherapy.

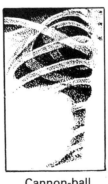 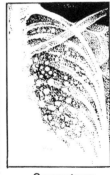

Cannon-ball   Snowstorm

Treatment

Invasive mole usually dies within 9 months, but there are 3 risks which make treatment imperative:
1. Severe haemorrhage which may be intra-abdominal, uterine or pulmonary.
2. Metastatic spread.
3. Conversion to chorio-carcinoma.

If no more children are wanted, the uterus should be removed. If the patient is young and desires children, or if there is metastatic spread, chemotherapy should be employed as for chorio-carcinoma.

419

CHORIO-CARCINOMA

The tumour spreads rapidly both locally and to distant organs. Sometimes metastases are the most prominent feature and the tumour may appear to be wholly outside the uterus.

Treatment

In chorionic malignancy or suspected malignancy, chemotherapy is the only effective therapy. Cytotoxic drugs of the antimetabolite type are used. These are similar to chemical groups required for the formation of DNA. They are taken up preferentially by the enzymes involved in the DNA process and thus prevent its formation and replication of cells.

Several types of drug are used e.g.

1. **Methotrexate**. This is an antimetabolite and on its own is the most effective agent.
2. **Actinomycin D**. By combining with single strands of DNA protein synthesis is prevented.
3. **Vinca alkaloids**. These interfere with mitosis and therefore cell proliferation.

Rationale of drug therapy

Tumour cells multiply more slowly than normal cells. Both are affected by chemotherapy, therefore the drug is only given in short bursts. This allows normal cells to recover in between. One of the key factors in recovery of cells is the provision of folinic acid, the formation of which is prevented by the drug. The following regime is recommended.

Initial therapy	Non-metastatic disease	Metastatic disease
Methotrexate at 48 hr intervals for 4 doses	1mg/kg intramuscularly	1.5mg/kg intramuscularly
Folinic acid on alternate days	0.1mg/kg intramuscularly	0.15mg/kg intramuscularly

Subsequent therapy

Monitor by ßHCG estimations:

1. If the urinary level of ßHCG falls by 20%, indicating a response, repeat regimen until ßHCG excretion disappears.

2. If there is no response, increase the methotrexate by 0.5mg/kg and folinic acid by 0.05mg/kg.

3. In the absence of a response after 2 courses, change the therapy to Actinomycin D for 2 courses.

4. If there is still no satisfactory response, add Vinca alkaloids and use all three drugs. Synergism develops and the combined effect is greater than with any one alone.

There are dangerous side-effects.

CHORIO-CARCINOMA

Side-effects of treatment

Bone marrow . . Leucopenia, anaemia, agranulocytosis.
Gut . . . . Stomatitis, glossitis, nausea, vomiting, diarrhoea.
Liver . . . . Jaundice.
Kidney . . . . Proteinuria, renal impairment. Methotrexate is excreted unchanged and can damage the kidney tissue directly. Make certain that fluid intake is adequate
Skin . . . . Alopecia, rashes.

Tests to be carried out during therapy

1. Full blood count including platelets every other day during therapy.
2. Estimation of liver transaminase level prior to beginning therapy and every 2 days during treatment.
3. Test urine regularly for protein.

PROGNOSTIC FACTORS IN CHEMOTHERAPY FOR TROPHOBLAST NEOPLASM

ADVERSE

1. Histological evidence of chorio-carcinoma.

2. Large tumour masses or widespread secondaries.

3. Delay in detection of persisting tumour cells.

4. Very high HCG levels.

5. Previous unsuccessful chemotherapy.

FAVOURABLE

1. Evidence of invasive mole only.

2. No evidence of recurrence or spread: small tumour mass.

3. Early diagnosis of persistence.

4. Relatively low and falling HCG levels. (HCG excretion is roughly quantitative of the amount of tumour.)

IMMUNOLOGICAL FACTORS

Trophoblast tissue is in the nature of an allograft, and one would expect an immunological reaction between the host and her tumour. In 90% of cases the tumour shows reactive signs consisting of lymphocytes, plasma cells and histiocytes, and the more marked this immunological reaction, the better the prognosis. The ABO system also influences prognosis which is worst in women of groups B and AB whose husbands are O or A.

PREGNANCY AFTER CHEMOTHERAPY

Methotrexate can be retained in the body for up to 8 months, and the theoretical risk is of cytotoxic damage to oocytes resulting in an increased incidence of fetal abnormality. However this does not seem to be borne out in practice, although patients are advised to delay conception for a year so that possibly damaged ova may be shed. Barrier methods of contraception should be used rather than oral contraception, or the IUD which may cause misleading irregular haemorrhage. The steroids of oral contraceptives prolong the persistence of trophoblast cells and delay the fall in HCG production.

421

CHAPTER 17

SEXUALITY AND CONTRACEPTION

PHYSIOLOGY OF COITUS

Response to sexual stimulation is primarily an autonomic nervous reflex which is reinforced or inhibited by psychological and social factors. These factors are infinitely variable; but as a generalisation it may be said that the female responds to the consciousness of being desired as a whole person, while the satisfaction of the male depends to a greater extent on visceral sensation.

EXCITEMENT PHASE

This takes most of the time needed for coitus and, in the male, becomes longer with experience, while the female learns to respond in a shorter time.

Female:

Vasodilatation and vasocongestion of all erectile tissue. Breasts enlarge, the vaginal ostium opens and secretion from the vestibular glands and vaginal exudations cause "moistening".

Male:

Penile erection occurs and may be transient and recur if this stage is prolonged. Scrotal skin and dartos muscle contract and draw testes towards the perineum.

INTROMISSION

The couple assume the chosen coital position and the penis is inserted into the open vagina. Although this is the irrevocable commitment to intercourse, it is still in the excitement phase until thrusting begins, and the male still has some control over the timing of orgasm.

PLATEAU PHASE

The pulse rate is doubled and blood pressure and respiratory rate are beginning to rise. Both partners make involuntary thrusting movements of the pelvis towards each other.

Female:

Vasocongestion increases, and contraction of the uterine ligaments (which contain muscle) lift the uterus and move it more into alignment with the axis of the pelvis. The cervix dilates. There is engorgement of the lower third of the vagina and ballooning of the upper two thirds.

Male:

The intensity of penile erection increases and the testes are enlarged by congestion. Seminal fluid arrives at the urethra as a result of sympathetic nervous stimulation of the vas deferens, seminal vesicles and prostate. There is some pre-ejaculatory penile discharge which may contain sperm.

PHYSIOLOGY OF COITUS

ORGASM

Pulse and respiration rate are at double the resting rate and blood pressure may reach 180/110. Pelvic and genital sensations are completely dominating, and there is a noticeable reduction in sensory awareness in other parts of the body. The pelvic floor contracts involuntarily, with rhythmic contraction of vagina, urethra and anal sphincter.

Female:

Climactic sensations appear to be caused by spasmodic contractions of uterine muscle. The female is potentially capable of repeated orgasm.

Male:

Strong contractions pass along the penis causing ejaculation of seminal fluid. The greater the volume of ejaculate (after several days' continence) the more intense the sensations of orgasm.

POSTCOITAL PHASE or RESOLUTION PHASE

Pulse, respiratory rate and blood pressure rapidly return to normal and there is marked sweating. Vasocongestion recedes over about 5 minutes and there is complete relaxation of all muscles and detumescence of erectile tissue. In the male, but less so in the female, there occurs a refractory period which varies with individuals, from a few minutes to several hours when there is no response to further stimuli.

SEXUAL PROBLEMS AFFECTING THE FEMALE

FAILURE TO ACHIEVE ORGASM

It is common in gynaecological practice to meet women who profess never or seldom to have experienced orgasm and yet appear to enjoy sexual fulfilment. This is never the case with the male. The psychological gratifications of coitus must never be underestimated in the female, but the physical elements dominate and orgasm is the natural response of the female to adequate erotic stimulation.

The cause of anorgasmia is therefore failure of stimulation, either to receive it or to respond to it.

FAILURE TO RECEIVE STIMULATION

This is theoretically the more easily dealt with since its correction requires 'only' some education and instruction of the male. However the barriers to communication are formidable, and a deficiency in the male (premature ejaculation for example) may arise from some deficiency in the female.

FAILURE TO RESPOND TO STIMULATION

Primary Failure	Secondary Failure
Early psychological trauma.	Puerperal depression.
Early inculcation of social or religious taboos.	Fear of another pregnancy.
	Marital stress.
Profound defect of personality.	Dyspareunia (q.v.).
Lesbian tendency, unrecognised or undisclosed.	Endocrine disease.
	Any debilitating illness.

FRIGIDITY

This term, now outmoded, implies a failure by the wife to provide a satisfying coitus for the husband, and it embodies an attitude to woman's sexuality which is not now acceptable. Women will, in consultation, declare a condition which might be described as frigid: "I have no interest in my partner; I wouldn't mind if I never had sex, but I go through with it to keep him happy". Such women are conscious of and resent the absence of physical satisfaction, and are far better regarded as suffering from failure to achieve orgasm. The male's attitude may well be at fault, but he may fail to be aware of or admit to this.

ANORGASMIA

MANAGEMENT OF ANORGASMIA

Mechanical and Clinical Causes

Conditions such as puerperal depression, fear of pregnancy and local vaginal lesions can usually be diagnosed and treated by the gynaecologist in the appropriate manner.

Psychological and Personality Causes

These must be correctly identified by a clinical psychologist, and the treatment is likely to be in his hands. Ideally both parties should attend.

TREATMENT

If the treatment indicated is basically a matter of achieving communication and confidence between sexual partners and gradually allaying their apprehensions, the gynaecologist or the general practitioner may have to function as a therapist and, for such work, experience both sexual and therapeutic is essential.

The couple must face the situation and discuss it in detail without inhibition, much as in the manner of the alcoholic. They must accept that the object of treatment is to provide *both* parties with a satisfying and affectionate copulatory relationship *as an end in itself*, and once free communication is achieved the couple proceed gradually to give and receive pelvic and genital stimulation, the female learning to welcome arousal, the male to control his own response. Progress must be discussed in detail with the therapist, and it will be appreciated that this intensive treatment requires a properly motivated couple, a dedicated and experienced therapist, and a good deal of time and patience.

DYSPAREUNIA

DYSPAREUNIA (Painful coitus)

SUPERFICIAL DYSPAREUNIA

Vaginal pain during intromission of the penis. It is usually a genuine complaint and not simulated with the intention of avoiding coitus.

Causes include:

1. Vulvovaginitis (especially infection by trichomonas or candida).

2. Vaginal cysts. Small ones are usually symptomless.

3. Infection of Bartholin's gland.

4. Post-menopausal shrinkage.

5. Rarely there is a congenital smallness of the ostium or a thick hymen.

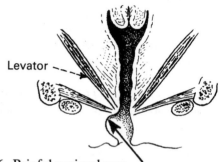

Levator

6. Painful perineal scar.
   This may be due to an inflamed or fibrous scar following childbirth, or to an imperfectly repaired episiotomy or tear which allows the formation, by attempts at coitus, of a small very tender 'blind alley' just inside the vagina below the levator muscle.

DEEP DYSPAREUNIA

Pain due to penile pressure on an area of tenderness near the vaginal vault. The cause is often difficult to identify and there may be no obvious disease. If the pain complained of cannot be reproduced by the examining fingers the gynaecologist should consider the possibility of a functional complaint.

Causes include: 1. Retroverted uterus with prolapsed ovaries, the 'ovarian entrapment' syndrome.
2. Chronic pelvic infection.
3. Endometriosis.
4. Pelvic tumours including ectopic pregnancy.

PELVIC CONGESTION

Some women complain of congestive pain developing after coitus and lasting several hours. It has been suggested that this is a result of sexual frustration following failure to achieve orgasm, and there is often some functional element to be identified. No specific treatment is known.

VAGINISMUS

VAGINISMUS

A partly voluntary contraction of the pelvic muscles which takes place when introduction of the penis is attempted, making coitus impossible.

Mild Vaginismus

The patient has erotic desires, takes part in preliminary love play and is aroused by manual stimulation of the genitals. Vaginismus occurs only when intromission is attempted.

Severe Vaginismus

No touching of the vulva is allowed, and attempts are met with an arching of the back and strong apposition of the thighs. Some reluctance or tenseness is usually apparent in the preliminary love play.

Causes are those of other forms of sexual dysfunction. Mild degrees are usually the result of apprehension, severe degrees to some profound disturbance of personality.

Treatment

1. An examination under anaesthesia should be carried out to exclude organic causes and to reassure the patient that there is no anatomical abnormality.

2. Male and female should be interviewed together and the use of vaginal dilators of graduated sizes explained. The purpose is not to dilate a narrow vagina but to give the patient confidence that her vagina can easily accommodate the penis. Once the patient can use them up to the largest size, the male partner should be instructed in their insertion in the vagina and from there the couple should achieve intromission.

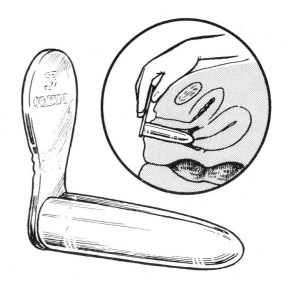

Failure of this treatment is an indication for more extensive psychiatric investigation. Mild vaginismus usually responds well to these simple measures, but in severe cases the results are poor.

The clinical psychologist and the medical hypnotist can often be helpful in treating vaginismus.

SEXUAL PROBLEMS AFFECTING THE MALE

The gynaecologist is not normally called upon to deal directly with the male, but he must be aware of these sexual problems and know something of their management.

PREMATURE EJACULATION

The male ejaculates before or immediately after intromission; and, if this prevents the female from achieving orgasm, it must be regarded as a disability.

Certain behavioural patterns seem to be associated:
1. Inexperience, producing undue haste and an inadequate excitement phase.
2. Pre-marital conditioning to rapid response – clandestine intercourse under fear of discovery, intercourse with prostitutes.
3. Any display of disinclination on the part of the female.

Treatment

If both partners genuinely seek improvement and can be induced to discuss the problem without inhibitions, treatment is generally successful. The male must be allowed to gain the confidence to prolong foreplay, and the female learns to respond more readily.

The 'squeeze technique' of Masters and Johnson

If the female squeezes the penis for a few seconds, the erection will decrease a little with a temporary loss of the stimulus to ejaculate. This can be repeated several times, extending the excitement phase and accustoming the male to delay ejaculation.

Perhaps the greatest advantage of this technique is the complete communication and awareness that develops between male and female.

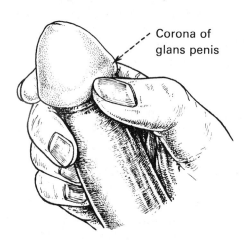

Corona of glans penis

Drug Treatment Reserpine (Serpasil) 0.1mg taken in the evening is said to retard the ejaculatory reflex, and sedative drugs such as diazepam (Valium) 2mg act by reducing the level of erotic response. When the nervous system is intact, drugs should not really be required in the treatment of this condition.

EJACULATORY FAILURE

EJACULATORY FAILURE

Inability to ejaculate although there is no loss of erotic drive and erection and intromission are normal.

The ejaculatory reflex requires intact pathways in both autonomic and somatic systems. Somatic nerves receive the sensory stimuli of coitus and pass impulses to the sympathetic nerves which stimulate the delivery of seminal fluid to the urethra by the vasa deferentia, seminal vesicles and prostate, and prevent retrograde ejaculation into the bladder by causing contraction of the internal urinary sphincters. Sympathectomy from T12 to L3 will abolish ejaculation without affecting erectile ability or the sensations of orgasm, a phenomenon known as 'dry sex'.

Aetiology is nearly always psychological, although some drugs are known to cause the condition.

Psychological Factors

1. Influence of repressive religious teaching on a susceptible personality. Coitus comes to be regarded as an act of sin.
2. Excessive maternal domination. There may be a subconscious oedipal conflict.
3. Some traumatic episode such as a humilitating sexual rejection; or the discovery of infidelity by the female partner.
4. Fear of pregnancy.
5. Dislike of the female partner.
6. Repressed homosexuality.

Drugs   Any drug with psychotropic action or which interferes with the autonomic system may cause impotence. Ejaculatory failure alone is known to occur with thioridazine (Melleril) and guanethidine (Ismelin) and especially with Indoramin, an alpha-adrenergic blocking agent.

Treatment   A complete analysis of the problem, involving both partners, must be made and this requires the skills of the psychotherapist.

If there is no serious psychological inhibition, treatment becomes essentially a matter of restoring the male's confidence, like the treatment of premature ejaculation in reverse. The female must manipulate the penis in the manner which is most acceptable to her partner, until extravaginal ejaculation occurs. Thereafter it becomes possible by degrees to achieve ejaculation after intromission.

Intercourse with another woman (a 'replacement partner') may well be more effective if the female has no interest in her partner's ejaculation or if her sexual approach is inadequate, but such single-minded therapy would, of course, introduce other problems.

IMPOTENCE

IMPOTENCE – Inability to achieve or sustain an erection.

PRIMARY IMPOTENCE
Physical causes due to some form of intersex abnormality are extremely rare, and primary impotence is nearly always due to psychological inhibition arising from abnormal influences in upbringing (medical, religious, homosexual, etc.).

SECONDARY IMPOTENCE
This may have either a physical or psychological basis.

Psychological
1. Developing from ejaculatory failure and having the same causation.
2. Social and domestic stress. The patient is typically successful, overworking and probably overdrinking. He is under stresses which affect his confidence and the harmony of his relationship.

Drugs
1. Alcohol in excess.
2. Hypotensives – beta blockers, methyldopa, guanethidine.
3. Phenothiazines – chlorpromazine.
4. Tricyclic antidepressants – imipramine, amitryptiline.

Endocrine Disease
Pituitary tumour may present as impotence.
Diabetes mellitus commonly causes impotence.

CNS Disease
Multiple sclerosis, paraplegia.

Vascular Disease
Iliac and pudendal thrombosis.

Postoperative sequel
Usually after radical pelvic operations such as abdomino-perineal resection or extended prostatectomy.

Urological Causes
These include congenital abnormalities such as hypospadias, chordee, congenital short urethra and Peyronie's disease, a fibrosis of the erectile tissue or the tunica albuginea. Such conditions are classed as 'mechanical' causes of impotence because the penile deformity gradually makes coitus impossible, but psychological impotence may be superimposed.

IMPOTENCE

TREATMENT OF IMPOTENCE

PSYCHOTHERAPY

This is seldom successful in primary impotence, but in secondary impotence, if a cause can be identified, psychotherapy may be successful. The management of the couple should be in the hands of the psychiatrist and the psychotherapist.

PHYSICAL CAUSES

These may be reversible as in endocrine lesions and drug impotence, or irreversible as in vascular and CNS disease.

Drugs acting on the autonomic nervous system, mainly antihypertensive and psychotropic drugs (including all the major tranquillisers) are recognised causes of impotence or ejaculatory failure.

SEX HORMONES

Simple prescription of male sex hormone is seldom successful and its part in the physiology of erection and ejaculation is not yet known. It seems reasonable to suppose that complete absence of male sex hormone would result in impotence; but castrated males can achieve erections. Sex hormones in such cases are presumably supplied by the adrenal glands.

PAPAVERINE

This is a smooth muscle relaxant. Intracavernosal injection of 7.5mg initially, increasing to 30–60mg according to response, is the most effective treatment for impotence. Phentolamine 0.25–1.25mg may be added if the response to papaverine is not adequate.

N.B. Papaverine, and *NOT Papaveretum* (hydrochlorides of alkaloids of opium), must be prescribed and dispensed!

When the gynaecologist is consulted by a female patient about her real or supposed sexual inadequacy, it is essential that he bears in mind the possibility that the cause may lie with her partner. For example, failure of intromission is less likely to be due to a small vaginal introitus than to an imperfect or absent erection, but the female, from embarrassment, loyalty or ignorance, may not raise this possibility.

433

MEDICO-LEGAL PROBLEMS

RAPE

The doctor may on occasion be asked to examine a victim of alleged rape.
This crime has heavy penalties and examination must be thorough and careful.
The following preliminary notes should be made:
1. Authority for examination.
2. Consent for examination.
3. General appearance of person and clothing.
4. History of circumstances of crime.

Rape is defined as unlawful sexual intercourse with a woman by force and against her will.

Sexual intercourse is described as the slightest degree of penetration of the vulva by the penis and entry of the hymen is therefore not necessary. (Use of vaginal tampons by virgins may confuse the issue.)

The vulva should be inspected for signs of bruising, scratching or tearing. The hymen may be torn and bleeding.

When the orifice is small or the hymen vestigial, bruising may be present because of the force needed to penetrate against the resistance of the victim. The presence of seminal fluid in the vagina and cervix may be the only sign. This fluid is removed and examined microscopically.

General examination of the patient may show injuries and bruising confirming a story of resistance overcome by violence.

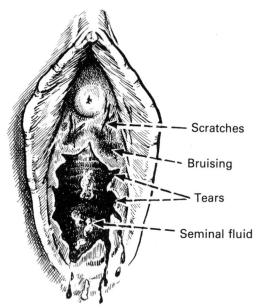

Scratches

Bruising

Tears

Seminal fluid

Major police forces have specially trained rape investigation teams whose expertise may be invaluable.

Careful record keeping is essential.

MEDICO-LEGAL PROBLEMS

SIGNS OF RECENT DELIVERY

Pregnancy and birth have usually been concealed when a medical opinion is sought. The patient is usually primiparous and looks exhausted and pale. The breasts, their veins prominent, are enlarged, tense and knotty, and pressure will express milk and colostrum.

The abdomen is lax and there may be fresh striae gravidarum – especially in the flanks.

The uterus is firm and remains 5–6 inches above the pubis in the first day or two, is behind the pubis by the 10th day and in 6 weeks is completely involuted and of normal parous size.

The labia and perineum may be lacerated and bruised.

The cervical os is torn and soft and will admit two fingers for a few days and one finger for another week or so. At 2 weeks the os is closed.

The lochial discharges are of blood and mucus for about 5 days, becoming brown, yellow and finally serous, and drying up in 4 weeks.

A pregnancy test is normally positive for a few days in the puerperium.

CRIMINAL ABORTION

Expulsion of the uterine contents by unlawful means is a crime in Scotland and in England and Wales. If death occurs the crime becomes at least culpable homicide (manslaughter in England and Wales) and may be murder.

The history may help. Examination of the woman is important. The cervix is soft and partly patent with recent abortion. The abortion may be incomplete.

Visual examination of the cervix may show signs of injury, e.g. forceps marks. There may be signs of uterine infection or of peritonitis.

Confidentiality is maintained as far as possible, but if the patient becomes seriously ill, the proper legal authorities must be notified. Careful record keeping is essential.

METHODS OF CONTRACEPTION

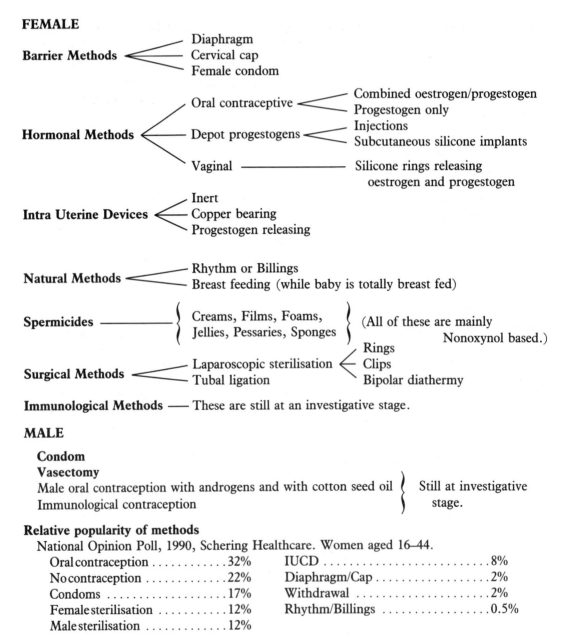

FEMALE

Barrier Methods — Diaphragm
— Cervical cap
— Female condom

Hormonal Methods — Oral contraceptive — Combined oestrogen/progestogen
— Progestogen only
— Depot progestogens — Injections
— Subcutaneous silicone implants
— Vaginal — Silicone rings releasing oestrogen and progestogen

Intra Uterine Devices — Inert
— Copper bearing
— Progestogen releasing

Natural Methods — Rhythm or Billings
— Breast feeding (while baby is totally breast fed)

Spermicides — { Creams, Films, Foams, Jellies, Pessaries, Sponges } (All of these are mainly Nonoxynol based.)

Surgical Methods — Laparoscopic sterilisation — Rings, Clips, Bipolar diathermy
— Tubal ligation

Immunological Methods — These are still at an investigative stage.

MALE

Condom
Vasectomy
Male oral contraception with androgens and with cotton seed oil } Still at investigative
Immunological contraception } stage.

Relative popularity of methods

National Opinion Poll, 1990, Schering Healthcare. Women aged 16–44.

Oral contraception	32%	IUCD	8%
No contraception	22%	Diaphragm/Cap	2%
Condoms	17%	Withdrawal	2%
Female sterilisation	12%	Rhythm/Billings	0.5%
Male sterilisation	12%		

Even the most intelligent, articulate people are often ill-informed about contraception and fears about possible ill-effects, together with problems experienced by friends and relatives, may play a greater role in influencing choice than medical advice and statistics. Many doctors are surprisingly poorly informed and therefore unable to give appropriate advice. Adequate, correct information and counselling are essential, and written details should, ideally, be supplied as well as verbal.

ORAL CONTRACEPTION

About three million women in the United Kingdom are said to be 'taking the pill'. The pill is a mixture of oestrogen and progestogen, or a progestogen alone, and its most serious disadvantage is the increased risk of cardiovascular disease, though this is lower with modern low-dose preparations.

Mode of Action

The pill prevents ovulation. FSH secretion is depressed and the LH peak is abolished. Urinary androgen excretion is much increased and this must add to the contraceptive effect.

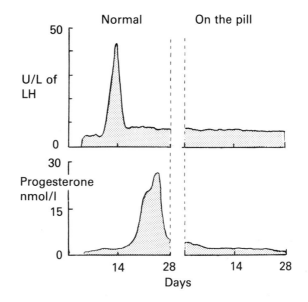

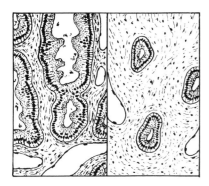

Normal   'Pseudo-atrophy'
endometrium

Absence of a corpus luteum inhibits preparation of an endometrium suitable for implantation, and a 'pseudo-atrophy' develops.

Changes in cervical mucus make sperm penetration less likely.

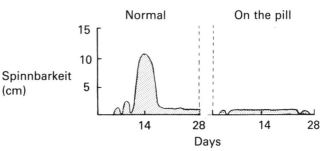

All these effects are the result of synergistic action between the oestrogen and progestogen. Progestogens when used by themselves have varying degrees of oestrogenicity.

ORAL CONTRACEPTION

Constituents

Oestrogens	Progestogens
Ethinyloestradiol Mestranol (ethinyloestradiol- 3-methyl-ether)	Levonorgestrel Norethisterone Ethynodiol diacetate Desogestrel Gestodene Norgestimate

Choice of Pill

There are over 30 brands available, using different drugs in different proportions.

High O, high P

ethinyloestradiol 50μg
norethisterone acetate 4mg

Medium O, low P

ethinyloestradiol 30μg
L-norgestrel 150μg

Low O, low P

ethinyloestradiol 20μg
norethisterone acetate 1mg

P only

L-norgestrel 30μg
norethisterone 350μg

O/P and triphasic pills are taken from the 5th to the 25th day of the cycle. P only pills are taken every day, at exactly the same time each day.

Triphasic pills

O/P proportions vary
roughly according to
the phase of the cycle.

	days	1–6	7–11	12–21
ethinyloestradiol	(μg)	30	40	30
L-norgestrel	(μg)	50	75	125

1. As a general rule, since both O and P constituents are responsible for unwanted side-effects, use the pill with the lowest amount of steroid drug. None is perfect and several may have to be tried to find one that is acceptable to the patient.
2. P-only and low-O pills are less reliable as contraceptives than those with 50μg of O, and tend to cause more breakthrough bleeding. P-only pills may be accompanied by depression.
3. O-dominant pills are required for women with greasy skins or acne.
4. Triphasics have the lowest amount of steroid and are indicated in the older age group who have a higher risk of thrombosis than younger women. They are O-dominant and may cause fluid retention and pre-menstrual irritability.

ORAL CONTRACEPTION – RISKS

A great deal of clinical and laboratory research and epidemiological analysis all go to support an association between OCs and myocardial infarction, thrombo-embolism and stroke. This evidence of association is not universally accepted (a verdict of 'not proven' has been suggested) and there is as yet no readily available and standardised test for hypercoagulability. Nevertheless OCs have been shown to increase many of the factors related to coagulation of the blood, and the clinician must take note of the probable risks. Modern low-dose preparations probably carry less associated risk.

THROMBOEMBOLISM

This appears to be due to the oestrogen component and is dose related, hence the introduction of low-dose oestrogen or progestogen-only. Even the low-oestrogen pills are associated with a significantly higher risk in women over 25, and hypertension and obesity are predisposing factors.

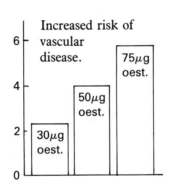

MYOCARDIAL INFARCTION AND STROKE

It has been claimed that OC users run a fourfold risk of these diseases, especially women over 35 who smoke. Arterial disease is attributed mainly to the effects of the progestogens. It has been known for some time that OCs alter the characteristics of lipoproteins in the direction of vascular disease. Low levels of high density lipoprotein-cholesterol (HDL-C) are produced by many of the progestogens used (oestrogens appear to increase HDL-C), and new progestogens have been introduced in which this effect has been reduced. Androgen-derived progestogens reduce lipoprotein 'a' (LP_a), a favourable effect.

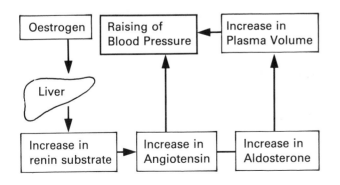

HYPERTENSION

OCs gradually raise the blood pressure, sometimes to the hypertensive range. The blood volume is increased by fluid retention, and the secretion of angiotensin is increased.

ORAL CONTRACEPTION – RISKS

MINOR SIDE-EFFECTS OF OCs

Oestrogen	**Oestrogen and Progestogen**	**Progestogen**
Breakthrough bleeding		Acne Depression
Nausea	Weight gain	Dry vagina
Painful breasts	Post-pill	Loss of libido
Headache	amenorrhoea	Insulin resistance
		(This is not a minor complication in diabetes.)

ORAL CONTRACEPTIVES AND NEOPLASIA

No causal link has yet been established between OC and any kind of neoplasia, but there has been much epidemiological controversy.

BREAST CANCER

Progesterone stimulates mitotic activity in breast epithelium, and evidence has been published which suggests that long-term OC users before age 25, especially with the more potent progestogens, may incur an increased risk of subsequent breast cancer.

CERVICAL CANCER

Evidence has been offered to suggest that long-term OC users run a greater risk of cervical cancer and dysplasia, perhaps because the steroid hormones reduce immunity to antigenic causal factors. Long-term users should certainly have regular cervical cytology examinations.

ENDOMETRIUM AND OVARY

Prolonged OC use depresses mitotic activity in the endometrium and follicular maturation in the ovary, and these effects are considered to offer some protection against cancer of these tissues.

CONTRAINDICATIONS

History of cardiovascular disease
Hypertension
Heavy smoking
Obesity
Chronic hepatitis
Endogenous depression

SPECIAL PRECAUTIONS

Collagen diseases
Otosclerosis
Diabetes mellitus
Sickle cell anaemia
Severe varicose veins
History of depression
Migraine

ORAL CONTRACEPTION – RISKS

CONTRACEPTION BY INJECTION OF PROGESTOGEN

Two long-acting compounds are used:

Medroxyprogesterone acetate
(Depo-Provera) – 50mg
    every 3 months.

Norethisterone oenanthate
(Noristerat) 200mg

Depo-Provera is now licensed for long-term use in the United Kingdom. It tends to have side-effects such as irregularity of the menstrual cycle, depression and loss of libido, and has induced breast tumours in experimental animals when given in large doses. The only significant metabolic effect appears to be a reduction in HDL-cholesterol which also occurs with oral progestogens. Three-monthly injections offer a simple and effective method of contraception in some circumstances, but in this country they are usually on a short-term basis.

FAILURE OF THE PILL

The failure rate of the combined pill is very small, between 0 and 1%, and there is often an avoidable factor.

1. The patient may forget to take the pill. Packing by the pharmaceutical firms is ingenious but not foolproof. If one pill is missed, two are taken the next day.

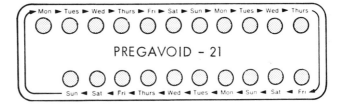

2. Gastroenteritis, perhaps following dietary indiscretion, may impair absorption.

3. Certain groups of drugs such as anticonvulsants, usually phenytoin and phenobarbitone, and the antibiotic rifampicin are known to increase the metabolic activity of hepatic enzymes, and increase the rate of excretion of contraceptive steroids. (Cf. the treatment of neonatal jaundice with phenobarbitone.)

4. Several antibiotics including ampicillin are associated with an increase in breakthrough bleeding, and pregnancy has been reported. Oral contraceptives are conjugated in the liver, excreted in the bile, and partly reabsorbed. If gut bacteria are inhibited by antibiotics, reabsorption may not occur, leading to increased bowel excretion but lower circulating levels of steroids.

CONTRACEPTION BY THE INTRA-UTERINE DEVICE (IUD)

An IUD is made of polythene and copper (gold, silver and stainless steel have also been used) and is sufficiently flexible to be drawn into an introducer for insertion into the uterine cavity.

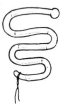

Lippes Loop

Saf-T-Coil

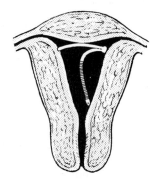

Copper-7 IUD in place.

These are polythene ('inert') IUDs, a little bulkier than copper-and-polythene, and therefore perhaps more likely to cause heavy periods. There have been reports of pelvic actinomycosis in association with inert IUDs, and recent results suggest that these inert devices predispose to colonisation with actinomyces-like organisms, especially actinomyces israeli, notably in long-term users. Inert IUDs should be changed every 3 years or so, even in the absence of side effects.

Copper-containing IUDs incorporate a winding of copper wire which is said to increase contraceptive efficiency. Their thinner diameter makes them easier to insert, and it is claimed that the menstrual loss is smaller.

Because of the gradual absorption of copper, these IUDs are renewed every 2 or 3 years. Copper IUDs produce local concentrations of copper salts which apparently give some protection against bacterial contamination.

Some IUD's are licensed for 5 years and there may be devices licensed for 10 years eventually.

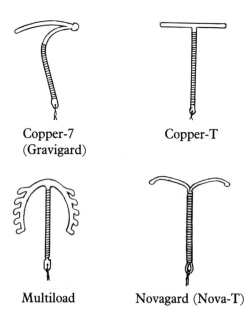

Copper-7 (Gravigard)

Copper-T

Multiload

Novagard (Nova-T)

Progesterone-releasing IUD's exist but none is licensed in the UK.

INTRA-UTERINE DEVICES (IUD)

MODE OF ACTION

This varies in experimental animals, and in the human it is not yet certain whether it prevents implantation or fertilisation. An inflammatory reaction is certainly induced in the endometrium, and there is an increase in serum immunoglobulins, suggesting an immune reaction. Endocrine patterns are unchanged, but the luteal phase is often shortened by about 2 days, perhaps because of an increased secretion of prostaglandin. Yet IUDs do not, as a rule, cause dysmenorrhoea.

PRINCIPLE OF INSERTION OF IUDs

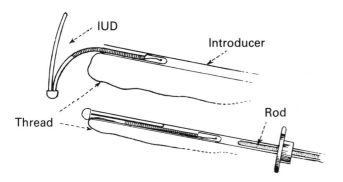

1. The IUD is first of all folded and pulled into a plastic tube called the introducer.

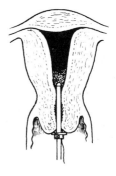

2. The introducer is then inserted into the uterus.

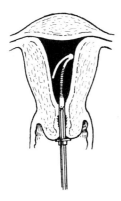

3. The IUD is forced out of the introducer by a rod . . .

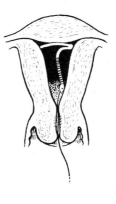

4. . . . and takes up its position in the uterus.

INTRA-UTERINE DEVICES (IUD)

TECHNIQUE OF INSERTION

1. The cervix is exposed, swabbed and grasped with a tenaculum forceps.
2. The introducer is inserted and the IUD expelled into the cavity. The thread is then cut, leaving about 2 inches in the vagina.

   With very nervous women some sedation or even an anaesthetic may be required.

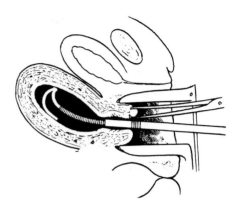

COMPLICATIONS OF IUDs

1. **Increased menstrual loss**

   The cause may be the increased fibrinolytic activity which occurs round the IUD. It can be minimised by the use of antifibrinolytic agents such as tranexamic acid. Antiprostaglandin agents such as mefanemic acid or diclofenac are also effective.

2. **Infection**

   There is an increased risk of pelvic inflammatory disease, especially during the first year, and inert IUDs are associated with actinomycosis infection if retained for long periods. There is disagreement about how long an IUD should be left if symptomless, but extraction is often more difficult after several years *in situ*, and changing the IUD at 3-yearly intervals seems sensible.

3. **Pregnancy**

   This is about 1 to 1.5 per 100 woman years, and is most likely in the first 2 years. The risk of ectopic pregnancy is greater in IUD users and has been calculated as 1.2 per 1000 woman years.*

4. **Expulsion**

   There is a 5 to 10% incidence, usually in the first 6 months.

5. **Translocation**

   The IUD passes through the uterine wall into the peritoneal cavity or broad ligament. It is thought that this begins at the time of faulty insertion, and once diagnosed by X-ray the IUD should be removed at laparoscopy.

   * Vessey M.P. et al. *Lancet* (1979) ii, 501

CONTRAINDICATIONS TO IUD CONTRACEPTION

1. Existing pelvic inflammatory disease.
2. Menorrhagia.
3. History of previous ectopic pregnancy.
4. Severe dysmenorrhoea.

IUD's inserted at or after age 40 do not require to be replaced.

THE VAGINAL DIAPHRAGM ('DUTCH CAP')

This is a rubber diaphragm which when smeared with spermicidal cream will prevent sperms from reaching the cervical canal. It is less efficient than oral contraceptives or IUDs unless used strictly according to instructions; but it has no side-effects.

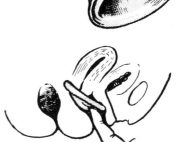

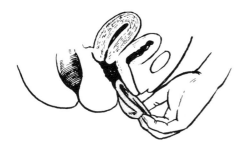

1. The diaphragm is smeared with spermicidal cream round the edges and on both sides, and guided into the posterior fornix.

2. The front end is tucked up behind the symphysis.

The diaphragm must not be removed until 6 hours after intercourse, and if intercourse is repeated in that period more cream must first be injected with an applicator.

A female condom, 'Femidom', has recently become available.

VAGINAL SPERMICIDES

Spermicidal agents are inserted into the vagina in the form of creams, pessaries, gels or aerosols. One dose of spermicide must be injected before each act of coitus. The method is simpler in practice than the diaphragm, but probably less reliable.

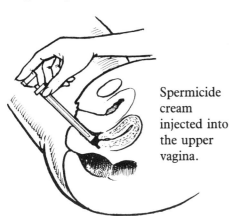

Spermicide cream injected into the upper vagina.

The COLLATEX SPONGE

A disposable plastic sponge is inserted into the vagina and can be left in situ for at least 24 hours. Sponges need no fitting, are comfortable and, when smeared with spermicidal cream, offer an effective barrier.

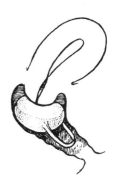

CONTRACEPTION BASED ON TIME OF OVULATION

THE RHYTHM METHOD ('Safe Period')

The woman must take her temperature every morning and watch for the sustained rise which indicates ovulation. Such graphs are not now accepted as being very precise indicators, but women with regular periods can usually identify the peri-ovulatory time with a fair degree of accuracy.

If the evidence suggests ovulation, say between the 12th and 14th days, 24 hours are allowed for ovum survival and 3 days should be allowed for the survival time of sperms in the genital tract, these times being all suppositious. This means that coitus must be avoided from the 9th to the 15th day and a 24 hour safety margin at either end increases the avoidance period from the 8th to the 17th day inclusive.

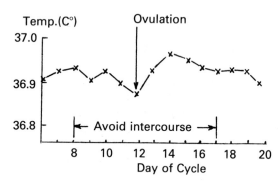

THE OVULATION METHOD (The Billings' Method)

The woman is taught to identify the peri-ovulatory phase by noting the vaginal sensations associated with changes in cervical mucus.

This method provides the same opportunities for coitus as the Rhythm method, but should be more accurate.

In practice, more protection would be afforded by a combination of arbitrary distinction between safe and unsafe days, and a close observation of physical signs and symptoms.

Say 5 days	Menstruation	
2–3 days	'Early Safe Days'	Sensation of vaginal dryness
4–5 days	Moist Days – **Not Safe**	Increasing amounts of sticky mucus
2 days	Ovulation Peak – **Not Safe**	Copious, clear 'slippery' mucus
3 days	Post-ovulation Peak – **Not Safe**	Gradual decrease in secretion
11 days	'Late Safe Days'	Minimal secretion

POSTCOITAL CONTRACEPTION

POSTCOITAL CONTRACEPTION ('Morning After' Contraception; 'Intraception')

Effective postcoital contraception has been sought for many years, usually in the form of douching with various liquids which have been unsuccessful because of the rapidity with which the sperms leave the vagina for the cervical canal and uterus. Modern methods are extremely effective if started early enough.

High Dosage Oestrogens

Ethinyloestradiol 5mg, or diethylstilboestrol 50mg taken daily for 5 days in divided doses starting within 72 hours of coitus. These dosages cause nausea and vomiting which may be so severe that the patient cannot continue with treatment, and it is possible that levels of antithrombin III may be reduced, contributing to an increased risk of thrombo-embolism.

Method of Action

Corpus luteum function is depressed and the preparation of the endometrium for implantation is prevented.

Double Dose of OC Pill

Two tablets of $50\mu g$ ethinyloestradiol and $500\mu g$ levonorgestrol (Eugynon-50 or Ovran) are taken within 72 hours and repeated in 12 hours. This treatment is very much better tolerated.

Complications of Hormone Treatment

1. Pregnancy may not be prevented and there is a theoretical risk that the embryo may be affected.
2. If pregnancy occurs, there is an increased risk of ectopic pregnancy.

Insertion of IUD

This method can be used for up to 5 days after coitus. It offers the advantage of being free from patient failure and should be offered when hormonal treatment is contraindicated, but like steroid hormones it should not be used if there is a history of previous ectopic pregnancy.

ETHICAL CONSIDERATIONS

The distinction between contraception and abortion depends on the stage at which the individual is considered to have come into existence – at fertilisation or nidation – and whatever method of postcoital contraception is used, there can be no certainty as to the point at which interference with the natural process took place.

FAILURE RATES IN CONTRACEPTION

There are 4 factors affecting the failure rate for any method of contraception:

1. **Inherent Weakness of the Method**
   For example, the rhythm method which depends on the accurate determination of the time of ovulation can never be as reliable as OC.

3. **Motivation**
   Every method depends on the determination of the woman to use it correctly. Thus pills may be forgotten, diaphragm users 'take a chance', even with IUDs a suspicion that the device is out of place may be ignored. Social class affects motivation.

2. **Age**
   With all methods, the failure rate declines as age increases.

4. **Duration of Use**
   The failure rate, especially with occlusive methods, declines as duration of use and therefore habit, increase. This observation is also true of IUDs, perhaps because the IUD becomes more effective the longer it is in place. Prolonged use is itself an indication of good motivation.

TABLE OF FAILURE RATES

The following table is taken from Vessey et al (1982) and their figures are based on the prolonged observation of over 17000 women, all 25 and over, and about 40% of whom were in social class I or II.

Method	Number of accidental pregnancies	Number of woman-years of observation	Failure rate per 1000 woman-years
OC			
$\quad$ 50μg oestrogen	61	37412	0.16
$\quad$ Progestogen only	21	1756	1.2
IUDs			
$\quad$ Saf-T-Coil	85	6791	1.3
$\quad$ Copper-7	34	2200	1.5
Diaphragm	485	25146	1.9
Condom	449	12492	3.6
Coitus Interruptus	45	674	6.7
Chemicals alone	36	303	11.9
Rhythm Method	25	161	15.5

CONTRACEPTION IN THE MALE

COITUS INTERRUPTUS

This means withdrawal of the penis just before ejaculation. It is widely practised and probably adequate for couples of low fertility, but some sperms must enter the vagina, and withdrawal at the point of orgasm is unnatural.

SHEATH (Condom, 'French Letter')

A thin rubber sheath fits over the penis. It interferes with sensation and is liable to come off as the penis is withdrawn after the act, but it is a very efficient method if used correctly.

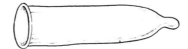

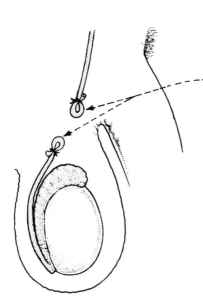

VASECTOMY

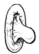

The vasa deferentia can be divided by a simple operation done under local anaesthesia.

1. It takes several months for the storage system to become clear of sperms and a few non-motile ones may persist whose significance is uncertain. It may take a year before the ejaculate is completely sperm free.
2. About 5% of patients demonstrate minor complications, including vaso-vagal reactions, haematoma and mild infection. There are occasional reports of severe infection.
3. Possible long-term complications include the development of sperm autoantibodies, and there is often great difficulty in reversing the operation if this should be required.

CHAPTER 18

INFERTILITY

INFERTILITY

The causes of infertility are numerous, especially in the female. Some are obvious, but others are obscure and require extensive investigation. Although abnormalities in the female provide the majority of reasons for failure to achieve pregnancy (almost 70%), in a significant proportion of cases (32%) male factors are responsible. It is therefore important that in all instances the couple should be investigated.

Clinical Investigation

In the case of the female partner a detailed menstrual history must be obtained. Oligomenorrhoea or irregular periods would tend to indicate problems related to ovulation. Some amenorrhoeic patients may complain of infertility but the patient in these circumstances is more likely to be concerned about the immediate problem – lack of menstruation – than infertility. However the investigation of the amenorrhoea will follow the same lines as are used in infertility and both problems may be overcome.

Pain during menstruation or intercourse may reflect the presence of pelvic inflammation or endometriosis.

Examination of the patient may also suggest reasons for the infertility. The secondary sex characteristics, distribution of sexual hair, should be assessed. Metabolic changes, such as the presence of obesity, glycosuria and altered thyroid status, should be noted. Pelvic examination must be carried out and any tenderness, enlargements of pelvic structures etc. should lead to other methods of investigation such as laparoscopy.

In many patients the infertility is the result of more subtle changes in the physiology of reproductive function. The first and most important of investigations is to determine whether the patient is ovulating.

EVIDENCE OF OVULATION

Regular menstruation is usually associated with regular ovulation, but pregnancy is the only certain proof, and other evidences must be looked for in the investigation.

1. CLINICAL SYMPTOMS and SIGNS

Mid-cycle pain is a pre-ovulatory event and is evidence of follicle development but not necessarily of ovulation.

An increased sensation of 'wetness' which is the basis of the Billings' method of contraception is a pre-ovulatory phenomenon but not a completely reliable evidence of ovulation.

2. VAGINAL CYTOLOGY

The cyclic oestrogen/progesterone effect on vaginal squames is good presumptive evidence that ovulation has occurred, but it is too imprecise for the timing of ovulation. It is a time-consuming procedure for the patient as daily smears are required over about a week.

EVIDENCE OF OVULATION

Vaginal Cytology (*contd*)

Pre-ovulatory squames

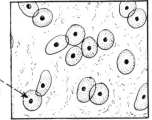

A large cell with a small nucleus shows oestrogen stimulation

Post-ovulatory squames

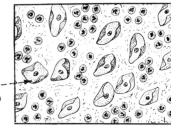

Progesterone matures the squames which develop rolled edges

Note the 'shower of leucocytes'

The secretion of progesterone by the corpus luteum induces a slight rise of about 0.2°C in basal body temperature (BBT) and such charts will usually distinguish between ovulation and non-ovulation, but the events of ovulation – LH surge, rupture of follicle, formation of corpus luteum, secretion of progesterone – cannot be accurately timed from a BBT chart.

Normal BBT chart ───────▶

There is a slight fall in temperature (the 'thermal nadir') just about the time of the LH surge (arrowed) and ovulation occurs about 24 hours later.

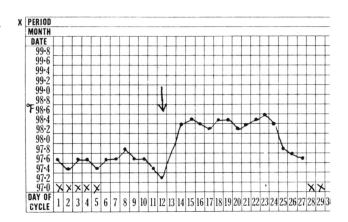

Abnormal BBT chart ───────▶

This kind of chart is often produced by infertility patients. The LH surge is arrowed and occurs 5 days after the thermal nadir, and apart from a gradual rise in temperature there is no evidence of the ovulation which did occur.

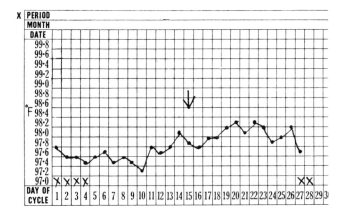

453

EVIDENCE OF OVULATION

In spite of their unreliability, BBT charts are widely used in infertility work. They allow the patient to participate in what she feels to be a meaningful investigation, and they provide a reliable record of the menstrual cycle, frequency of coitus, and the timing of any hormone treatment. The patient is instructed to take her axillary temperature every morning about the same time before getting up.

3. CERVICAL CHANGES

These are the basis of the Billings' method of contraception.

Cervical mucus is under oestrogen/progesterone control, relating to the phase of the cycle, and there are well-differentiated signs of imminent ovulation.

(a) Pre-ovulatory mucus is clear, cellular, watery and copious (the 'cervical cascade').

(b) The 'spinnbarkeit' phenomenon is marked. A drop of mucus placed between two points can form threads of up to 15cm in length.

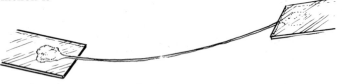

(c) When dried on a microscope slide the mucus displays a ferning pattern.

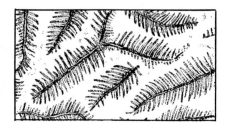

(d) The cervical os is gaping slightly and allows free access to sperm. These changes can be detected by the woman from the increase in watery discharge.

After ovulation the progesterone effect dominates, the cervical os closes and the mucus becomes scanty, viscous and impenetrable to sperm.

Scoring System for Cervical Mucus

Various attempts at a semi-quantitative description of cervical mucus have been published, and the one described here is modified from the scoring system of Insler.

Quality of mucus measured	Scoring Points			
	0	1	2	3
Volume	None	Scanty	Dribbling	Cascade
Spinnbarkeit	None	<3cm	<8cm	>8cm
Ferning	None	Slight	Partial	Complete
Cervix	Closed. Pale pink mucosa.		Partially open	Gaping os. Hyperaemic mucosa.

Day 0 = ovulation; and on days -1, 0 and +1 the score should be over 8.

The examination of cervical mucus can be done on a post-coital specimen any time up to 24 hours after intercourse in the pre-ovulatory period. Not only can the spinnbarkeit phenomenon be demonstrated but microscopic examination will reveal the character of the cell content and whether the sperms are normal in shape and forwardly motile.

EVIDENCE OF OVULATION

The lack of reliability of these tests makes more intrusive methods unavoidable.

4. ENDOMETRIAL BIOPSY

Premenstrual endometrium is strong presumptive evidence of an ovulatory cycle, but curettage or aspiration is uncomfortable for the patient, and not always feasible through a nulliparous cervix. 'Post-ovulatory' secretory endometrium is almost certain evidence that ovulation has taken place.

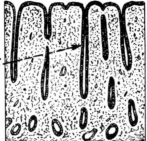

Pre-ovulatory endometrium showing oestrogen stimulation. Note the narrow non-secreting glands. The epithelial and stromal cells show proliferative activity.

Post-ovulatory endometrium showing the effect of progesterone. Note the dilated secretory glands.

5. HORMONE TESTS

Mid-cycle peak of LH

This is nearly always well marked and is the commonest reference point for ovulation. Oestradiol levels rise as the follicle matures, and at the pre-ovulatory point are high enough to stimulate a secretion of LH which leads to ovulation.

FSH Estimations

The peak is less marked than for LH, and FSH estimations are used mainly for diagnostic purposes. Low values indicate a hypothalamo-pituitary failure, while high values are evidence of ovarian failure, as in the menopause.

Oestrogen Assays The oestrogen peak is usually about day 11 and well defined. Daily estimations over a cycle ('tracking profile') give a good assessment of ovarian activity.

PITUITARY GONADOTROPHINS

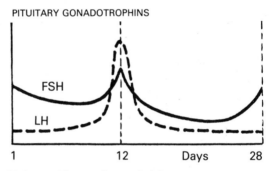

Values will vary for each laboratory, depending on the antisera and reference standards used in the radioimmunoassay technique.

	Plasma Oestradiol *p*mol/litre	Plasma Progesterone *n*mol/litre
Follicular Phase	200 – 400	<2
Ovulation Peak	300 – 800	2
Luteal Phase	400 – 600	>40

Progesterone Levels can be estimated in the plasma. An increase in plasma progesterone secretion is observable beginning about 24 hours before ovulation, rising from about 0.1 *n*mol/litre in the follicular phase to over 40 *n*mol/litre in the developed luteal phase, about the 19th day. In most women this constitutes the most reliable evidence of ovulation. However, in some patients, despite an LH peak and some rise in progesterone levels, ovulation does not occur and further investigation is required. Sometimes this is associated with a condition known as 'Luteinised unruptured follicle'.

INVESTIGATION OF INFERTILITY

Infertility may be defined as failure to conceive after a year of unrestricted intercourse, and investigations, which usually are prolonged and involve expensive tests and staff, should not be commenced before that time has passed.

The investigations are now so complex and specialised that the creation of special Departments of Infertility has become inevitable. The preliminary stages are in the hands of general practitioners who, because of their knowledge of the patients and their family circumstances, can instil a feeling of confidence and explain the various aspects of the situation, thus preparing the couple for what is likely to follow. The practitioner can obtain a detailed history from both parties with special reference to coital factors such as attempts at timing of coitus in relationship to the menstrual cycle, frequency of coitus, occurrence of pain, etc. Subsequently the general practitioner can direct them to the appropriate hospital department.

Aetiology – The FEMALE

The causes of infertility in the female can be divided into 5 groups which indicate the main areas requiring investigation. The incidence of these causes is as follows:

1. Hormonal factors controlling the process of ovulation – 41%.
2. Abnormalities involving the Fallopian tubes – 32%.
3. Uterine factors – 16%.
4. Cervical factors – 4.7%.
5. In some patients no abnormality can be found. At present the incidence of these cases is around 5%, but as research continues and techniques improve this figure is diminishing.

Each of these groups requires definition, different techniques of investigation and treatment.

HORMONAL FACTORS

In normal circumstances the control of these factors is initiated at hypothalamic level but in the clinical field there is often the extra uncertain factor of cerebral reaction.

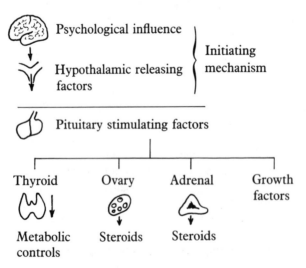

Primary hypothalamic failure is rare and only occurs as a congenital autosomal condition – Kallman's syndrome – characterised by anosmia, colour blindness and deficient secretion of releasing factors especially gonadotrophic.

Secondary hypothalamic failure is comparatively frequent. In the majority of cases it is a functional condition, the result of a psychological upset e.g. anorexia nervosa, mental fixations, fears, anxiety etc. These mental changes are important.

Iatrogenic causes: Some pharmaceutical preparations interfere with hypothalamic reactivity e.g. ganglion blockers, reserpine and phenothiazines.

Very occasionally the hypothalamus may be damaged by infection, injury or tumour growth.

INVESTIGATION OF INFERTILITY

Hormonal Factors (*contd*)

Pituitary Factors

These are not so common and are usually limited to two situations:

1. Hyperprolactinaemia may be caused by an adenoma of the pituitary, pregnancy or drugs which are antagonistic to dopamine. The patient frequently complains of amenorrhoea, loss of libido and occasionally may show signs of acromegaly.

2. Pituitary damage by injury or ischaemia. Gonadotrophin secretion becomes deficient but more commonly secretion of all pituitary hormones ceases. The best known clinical example of this is Sheehan's syndrome caused by shock due to gross haemorrhage in pregnancy.

Ovarian failure

This group of patients often present the greatest difficulty in determining where the fault lies. In some the causes of anovulation are obvious and unfortunately little can be done to overcome the abnormality. Examples are ovarian damage by radiotherapy or chemotherapy, congenital or genetic disorders such as 'streak' ovaries. Premature menopause is another such condition.

Anovulation is responsible for around 25% of cases of infertility. The most important ovarian abnormality is the polycystic syndrome (see page 104). In approximately 80% of cases menstruation is irregular or absent. It is difficult to determine whether the initiation of this syndrome is due to a defect in pituitary or ovarian function. There appears to be an excess of LH production plus a diminished FSH secretion. The result is a lack of oestrogen and an excess of androgenic substances.

Two other conditions have been suggested as ovarian causes of infertility. The first is the 'Luteinised unruptured follicle syndrome' (LUF). In this condition the cyclical changes in endocrine values are apparently normal, the granulosa layer undergoes luteinisation but the follicle fails to rupture. The clinical significance of this is doubtful especially since a luteinised unruptured follicle can be found in an ovary containing a fresh corpus luteum. Another questionable cause of infertility is 'Luteal phase deficiency', either deficient in length or deficient in progesterone production. To prove the case, intensive investigation is necessary.

ABNORMALITIES OF THE FALLOPIAN TUBE

There are two prominent aetiological factors producing changes in the fallopian tubes leading to infertility. The main factor is infection. This may be sexually transmitted. Two of the commonest organisms are chlamydia and gonococci. In many cases, however, the infection arises as a result of termination of pregnancy, abortion, wearing an intra-uterine contraceptive device and inflammatory conditions in other abdominal organs. The damage to the tube may be mild, consisting of destruction of the epithelial cilia, but more commonly the changes are gross such as salpingitis isthmica nodosa, hydrosalpinx or widespread pelvic adhesions often smothering the ovaries so that the ovum cannot escape (see page 167).

The second factor is endometriosis. It is said that treatment of endometriosis does not increase the pregnancy rate. However it is not endometriosis *per se* which is important, it is the adhesions formed during the healing of the haemorrhages, especially if these affect the ovary (see page 130).

One other cause is careless surgery e.g. failure to rinse powder off gloves prior to laparotomy.

INVESTIGATION AND DIAGNOSIS OF INFERTILITY

UTERINE FACTORS

There are several uterine lesions which on occasion seem to interfere with fertility but whether the association is really causal is still questionable. Sometimes fibroids can cause gross distortion of the cervical canal, the uterine cavity or tubal ostia and careful removal will relieve the infertility. Adenomyosis by causing uterine fibrosis also reduces fertility. Endometritis is another condition which certainly results in infertility and, if chronic, can lead to 'Asherman's syndrome' in which the cavity is obliterated by internal adhesions.

CERVICAL FACTORS

These are very questionable causes of infertility. The main problem is damage to the cervix due to childbirth or surgery. Thick mucus has been blamed for obstructing the passage of sperm.

Some women have antibodies to their husband's sperm and positive tests can be demonstrated in both plasma and cervical mucus. These cases are rare.

GENERAL FACTORS

Poor general health due to social behaviour may be important. Drugs, alcohol, smoking, caffeine and obesity will all affect fertility. Similarly, exposure to toxic chemicals as in paints and pesticides at work will influence fertility although this is more likely in the case of men.

Hormonal Tests

It is possible to some extent to relate the investigation to the group mentioned in the paragraphs on aetiology.

1. Progesterone 21 day Test: If the patient is menstruating normally, an estimation of blood progesterone on day 21 of the cycle is made. If the level is >30 $n$mol/litre this indicates ovulation in that cycle.

2. If there are signs of abnormal follicular development, such as some irregularity of cycle, a full hormone profile during one cycle should be carried out. This would include daily estimation of ovarian steroids, FSH and LH, prolactin and thyroid hormones.
   In addition, daily ultrasound tests should be made to judge follicular growth.

3. If prolactin levels are high, X-ray examination of the skull, CT scan and tests of visual fields are necessary. If no abnormality is detected, bromocriptine should be prescribed.

4. FSH and LH levels: Very high levels of these hormones would indicate ovarian failure, possibly premature menopause. In such cases oestrogen levels are likely to be low.
   Slightly raised levels of LH or a relative increase compared with FSH would suggest polycystic disease of the ovaries.

Laparoscopy and Hysterosalpingoscopy

Where the cause of infertility is obscure laparoscopic examination of the pelvic organs can be helpful. The presence of adhesions, fibroids, endometriosis or distortions of the organs can be confirmed and assessed. If it is performed in conjunction with curettage it may be possible to assess follicular growth in relation to the stage of the endometrial cycle. Cervical injection of methylene blue will demonstrate patency of the tubes.

HYSTEROSALPINGOGRAPHY

The radiological visualisation of the genital tract by the injection of contrast medium through the cervix. It has been largely displaced by laparoscopy and hydrotubation (page 88) but it is the only way of demonstrating internal uterine abnormalities and the site of tubal blockage.

Technique

The fluid is usually injected with the conscious patient lying on the X-ray table, but some nervous women will require an anaesthetic. The cervix is exposed with a speculum, the anterior lip grasped with a single-toothed forceps, and the cannula pressed into the cervical canal. Image intensification apparatus is preferable, connected to a television screen. This reduces the amount of radiation to the patient's ovaries, and allows the radiologist to observe the fluid as it flows rapidly through uterus and tubes to the peritoneal cavity. Indeed correct interpretation of radiograph stills may otherwise be impossible.

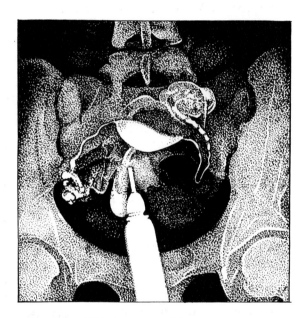

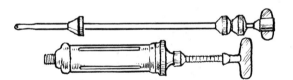

This is the Green-Armytage cannula. The syringe has a screw plunger and one turn delivers 1 ml. Any cannula and syringe will serve. Up to 20 ml may be needed.

This is a normal hysterosalpingogram. Note:
1. The anteverted uterus is foreshortened.
2. The long thin tubal outline.
3. The ill-defined shadow of peritoneal spill.
4. Cervico-vaginal leakage.

Hysterograms often require expert interpretation.

HYSTEROSALPINGOGRAPHY

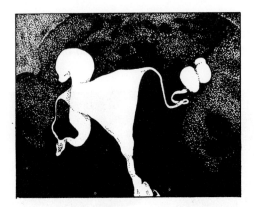

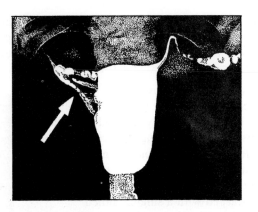

Hysterosalpingogram showing smoothly outlined bilateral hydrosalpinges, very suitable for surgery. The uterine cavity is normal. The test should be carried out during the first 2 weeks of the menstrual cycle in case a very early pregnancy is present. Abortion may occur otherwise.

Indications for Hysterosalpingography

1. If tubal insufflation or dye injection at laparoscopy have failed to demonstrate patent tubes.
2. To demonstrate the site of blockage.
3. If some intracavitary anomaly is suspected.
4. If the patient is unsuitable for laparoscopy.

Contraindications

1. Active pelvic infection.
2. Cervicitis or purulent vaginal discharge.
3. If pregnancy is suspected.

Hysterosalpingogram showing abnormal cavity with adhesions (Asherman's syndrome) at the right cornu. This woman had been left with a diagnosis of unexplained fertility for 7 years. Following this X-ray and hysteroscopy with adhesion division, successful pregnancy occurred later.

Complications of Hysterosalpingography

1. In a few cases severe pelvic pain and vomiting may occur an hour or two after injection for reasons unknown. Recovery is within 12 hours but admission to hospital is required for sedation and observation.
2. Infection, or exacerbation of already present infection.
3. With oily radio-opaque media there is a risk of embolism following intravasation. Watery media are safest and are quickly absorbed and excreted.
4. The procedure is something of an ordeal for the conscious patient.

TREATMENT OF INFERTILITY

Approximately 23% of cases of infertility are due to polycystic change in the ovaries. One of the almost constant features of this condition is obesity. Sometimes dietary control will restore fertility and this line of treatment should be pursued before turning to more sophisticated methods of investigation and treatment.

Clomiphene Treatment

This non-steroidal substance should be used for patients suffering from oligomenorrhoea plus infertility. It was originally developed as a chemical contraceptive and influences the hypothalamic cells producing gonadotrophin releasing hormone. If it is given to patients who menstruate normally it is possible that normal function will be upset and infertility be induced.

There is still a great deal of controversy regarding the mode of action of clomiphene. It appears to influence the activity of the hypothalamus, pituitary and ovary in varying degrees. The following is a favoured explanation of the way in which it induces ovulation.

1. Clomiphene, although not an oestrogen, binds to the oestrogen receptor sites in the cytoplasm of the hypothalamus target cell.
2. From the cytoplasm the clomiphene-receptor complex is transferred to the nucleus.
3. The cytoplasm is thus denuded of oestrogen receptors.
4. The hypothalamic cell is no longer aware of any change in circulating oestrogen.
5. It reacts by increasing the output of releasing factor which in turn increases the secretion of FSH and LH, leading to ovulation.

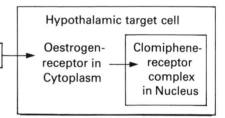

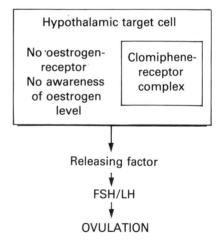

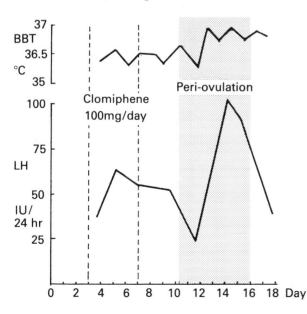

Clomiphene given about the 3rd to the 7th day of the cycle should produce ovulation about the 12th to the 14th day, but there is some variation which may be important.

INDUCTION OF OVULATION

ADMINISTRATION of Clomiphene

1. A progesterone challenge test is given first – 5mg norethisterone daily for 5 days. If oestrogen is present, withdrawal bleeding occurs when the drug is stopped. Clomiphene stimulation is much more likely to be successful in the presence of high oestrogen levels.

2. Clomiphene 50mg tablet is taken daily for 5 days from day 3 to day 7 of the cycle.

3. Ovulation may be expected about day 12–14, and this should be confirmed by estimating the plasma progesterone about day 19. If this test is not available, a temperature chart may be used but is much less reliable.

4. If ovulation does not occur, the dose of clomiphene should be increased over several months to 200mg daily for the 5 days in each cycle.

5. If there is still no response, some luteal inadequacy must be suspected, and 5000 IU of HCG should be given intramuscularly about the 14th day. If no proof of ovulation is obtained after three cycles of this treatment, clomiphene stimulation must be considered to have failed.

Side-Effects

1. 'Hot flushes' are the commonest, due to the anti-oestrogenic property of clomiphene.
2. Mild depression.
3. Mild nausea (rare).
4. Visual symptoms such as flickering or blurring. These are transient and very rare.
5. Hyperstimulation.   This is very rare but more likely when HCG is given as well. There is abdominal pain due to ovarian enlargement which may cause ascites and even hydrothorax. This leads to haemoconcentration, hypovolaemia and thrombosis, and haemorrhage if the ovarian cysts rupture. Treatment includes removal of ascitic fluid and restoration of plasma volume.

Ovulation following Cyclofenil (Rehibin)

This drug is a weak oestrogen which has also been used for inducing ovulation. It has the advantage over clomiphene of possessing no anti-oestrogenic effects and has even fewer side-effects. It has been recommended for use in patients with anovulatory cycles but it is less widely used than clomiphene in this country.

Results of Clomiphene Treatment

This depends on the cause of the ovulation failure, but in the absence of other disease an ovulation rate of 50% can be achieved. Pregnancy rate is half that figure. Multiple pregnancy sometimes occurs.

INDUCTION OF OVULATION

GONADOTROPHINS

The initiation of ovulation in patients with other infertility problems requires more intrusive methods of investigation and treatment. Briefly, the patients most likely to benefit fall into two groups:

1. Those with amenorrhoea and abnormal hormone levels, and
2. Patients who have relatively normal hormone levels and have failed to respond to clomiphene.

Basically the treatment consists of stimulating the ovaries with gonadotrophins to induce ovulation. Two methods are used:

1. A straightforward stimulation of the ovary is carried out using FSH and LH.

Gonadotrophin is expensive and requires close laboratory supervision to avoid overdosage and consequent hyperstimulation.

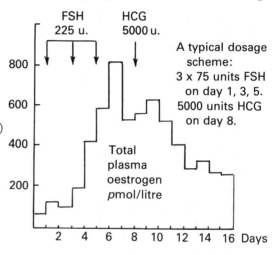

Scheme of Treatment

The object is to ripen a follicle with repeated doses of FSH, and then to bring the follicle to the point of ovulation with an injection of luteinising hormone.

Drugs commonly used are:
HMG (Human Menopausal Gonadotrophin) (FSH/LH ratio 1:1). This is a commercial preparation containing 75 IU of each hormone per ampule.
HCG (Human Chorionic Gonadotrophin) in ampules of 1000 to 5000 IU. This hormone is biologically the same as LH and much cheaper to prepare.

A typical dosage scheme:
3 x 75 units FSH on day 1, 3, 5.
5000 units HCG on day 8.

The dose varies from patient to patient and even from cycle to cycle, and much the best results are obtained with daily assays of urinary oestrogens. The timing of the HCG is particularly important.

ASSISTED FERTILISATION TECHNIQUES

2. A more controlled approach is to render the patient anovulatory and then induce growth of follicles up to approximately 20mm i.e. immediately before ovulation. The eggs are harvested and placed in a culture medium in an incubator. Several hours later they will be used in fertilisation processes.

Indications for assisted fertilisation techniques:

1. In cases of unexplained infertility when anatomy and function appear to be normal, and treatable causes of infertility have been eliminated.
2. Patients showing evidence of cervical hostility to sperm.
3. For patients with endometriosis when other treatment has been unsuccessful and when the ovaries are free of adhesions and capable of yielding eggs.
4. When tubal lesions which cannot be eliminated are the reason for infertility.
5. When the sperm count is low but not so low that fertilisation is impossible.

463

INDUCTION OF OVULATION

Assisted Fertilisation Techniques (*contd*)

Tests of suitability

Sperm counts, thorough physical examination including assessment of the uterus and a complete hormone assessment are all necessary.

SYSTEM OF TREATMENT

Day 20 of menstrual cycle

The patient starts to take intranasal doses of an LHRH analogue, 100μg five times a day. (Buserelin is one example of these analogues.) This blocks the LHRH receptors in the pituitary and stops the normal production of LHRH. FSH/LH levels rise suddenly, thus exhausting the pituitary content of FSH and LH, and then return to normal luteal levels. Menstruation occurs. Dosage of the LHRH analogue is continued. LH and FSH levels do not rise again.

Day 10 of the succeeding cycle

Daily injections of human menopausal gonadotrophin are started. LHRH analogue treatment is stopped. Follicular growth is monitored by daily ultrasound.

When follicles reach 20mm in diameter ovulation is imminent. An injection of HCG is given at this point. The timing of the injection is important. If given too early it may upset maturation processes. Some observers repeat this injection at 3-day intervals.

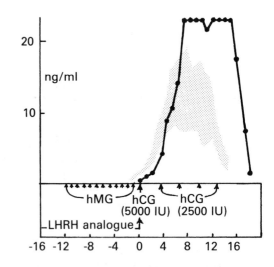

The diagram shows the sequence of hormone treatments, and the much improved luteal progesterone profile (●) compared with the normal (shaded).

Collection of eggs

Some operators collect eggs by laparoscopy. This involves general anaesthesia. Usually needle suction is used with the help of ultrasound. Light general anaesthesia may occasionally be required but in most cases local anaesthetic is all that is necessary. Repeated ultrasound examinations and daily hormone estimations are needed to be sure of follicle development.

Methods of utilising collected eggs

There are two main methods of achieving pregnancy:

1. The egg or eggs are injected together with prepared sperm into any one of 3 sites:
   (a) The Fallopian tube [Gamete Intra-Fallopian Transfer (GIFT)].
   (b) Pelvic peritoneal cavity [Direct Intra-Peritoneal Insemination (DIPI)].
   (c) In another procedure sperm are injected into the uterus at the time of ovulation [Intra-Uterine Insemination (IUI)].

Usually several eggs are introduced at the same time.

ASSISTED FERTILISATION TECHNIQUES

Methods of utilising eggs (*contd*)

2. *In vitro* fertilisation (IVF) of one egg, which is then grown in culture medium to the 4 to 8 cell size when it may be replaced in the fallopian tube or the uterus. A variation of this method is to replace the fertilised egg at the pronuclear stage – usually into the fallopian tube [Zygote Intra-Fallopian Transfer (ZIFT)].

Human egg 18 hours after fertilisation.

Two pronuclear bodies (one from the sperm and one from the egg itself).

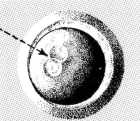

Normal human embryo at the 4 cell stage 48 hours after fertilisation. (Ready for transplant to the uterus.)

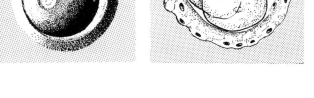

The ability to freeze fertilised ova successfully has altered the approach to artificial methods of inducing pregnancy. By this means multiple ovulation is induced and the ova fertilised. These ova are then frozen. They can be used one at a time. If the first attempt at re-introducing the fertilised ovum fails then the process can be repeated.

Freezing of unfertilised eggs has so far been unsuccessful due to cytoplasmic damage.

Adopting this technique the results of the original *in vitro* technique have been improved from 10% success to 40% or more.

Another procedure which has recently been introduced is the use of ovarian hormones to induce the production of a secretory type endometrium independently of the phase of the current cycle. This has been used in cases where ova are donated by one woman for use by another. It had been thought that donor and recipient cycles required to be synchronised carefully, which is difficult to achieve. This difficulty has been overcome by administering 2mg oestradiol valerate orally 3 or 4 times daily, plus 100mg progesterone given intramuscularly once per day or the same dose orally 3 times daily to the woman who is to receive the donated egg. The progesterone is started on the day before recovering the donated oocytes. After fertilising the egg it is planted in the uterus of the recipient. When pregnancy is proven the same doses of hormones are maintained until the 20th week.

INFERTILITY IN THE MALE

It is only within relatively recent times that it was realised that there were male factors causing infertility. It is now known that in more than 30% of cases of infertility the cause is a disorder of sperm production or function.

In all cases of infertility the male partner should be interviewed. The points to be investigated are:

1. Can it be established that the male has been previously fertile?
2. Are there any coital problems?
3. Is there any history of genito-urinary infection?
4. Has the male been exposed to agents or procedures which might affect testicular function e.g. radiation, cytotoxic drugs or toxic chemicals, surgery or testicular injury?

In addition, a physical examination must be made to establish that male anatomical features are normal with no congenital defects. The testicular size and consistency should be estimated. Examine for varicocele and epididymal swelling. A rectal examination must be made to exclude prostatic disease.

Semen analysis

Samples of seminal fluid should be obtained by masturbation. Any other method may introduce factors which will nullify the results obtained. Ordinary condoms and lubricating jellies contain spermicidal agents. If specimens can only be obtained by coitus, special non-toxic condoms are available. Once the sample is obtained it is placed in a wide-mouthed sterile container and delivered to the laboratory. During that time it should be kept between 15 and 38°C.

Normal Values

1. *Volume*: 2–5ml.

2. *Liquefaction*: The ejaculate coagulates shortly after production but liquefies within 30 minutes.

3. *Concentration* of sperm: 20–200 million/ml.

4. *Motility*: If this is evident in more than 40% of sperm with forward movement, the sperms are normal. The examination should be carried out with a microscope which has a heated stage.

Abnormalities

1. If less than 0.5ml, it may indicate retrograde spill into the bladder. Examine the urine for sperm.

2. High viscosity and prolonged liquefaction period will interfere with counting the sperm.

3. If less than 10 million/ml, this is oligospermia and fertilisation may be very difficult.

4. If the sperms are slow in movement with little forward motion and if a coagulum is present, it suggests the presence of antibodies.

INFERTILITY IN THE MALE

Morphology of Sperm

At present this is not a very reliable method of judging the character of sperm. If the spermatocytes are grossly malformed, fertilisation is unlikely but judging minor changes tends to be a very subjective matter.

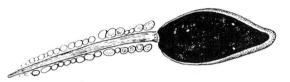 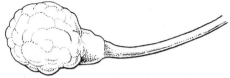

Human sperm (from transmission electron micrograph).
Its acrosome is intact.

Abnormal sperm (from scanning electron micrograph). If more than 20% of sperm in a sample show this kind of deformity, there is likely to be a major degree of male infertility.

A great deal of research is being devoted to study of morphology to define the detailed structure of the spermatocyte but so far the significance of results has not influenced the practical fields.

The causes of abnormalities in sperm production are only beginning to be understood. Unlike the female, few of them are due to functional abnormalities such as hormone deficiency. The main factors are:

1. **Acute and chronic infection** of the male genital tract occurs quite commonly. Gonococcal and coliform infections respond to antibiotics but chronic prostatitis can be difficult to treat. Spermatozoa are reduced in number and tend to be malformed and non-motile.

   Chlamydial infection may be found in both partners. Sperm motility is reduced, causing infertility. Both partners should be treated and follow-up examinations of ejaculate carried out.

   Viral infections can be important, especially mumps. Testicular atrophy may follow this infection and systematic immunoglobulin prophylaxis and corticosteroid treatment should be given as soon as there is the slightest hint of this infection.

2. **Immunological reactions** in the form of auto-antibodies occur in a variable number of men (3–12%). Formation of these anti-sperm antibodies may be stimulated by infection or injury but in most cases the cause is obscure. Steroids in short courses may be helpful.

3. **Environmental factors**

   These are a compound of social habits – smoking, alcohol and drugs. Reduction in smoking and alcohol consumption can generally be dealt with if the man is serious in his efforts to deal with the problem. Habit-forming drugs are a separate and more difficult issue but it is unlikely that the individual is very interested in fertility.

   Included under this heading are occupational hazards. Working with heavy metals, welding processes, exposure to high temperatures, pesticides and radioactive materials.

INFERTILITY IN THE MALE

Environmental factors (*contd*)

The list of occupations involving the substances mentioned in the previous page is remarkably long:

Agriculture and gardening: Pesticides, weed killers.
Car industry, painters, battery workers, domestic decorators, smelters – all using lead products.
Textile industry: Carbon disulphide.
Plastic manufacture: Chlorinated biphenyls.
Grain storage: Benzine hexachloride.

Equally disturbing is the large number of therapeutic agents which affect spermatogenesis.
1. Chemotherapeutic agents: These depress sperm production and cause germinal epithelial aplasia. Rising FSH levels are an indication of these changes. Mustargen, cyclophosphamide and chlorambucil have been incriminated.
2. Sulfasalazine used in the treatment of ulcerative colitis. Sperm motility is reduced, as is the number. These effects are reversed if treatment is stopped.
3. Cimetidine – used to reduce gastric acidity, spironolactone – used in oedema and ascites in renal and hepatic disease, and ketonazole – used in treating micotic infections of skin. These substances interfere with androgen action and may affect spermatogenesis.
4. Anabolic steroids depress spermatogenesis profoundly but the effect is reversible when the drug is withdrawn.
5. Anti-hypertensive drugs, anti-depressants and some sedatives cause impotence and may depress sperm count or motility.
6. Furadantin, anti-malarial drugs, corticosteroids, phenacitin and salicylic acid derivatives can depress spermatogenesis.

Preparation of Sperm for Fertilisation

Semen coagulates immediately on ejaculation. It liquefies within 30 minutes due to enzyme action. The sperm should be washed to get rid of traces of the seminal fluid. The various tests should be carried out quickly and if events have been arranged properly and the ovum is ready for fertilisation this procedure should be carried out immediately. If this is not possible, the sperms can be preserved by freezing but this reduces their activity somewhat.

INFERTILITY – COUNSELLING

COUNSELLING

This is difficult. The intimate nature of the problem makes it so. The questions which have to be asked are as disturbing as the idea of infertility. To the woman it is not just a medical problem, it affects her whole attitude to life and the purpose of marriage is almost completely destroyed. Without children she will be ostracised from a whole section of social communion which she has hitherto taken for granted. Great care must be taken to dispel any idea that the position is hopeless. She is probably going to face a series of investigations and the reasons for each one of these must be explained to her and the subsequent results discussed. It is very important that this explanatory process is not hurried. Time will be required to allow the patient to adjust to the problem. The term 'infertility' should be used sparingly and there is justification for the use of euphemisms in the early stages. Very often it requires several months before the couple will accept the position and begin to co-operate actively with the medical team. The members of the team must not be over-zealous in reassurance but rather accept the feelings of the couple as normal, however they are expressed.

Where the problem lies with the male partner the position can be more difficult. Traditionally, infertility in a marriage has always been regarded as a 'fault' in the female. For the male to be told he is infertile is devastating. His role as the dominant partner is gone and his ego destroyed. The sexual relationship is likely to be upset. There are apt to be periods of impotence due to the effects of psychological stress. This is a time when the question of donor sperm should not be discussed. Time must be allowed until the couple can view the position with some degree of objectivity.

CHAPTER 19

THE MENOPAUSE

THE MENOPAUSE

The word menopause means the cessation of menstruation, but is commonly used instead of 'climacteric', a wider term for events leading up to and following the menopause, the pre-, peri- and post-menopause. The terms menarche and puberty bear a similar relationship.

Menstruation may gradually decrease, suddenly cease or become irregular.

Oestrogen levels fall over the 5 years preceding ovarian failure, which occurs usually between 45 and 55 years of age, with an average around 50 years. The fall in oestradiol has a positive feedback on the pituitary, increasing production of FSH and LH.

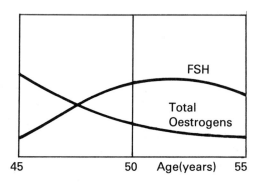

The ovary eventually produces only androstenedione, which is also produced by the adrenals, and is converted in peripheral fat to the weak oestrogen oestrone.

Causes of Menopause

Ovarian failure occurs when only a few thousand primordial follicles remain – insufficient to stimulate cyclical activity. Approximately one third of a woman's life is spent in the post-reproductive 'menopausal' phase.

Premature menopause may occur due to surgical removal of both ovaries, radiotherapy, chemotherapy or an unusually small number of primordial follicles present at birth. Conserved ovaries may fail following hysterectomy.

Differential Diagnosis

Before the days of immunological pregnancy tests and effective contraception, pregnancy and menopause could easily be confused.

Polycystic ovary syndrome may produce amenorrhoea in this group.

Prolactinoma should be borne in mind, especially in younger women.

Confirmation is by measurement of LH (raised disproportionately in PCO syndrome), FSH and oestradiol, ideally on 2 occasions 2 weeks apart to avoid a mid-cycle FSH peak. Prolactin assay and pregnancy testing are appropriate if clinically indicated.

| | | FSH | LH | Oestradiol |
		(U/litre)		($pmol/l$)
Principal changes in serum hormone levels:	Pre-menopausal	2–20	5–25	100–600
	Post-menopausal	40–70	50–70	60

THE MENOPAUSE

Signs and Symptoms

These are related to changes in circulating oestrogen levels, and subjective symptoms may occur some years before menstruation ceases, while physical changes are more long-term.

Climacteric Signs and Symptoms

ACUTE ⟶ CHRONIC
and/or early onset   and/or later onset

Vasomotor Symptoms	Psychological Symptoms	Urogenital Tract Symptoms	Skeletal Disease	Cardiovascular Disease
Hot flushes. Sweats – often associated with Palpitation. Panic attacks. Insomnia.	Emotional lability. Anxiety. Depressed mood. Poor memory and concentration. Irritability. Decreased libido.	Breast atrophy. Genital tract atrophy. Dyspareunia. Urethral syndrome. Trigonitis. Urinary urgency and frequency.	Osteoporosis. Vertebral crush fractures. Femoral neck fractures.	Ischaemic heart disease. Cerebro-vascular disease.

Changes in the Genital Tract

These changes are of atrophic type and affect the external genitalia as well as the internal organs. They take time to occur – over a number of years.

Not only are the main pelvic structures reduced in size but, more importantly, the fascial framework and intra-pelvic ligaments supporting the bladder and genitalia are weakened; this may lead to complications.

Vulva: This shows flattening of the labia majora, the minor labia becoming more evident. Sexual hair becomes grey and sparse. The clitoris shrinks.

Uterus: The uterus becomes small with a relatively large cervix – a return to infantile proportions.

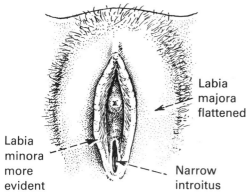

Labia majora flattened

Labia minora more evident

Narrow introitus

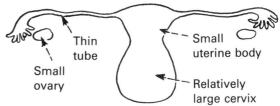

Thin tube

Small ovary

Small uterine body

Relatively large cervix

Tubes and Ovaries: These show great shrinkage, the tubes becoming thin, while the ovaries are reduced to small white wrinkled bodies 2–3cm in length.

473

THE MENOPAUSE

Changes in the Genital Tract (*contd*)
In addition to shrinkage of the vaginal introitus, the vagina diminishes in length and its secretions are limited, leading to sexual problems. Changes in the vaginal epithelium increase these problems.

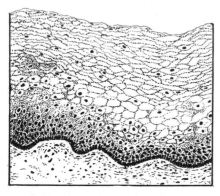

Normal pre-menopausal vaginal epithelium. Note the thick cornified layer.

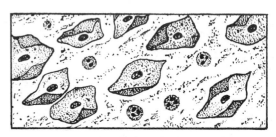

Smear of pre-menopausal vaginal epithelium. The cells are large with small nuclei and characteristic folded edges. Polymorphs are few in number.

Severity and Duration of Symptoms

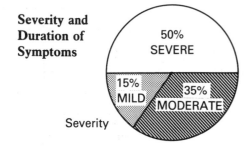

Severity

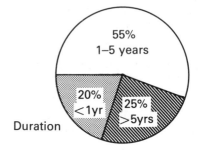

Duration

Menopausal Symptoms merit treatment

Vascular symptoms can be very distressing especially where night sweats prevent adequate sleep, and are the commonest reason for requests for treatment (65%). Psychological symptoms may cause problems coping with a job or running a home, and often cause friction with relatives, friends or work mates. Approximately 45% of requests for treatment are related to such problems.

Of 424 Glasgow women aged between 40 and 60 years, the number and percentage by age groups who had ever felt a need for treatment for the menopause were as follows:

Age	No.	%
40–45	105	38.1
46–50	120	49.2
51–55	114	65.2
56–60	85	40.0

The mean age of onset of need for treatment was 44.3 ± 5.1 years.

Those who suffer symptoms and succeed in obtaining hormone replacement are in fact the fortunate ones, since appropriate treatment for symptoms will reduce skeletal and cardiovascular disease.

THE GREENE CLIMACTERIC SCALE

Please indicate the extent to which you are troubled at the moment by any of these symptoms by placing a tick in the appropriate box.

SYMPTOMS	Not at all	A little	Quite a bit	Extremely	Score 0–3
1. Heart beating quickly or strongly					
2. Feeling tense or nervous					
3. Difficulty in sleeping					
4. Excitable					
5. Attacks of panic					
6. Difficulty in concentrating					
7. Feeling tired or lacking in energy					
8. Loss of interest in most things					
9. Feeling unhappy or depressed					
10. Crying spells					
11. Irritability					
12. Feeling dizzy or faint					
13. Pressure or tightness in head or body					
14. Parts of body feel numb or tingling					
15. Headaches					
16. Muscle and joint pains					
17. Loss of feeling in hands or feet					
18. Breathing difficulties					
19. Hot flushes					
20. Sweating at night					
21. Loss of interest in sex					

Psychological (1–11) = ☐   Somatic (12–18) = ☐   Vasomotor (19–20) = ☐
Anxiety (1–6) = ☐   Depression (7–11) = ☐   Sexual dysfunction (21) = ☐

[Greene, J.G. (1991), *Guide to the Greene Climacteric Scale*. University of Glasgow.]

This scale may be used to measure climacteric symptoms and the response to treatment or to compare different treatment regimes.

An Anxiety score of 10 or more indicates severe, possibly clinical, anxiety.
A Depression score of 10 or more indicates severe, possibly clinical, depression.

HORMONE REPLACEMENT THERAPY (HRT)

Do not confuse HRT with oral contraception.

Do not extrapolate real or imagined side-effects of oral contraception to apply to HRT.

HRT is very effective in treating menopausal symptoms, as proved by many placebo-controlled cross-over studies looking at vasomotor, psychological and sexual symptoms, giving an 80–90% success rate. Despite this, less than 10% of women receive HRT and, even after hysterectomy and bilateral oophorectomy, not all women receive oestrogen, although failure to prescribe in these circumstances could lead to litigation. HRT reduces the cardiovascular and skeletal effects of ovarian failure.

Factors Influencing Prescription of HRT

Indications for Therapy: Symptoms – shorter term
Prophylaxis – longer term. } Often both.

Personal and Family History: Osteoporosis – higher dose, longer term.
Cardiovascular disease – see Cardiovascular Disease and the Menopause (page 482).
Breast cancer – see HRT and the Breast (page 483).

Hysterectomy or not: Usually no progestogen after hysterectomy.

Patient's Preferences: Tablets, Implants, Transdermal patches, Local preparations.

Avoidance of Fluid Retention: Low dose HRT and low calorie diet may help to minimise fluid retention (bloating and breast discomfort) which occurs quite commonly during HRT. For some women, however, it is impossible to find a dose low enough to avoid fluid retention yet high enough to relieve other symptoms.

Concurrent Medication: With anti-epileptic or other liver enzyme inducing therapy, avoid oral HRT.

Duration of Therapy depends on:

Reason for therapy: Prophylaxis – long-term – 5 years plus.
Symptoms – could stop at intervals and recommence if symptoms recur.

Acceptability of therapy: If side-effects are unacceptable, or worse than symptoms, discontinue. Withdrawal bleeds, fluid retention and fear of breast cancer are common reasons for stopping.

History: No relative contraindications – longer therapy – perhaps till 65 years of age.
Family or personal risk of ischaemic heart disease – longer therapy.
Osteoporosis risk factors – longer therapy.
Family breast cancer history – shorter therapy – 5–10 years.

Screening

Screening before and on HRT is basically well-woman screening.

When a woman has had hysterectomy with conservation of one or both ovaries, it is sensible to measure FSH and oestradiol before commencing oestrogen as symptoms may occur in the presence of normal ovarian function – sometimes due to clinical anxiety.

HORMONE REPLACEMENT THERAPY (HRT)

Screening (*contd*)

Pre-treatment	*On treatment*
FBC. Biochemical screen (principally for liver function). Breast examination. Mammography if over 50 or if otherwise indicated. Pelvic examination. Papanicolaou smear. Endometrial sampling if indicated by abnormal bleeding. Blood pressure. Weight.	Breast examination regularly. Mammography every 3 years, 50–65 years. Papanicolaou smear every 3 years. Endometrial sampling only if abnormal bleeding occurs (before 10th day of progestogen). Blood pressure 6-monthly.

Contraindications to HRT

These are more theoretical and medico-legal than real. Contraindications have been extrapolated from the old high-dose oral contraceptive formulations to HRT and many contraindications appearing on UK data sheets are not significant. Some, however, such as elevated cholesterol and ischaemic heart disease are actually indications. Not all gynaecologists are aware of the change in attitude to contraindications which has developed in menopause clinics.

Hepatic: Acute Porphyria.

Cardiovascular: Uncontrolled or uncontrollable hypertension. (Controlled hypertension or hypertension not requiring treatment are not contraindications.)

Deep vein thrombosis or pulmonary thrombo-embolism which occurred during pregnancy or when on the oral contraceptive pill or HRT, with anti-thrombin III deficiency. (A past history of thrombo-embolic phenomena without such defect is not a genuine contraindication, but transdermal, percutaneous or implant therapy is preferred, to minimise oestrogen dose to the liver.)

Myocardial infarction and cerebrovascular accident. Once the patient is mobilised, these are indications, not contraindications.

Malignant Disease: Breast cancer is regarded by many surgeons as a contraindication, though there is no proof of adverse effect and breast cancer diagnosed during HRT has a higher cure rate. Caution is sensible and progestogens should be employed first.

Endometrial cancer is oestrogen sensitive and progestogens are usually employed first. Combined oestrogen progestogen therapy has been shown to be safe.

Melanoma is not now thought to be a contraindication.

477

HORMONE REPLACEMENT THERAPY (HRT)

Contraindications (*contd*)

There is no significant evidence that multiple sclerosis or otosclerosis are adversely affected by HRT, though anecdotal stories exist, based on extrapolation from effects of pregnancy.

Prolactinoma might be adversely affected and pregnancy is a contraindication, hence the need to exclude pregnancy before commencing HRT should any doubt exist.

Migraine can be adversely or beneficially affected by HRT and is not a reason for refusing to prescribe. Individuals may tolerate one preparation better than another.

Choice of Treatment
This involves the following considerations:
1. Presence or absence of uterus. – Usually, no uterus no progestogen.
2. Effectiveness.
3. Convenience – Convenience aids compliance.
4. Cost.
5. Patient preference – often related to the experience of friends.
6. Medical considerations – parenteral therapy has least effect on and is least affected by the liver.
7. Side effects – see below.

Routes of administration
1. Oral – tablets.
2. Transdermal – patches.
3. Percutaneous – gel.
4. Subcutaneous – implants.
5. Vaginal 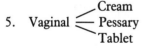 Cream / Pessary / Tablet

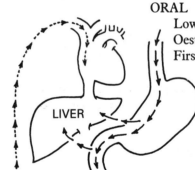

ORAL
Low bioavailability.
Oestradiol dose in mg.
First pass metabolism in liver.
Serum oestrone level > oestradiol level.

PARENTERAL
High bioavailability.
Oestradiol dose absorbed in μg per day.
No first pass liver metabolism.
Serum oestradiol level > oestrone level.

Pro's and Con's of different routes

Oral
1. Economical.
2. Wide choice of preparations and doses.
3. Only route available for progestogens in some countries.
4. Absorbed into portal system and passes through liver before reaching systemic circulation with metabolism to oestrone and liver enzyme induction.
5. May cause nausea.
6. Majority of data on prevention of osteoporosis and cardiovascular disease relate to oral therapy.

HORMONE REPLACEMENT THERAPY (HRT)

Pro's and Con's of different routes (*contd*)

Transdermal and Percutaneous

1. More physiological, with absorption into and distribution by systemic circulation, not hepatic portal system.
2. Minimum effect on liver.
3. More lipid-friendly route for progestogens.
4. Effective against osteoporosis.
5. High patient acceptability (if no skin irritation).
6. More costly.

Subcutaneous implants   (25mg or 50mg pure crystalline oestradiol).

1. Effective where other routes fail.
2. Possibly best therapy for decreased libido. Testosterone 100mg may be added for this.
3. Good skeletal effect.
4. Little effect on lipids.
5. Risk of escalation of oestradiol levels, so strict control of dose and frequency of implants is necessary.
6. Long-term effects on endometrium after stopping treatment, so best used after hysterectomy.

Vaginal preparations

Oestriol preparations and low dose oestradiol tablets do not have systemic effects, so do not induce uterine bleeding and can give local benefit in women with contraindications to systemic therapy.

Potent oestrogens given vaginally have systemic effects.

Vaginal preparations relieve atrophic vaginitis, trigonitis, vaginal dryness and dyspareunia.

Recommended Regimes

After Hysterectomy

Oral oestradiol, oestradiol esters or conjugated equine oestrogens.

Transdermal oestradiol. Oestradiol implants.

Combined oestrogen and progestogen (cyclical or continuous combined) may be employed when the hysterectomy was performed for extensive endometriosis. Norethisterone 5 or 10mg daily or medroxyprogesterone acetate 10 or 20mg daily may be employed after endometrial or breast carcinoma, deep vein thrombosis or pulmonary thrombo-embolism.

HORMONE REPLACEMENT THERAPY (HRT)

Recommended Regimes (*contd*)

With Intact Uterus

Oral oestradiol, oestradiol esters or conjugated equine oestrogens daily with norethisterone, norgestrel, medroxyprogesterone acetate or dydrogesterone added for at least 10 or 12 days per month. This will avoid endometrial hyperplasia and irregular, unpredictable bleeding and reduce the risk of the rare endometrial cancer.

Transdermal oestradiol and transdermal or oral norethisterone, as above. Norethisterone or medroxyprogesterone acetate may be employed after oestrogen-dependent tumours or thrombo-embolic phenomena as in hysterectomy patients.

Proprietary names and dosages are listed in MIMS and the National Formulary.

Alternatives to oestrogen

When systemic oestrogen is contraindicated, not tolerated or declined, the following may be useful:

1. Unopposed progestogens (norethisterone, medroxyprogesterone acetate).
2. Oestriol vaginal preparations.
3. Low dose oestradiol vaginal preparations.
4. Clinical psychology.
5. Hypnosis.
6. Bisphosphonates (for skeletal benefit only).

OSTEOPOROSIS

Osteoporosis is the commonest metabolic bone disease. Post-menopausal osteoporosis results from an excess of bone resorption over bone formation associated with loss of oestrogen. Women have 20% less bone than men at peak skeletal development, so women have less bone to lose before reaching the fragility threshold. More than 50% of Caucasian women suffer one or more osteoporotic fractures by the age of 70.

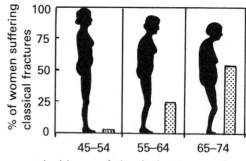

Incidence of classical osteoporotic fractures by decades of life (stipple).

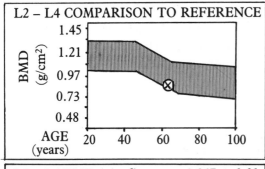

L2 – L4 BMD (g/cm²)	0.867 ± 0.01
L2 – L4 % YOUNG ADULT	72 ± 3
L2 – L4 % AGE MATCHED[3]	85 ± 3

Dual X-ray densitometry is the currently favoured technique for measuring lumbar spine and femoral neck density, though loss of height or radiological demonstration of vertebral crush fractures give clear evidence of osteoporosis.

OSTEOPOROSIS

Comparative cortical bone thicknesses:

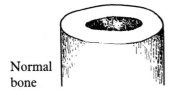

Normal bone

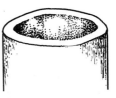

Osteoporotic bone

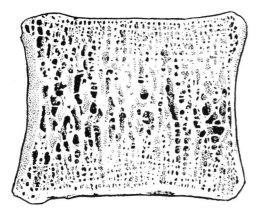

Normal vertebral body. Note the thick trabeculae of bone.

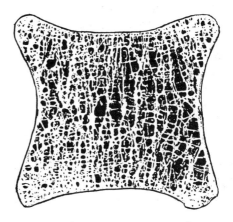

Vertebra from post-menopausal woman showing extreme rarefaction of the trabeculae.

Oestrogens have an anti-resorptive effect on bone.

Prevention of osteoporosis is preferable to attempted treatment once established. It is particularly important after premature menopause, whether natural or surgical, and oestrogen at an appropriate dose (at least 0.625mg conjugated equine oestrogen orally or equivalent; 50 μg oestradiol patch; oestradiol implants) will prevent development of osteoporosis in the great majority of women. Therapy for 5 years or more may reduce the incidence of Colles' fractures and hip fractures by 50% and vertebral crush fractures by up to 90% in those who take oestrogens.

Bone loss recommences on stopping therapy.

Risk factors for osteoporosis are:

1. Female sex.
2. White or oriental race.
3. Family history of osteoporosis.
4. Early menopause (natural or oophorectomy).
5. Sedentary life-style.
6. Low weight for height.
7. Tobacco and alcohol abuse.
8. Low calcium intake.

CARDIOVASCULAR DISEASE AND THE MENOPAUSE

In European countries, 40 to 45% of deaths are due to cardiovascular causes with a relative increase in risk in females after the menopause. (The actual risk is greater in males even after 75 years.)

Mortality rate for selected causes per 100,000 population in Scotland, 1988. (Source: Registrar General for Scotland.)

	Endometrial cancer	Cervical cancer	Breast cancer	Lung cancer	Fractured femur (estimated)	Ischaemic heart disease	Cerebro-vascular disease
All ages	4	7	48	52	<20	316	196
45 – 64	6	14	88	114	<10	170	62
65 – 74	12	22	130	206	<25	854	325

The risk of coronary heart disease is increased sevenfold by bilateral oophorectomy before 35 years of age or premature menopause at 35 years. Oestrogen replacement reduces ischaemic heart disease to less than 50% of the untreated incidence. The greatest reduction in deaths is in women with cardiovascular disease. There appears to be a reduction in deaths from cerebrovascular disease but this is less clear. Henderson et al., *Arch.Int.Med.* (1991), 151, 74, detail the decreased mortality on HRT which may amount to a 20% reduction in all causes of mortality after 15 years of HRT.

It has been feared that addition of a progestogen might reduce the cardiovascular protection afforded by oestrogens, but androgen derived progestogens lower the level of lipoprotein 'a' (LP_a) in women and animal work suggests that progestogens may not be harmful.

HRT may influence cardiovascular risk factors through effects on:

Lipid metabolism . . . . oestrogen increases HDL cholesterol and lowers LDL cholesterol.

Carbohydrate metabolism.

Body fat distribution . . . . oestrogen promotes gynaecoid fat distribution.

Coagulation and fibrinolysis.

Blood flow . . . . oestrogen increases arterial flow.

Blood pressure.

A number of studies have shown no hypertensive effect of HRT. Blood pressure rises with age and may reach levels requiring therapy in the early post-menopausal years, incorrectly attributed to HRT. The occasional idiosyncratic rise in BP may occur.

HRT AND THE BREAST

Fear of an increased risk of breast cancer is the main cause of concern about HRT in patients and in doctors.

Breast cancer is increasing in incidence and may affect one woman in 9 in a lifetime.

Alcohol use in young women may increase the risk and obesity, high socio-economic status and delayed first pregnancy are risk factors. Early menarche, late menopause and nulliparity are risk factors. Only 20% of subjects have a positive family history.

Early menopause decreases breast cancer risk (70% reduction with menopause before 35 years).

An increased risk of breast cancer related to HRT cannot be ruled out, but ever use of oestrogen is probably irrelevant, while current use or duration may be more relevant. Oestrogen may be promotive rather than causative. There is insufficient evidence to recommend adding a progestogen to decrease the risk of breast cancer.

The relative risk of breast cancer after 10+ years of HRT is 1.3–1.8, but breast cancer diagnosed while on HRT has a higher survival rate and it must be remembered that there are 9 times as many deaths from heart disease as from breast cancer, with more than 50% of the cardiovascular deaths potentially preventable by HRT. Perspective and patient choice are important.

Contraception in the Climacteric

Ovulation may occur after 6 months of amenorrhoea.

Most HRT preparations are not contraceptive.

Effective contraception is recommended until one year after menstruation ceases, in the absence of vasectomy or female sterilisation. Cyclical HRT makes it difficult to assess the one year criterion and some family planning doctors add a progesterone only oral contraceptive to cyclical formulations on the days when no progestogen is present.

After the age of 45, it is considered that IUCD's do not require to be renewed regularly and can be left in situ till there is no risk of pregnancy.

Barrier contraception has a low failure rate in climacteric women.

Future Developments

New progestogens may have more favourable metabolic effects.

Withdrawal bleeding may be avoided in a high percentage of genuinely post-menopausal (1 year or more) women by using a single molecule with oestrogen and progestogen effect (Tibolone), or continuous, rather than cyclical, combined oestrogen and progestogen.

Benefits and Risks of HRT

Appropriate hormone treatment:

Relieves vasomotor symptoms.
Relieves psychological symptoms.
Protects and restores collagen.
Prevents and improves osteoporosis.
Reduces cardiovascular disease.
Reduces all-cause mortality.

May increase breast cancer.
May cause fluid retention.
May cause 'premenstrual' syndrome.
May cause unwanted uterine bleeding.

In terms of both symptom relief and mortality statistics, the benefits greatly outweigh the adverse effects.